£4

ORDER AND DISORDER:

THE HEALTH IMPLICATIONS OF EATING AND DRINKING IN THE NINETEENTH AND TWENTIETH CENTURIES

ORDER AND DISORDER:
THE HEALTH IMPLICATIONS OF EATING AND DRINKING IN THE NINETEENTH AND TWENTIETH CENTURIES

Proceedings of the Fifth Symposium of the International Commission for Research into European Food History, Aberdeen 1997

Edited by
Alexander Fenton

TUCKWELL PRESS
In association with
The European Ethnological Research Centre, Edinburgh

First published in Great Britain in 2000 by
Tuckwell Press Ltd
Phantassie
East Linton
East Lothian EH40 3DG
Scotland

ISBN 1 86232 117 5

British Library Cataloguing-in-Publication Data
A catalogue record for this book is available from the British Library

Typeset by Brinnoven, Livingston
Printed and bound by the Cromwell Press, Wiltshire

Contents

Preface

This volume contains the proceedings of the fifth symposium of the International Commission for Research into European Food History, hosted by The Rowett Research Institute, Aberdeen, Scotland, from 18–21 September 1997. It was organised by The European Ethnological Research Centre, Edinburgh, with the financial support of:

The Russell Trust
The Scotland Inheritance Fund
Macphie of Glenbervie
The Wellcome Trust
Paterson Arran Ltd

Since four of the papers are concerned with the work of the late Sir John Boyd Orr, the Rowett Research Institute, under its Director Professor Philip James, was a very appropriate setting. The then External Affairs Manager, Mrs Christine Cook, was an energetic on-the-spot organiser who facilitated the smooth running of the Symposium.

Thirteen countries were represented and nineteen papers are presented here on aspects of the health implications of eating and drinking, a most important subject for the present day. The Guest Speaker was Professor Hugh Pennington, Head of the University of Aberdeen's Department of Medical Microbiology, who has been playing a national role in relation to current and recent food crises. Although the development of European food patterns from the early nineteenth century to the present day has virtually eradicated deficiency diseases related to poverty and lack of hygiene, nevertheless major health problems arise from the modern food pattern, such as obesity, cardiovascular diseases, diabetes mellitus and cancer, largely as a result of over-nutrition. The Symposium fulfilled one of the roles of the members of the International Commission for Research into Food History by looking in an interdisciplinary way at the development of food and nutrition in different countries of Europe, especially over the last two centuries. The papers, therefore, help for the most part to set the background against which present day problems can be judged, whilst that of Hugh Pennington brings us face to face with current harsh realities.

The papers are divided into broad headings. The Guest Lecture by Professor Pennington presents a somewhat frightening aspect of the modern scene. Four papers deal with questions of nutrition raised by the work of Sir John Boyd Orr and the Carnegie Survey. Eleven deal with food consumption and biological standards, the development of nutrition and health education, the development of food hygiene in domestic and in workplace contexts, the consumption of specific foods as a public health issue (such as sugar, fat, alcohol), and vegetarian nutrition and health. Two papers examine specific food and drink products in relation to health, and finally one throws light on the role of tobacco and on the ambivalence of the authorities in their attitude to it. General conclusions are drawn in the various papers from specific instances, and the volume, taken as a whole, gives an extremely useful background to the present day situation as regards food and health in many parts of Europe.

For relaxation, there was a short bus excursion through the fine farmland of Aberdeenshire to Glendronach Distillery, near Huntly, and a Symposium Dinner was followed by an entertainment, 'Songs of the Agricultural Revolution in North-East Scotland', by Dr Ian Olson of Aberdeen University, and Aileen Carr.

The previous volumes published by ICREFH are:

Teuteberg, Hans-J, ed. *European Food History. A research review*, Leicester 1992

Burnett, John and Oddy, Derek J, eds *The Origins and Development of Food Policies in Europe*, Leicester 1994

Den Hartog, Adel P, ed. *Food Technology, Science and Marketing: European diet in the twentieth century*, East Linton 1995

Schärer, Martin R and Fenton, Alexander, eds *Food and Material Culture*, East Linton 1998

I am indebted to Helen Kemp and to Susan Storrier for editorial assistance.

Alexander Fenton
Symposium Organiser

Contributors

DR PETER ATKINS, Department of Geography, University of Durham, Durham DH1 3LE

PROFESSOR EMERITUS JOHN BURNETT, 'Castle Dene', Burgess Wood Road, Beaconsfield, Bucks HP9 1EQ

JOHN E BURNETT, National Museums of Scotland, Chambers St, Edinburgh EH1 1JF

KATARZYNA CWIERTKA, van der Palmstraat 100, 3022 VZ Rotterdam, The Netherlands

PROFESSOR EMERITUS ALEXANDER FENTON, European Ethnological Research Centre, c/o National Museums of Scotland, Edinburgh EH1 1JF

DR MAJA GODINA-GOLIJA, Institute of Slovenian Ethnology, ZRC SAZU, Novi trg 5, 1000-Ljublana, Slovenia

DR DAVID J GUNNELL, Department of Epidemiology and Public Health Medicine, University of Bristol, Canynge Hall, Whiteladies Road, Bristol BS8 2PR

DR ADEL P DEN HARTOG, Division of Human Nutrition and Epidemiology, Wageningen Agricultural University, PO Box 8129, 6700 EV Wageningen, The Netherlands

DR ANNEMARIE DE KNECHT-VAN EEKELEN, Medical Faculty, Section Medical History, Free University of Amsterdam, van de Boechorststraat 7, 1081 BT Amsterdam, The Netherlands

INGER JOHANNE LYNGØ, Department of Cultural Studies, University of Oslo, PO Box 1010 Blindern, N-0315 Oslo, Norway

DR CHRISTOPH MERKI, Historisches Institut der Universität Bern, Längasstrasse 49, CH-3000 Bern 9, Switzerland

SABINE MERTA, Reeser Strasse 3, 47533 Kleve, Germany

PROFESSOR DEREK J ODDY, School of Social and Policy Sciences, University of Westminster, 309 Regent Street, London W1R 8AL

DR ANNEKE VAN OTTERLOO, Vakgroep Sociologie, Faculty of Political and Socio-Cultural Sciences, Oude Hoogstraat 24, 1012 CE Amsterdam, The Netherlands

AROUNA P. OUÉDRAOGO, INRA-Corela, 65 bd de Brandebourg, F-94205 Ivry-sur-Seine, Cedex, France

PROFESSOR T HUGH PENNINGTON, Department of Medical Microbiology, University of Aberdeen, Medical School Buildings, Foresterhill, Aberdeen AB25 2ZD

PROFESSOR DR PETER SCHOLLIERS, Vrije Universiteit Brussel, Pleinlaan 2, 1050-Brussels, Belgium

DR DAVID SMITH, Department of History, University of Aberdeen, King's College, Meston Walk, Old Aberdeen AB24 3FX

PROFESSOR DR JAKOB TANNER, Historisches Seminar, University of Zürich, Karl Schmid-Strasse 4, CH-8006 Zürich, Switzerland

PROFESSOR DR HANS-J TEUTEBERG, Historisches Seminar der Westfälischen Wilhelms-Universität, Domplatz 20-22, D-48143 Münster, Germany

ULRIKE THOMS, Ferdinand-Freiligrath-Strasse 25, D-48147 Münster, Germany

Guest Lecture: the modern scene

1 BSE and *E Coli* food crises

T Hugh Pennington

Every now and then events occur with a timing and impact that causes them to have major effects on public policy. The *E coli* O157 outbreak in central Scotland at the end of 1996 was such an event,[1] not only because twenty died and more than 500 fell ill, but because it was yet another dramatic food scare to add to the long list that has dominated the news at regular intervals over the last two decades. It is a widely held view that crises like this one, notably BSE, have not only seriously damaged popular trust in the ability of the present British institutional arrangements to work effectively to protect the public, but have also induced scepticism about the role of 'official' experts and beliefs in 'cover ups' and the notion that policy-making has been captured by vested interests. These negative perceptions about food policies and their effect on health have caused the UK Government to propose a radical reform of the way it approaches food policy and its implementation. This is to set up a Food Standards Agency which will operate more openly and at arm's length from Government departments.[2] The purpose of this paper is to put this development into its scientific context by considering *E coli* O157 and BSE in some detail.

Epidemiologists firmly believe in a hidden hand which causes major food poisoning outbreaks to start on a Friday afternoon and to develop their full horror over the weekend. The 1996 *E coli* O157 outbreak in central Scotland was no exception.[3] The first cases from Wishaw were reported to the Department of Public Health Medicine of Lanarkshire Health Board just after lunchtime on Friday, 22 November. By the evening, histories had been obtained from nine of the fifteen cases. The indications were that eight of these nine had consumed food obtained, either directly or at a church lunch, from a particular butcher's shop in Wishaw. The possibility of other common exposures could not at this stage be excluded, as a high proportion of the population of Wishaw might patronise this shop in any one week. The number of cases of suspected or confirmed infection continued to increase dramatically. By Sunday, 24 November reports indicated that the distribution of products from the butcher extended into other parts of central Scotland. Cases of infection were subsequently reported in Forth Valley, Lothian and Greater Glasgow. The distribution chain of meat and meat products was diverse and complex and it took some days for the details to be unravelled from a painstaking investigation of the company's

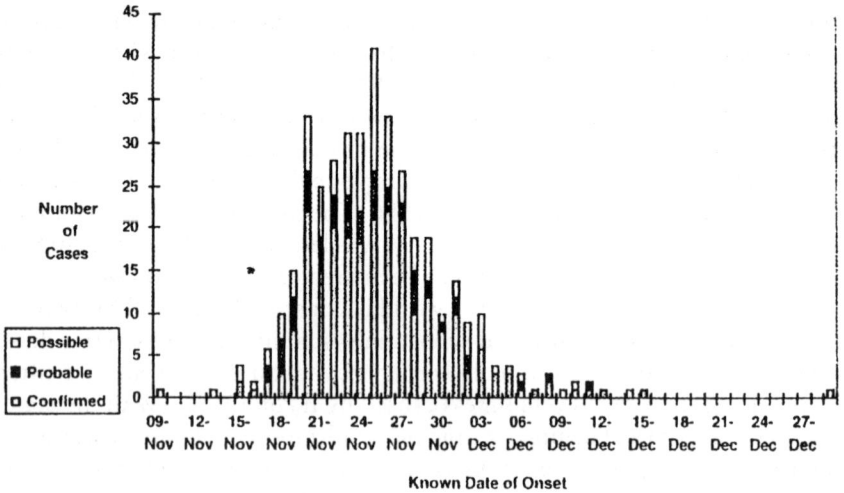

Fig. 1. E coli *O157 Central Scotland Outbreak Epidemic Curve by Date of Onset of Diarrhoea*

records. Some 85 outlets throughout central Scotland were eventually identified as being supplied by the company, making the task of outbreak management and control extremely difficult.

Epidemiological and subsequent microbiological evidence showed that the outbreak comprised several separate but related incidents relating to a lunch (attended by around 100 people) held in Wishaw Parish Church Hall, a birthday party held in a public house on 23 November 1996 and retail sales in Lanarkshire and Forth Valley. All isolates of *E coli* O157 from individuals in the outbreak belonging to phage type 2, had the verocytotoxin gene VT2, and showed indistinguishable profiles by pulsed field gel electrophoresis. At the end of the outbreak 501 cases had been documented. 151 patients had been hospitalised and twenty had died – all aged over 65. These figures make the outbreak one of the world's worst – certainly the worst in mortality, probably the worst in morbidity, and in the top three by number of cases.

The Wishaw outbreak is not the only major episode that has been caused by this organism in Scotland. The West Lothian milk outbreak in 1994 with 100 cases (68 confirmed) was also a world record and there have also been infections transmitted by cheese – with a 22-case outbreak in Grampian in the same year. Between 1989 and 1997 the Scottish Centre for Infection and Environmental Health (SCIEH) recorded 28 outbreaks – an unenviable record, particularly when account is taken of the fact that most cases of *E coli* O157 infection are sporadic (73 per cent of the 1744 cases reported to SCIEH between 1990 and 1996). Of even greater concern has been the long term trend in infection rates. A massive increase has occurred since 1984, when the organism was first seen in Scotland. In that year only three isolates were made. More than a hundred-fold increase has occurred since then and it continues. Annual infection rates for the whole country have risen from 2.24 per 100,000 in 1992 to 9.85 in 1996. That Scotland has a real and particular problem is shown by comparison with data from other countries. Wales probably has the most comprehensive surveillance system in the world. All acute faecal samples submitted from patients have been screened for *E coli* O157 since 1990. The average annual rate of laboratory confirmed infections for 1990–96 was less than 1.5/100,000. In Scotland for the same period the rate has been greater than 5/100,000.

Comparison with the rest of the world is not straightforward for two reasons. First, the surveillance and reporting system in the UK is better developed than just about anywhere else, and comparable data are not often available. Second, the severe illness caused by *E coli* O157 – with the major complication of the haemolytic uraemic syndrome as a notable feature – is sometimes caused in other countries by different *E coli* serotypes, such as O111. Routine selective detection methods for these organisms are not yet available. Those comparisons that can be made show, however, that Scotland stands out internationally because of its high incidence of infection.[4] Canada, which is the closest rival in incidence rates, approached Scottish levels with 5.3/100,000 in 1991. This fell back to 3.0/100,000 by 1993, but has increased again recently. A recent study there introduced a major caveat to these figures by estimating that for every symptomatic case reported, between 4–9 go unreported. In the USA more than 100 outbreaks have been reported since 1982. Country-wide laboratory-based surveillance is still being developed there – between 1993 and 1995 the annual average incidence across states was 0.74/100,000 – but under-reporting is known to be a significant problem, in part due to inadequate testing. In Japan the situation is very complex.[5] In 1996 9,451 cases were reported, 1,808 patients being hospitalised and 12 having died. Many strains of *E coli* O157 were involved and more than 200 pulsed field electrophoresis patterns have been identified. What about other smaller countries? Sweden had between zero and three cases per year up till 1995; since then there have been several outbreaks and an annual incidence of 0.1/100,000 from 1989 to 1996. Germany has a problem but is unsure about its scale because of the lack of a nationwide surveillance system. Australia has had two outbreaks, one in 1995 and one in 1996.

These statistics clearly indicate that on the one hand *E coli* O157 and its relatives are causing problems on an increasing scale in many parts of the world, and show on the other hand that a lot more work needs to be done to develop and set up systems to estimate accurately the size of the problem.

This is, of course, not the only unanswered question about the science of *E coli* O157. Indeed, as more infections are reported the more uncertainties are uncovered. It is because of this ignorance that no answer can be given to the question 'Why is *E coli* O157 such a problem in Scotland?' Although it is known that the organism can live in the intestines of cows and sheep (and a range of other animal species as well, although pigs and chickens do not appear to carry strains pathogenic for man) it is not clear whether the scale of the human health problem in Scotland relates to higher carriage rates in animals. The role played by other risk factors is equally uncertain – is the high human incidence due to features of the Scottish diet, or cooking practices? *E coli* O157 is a new organism – it appeared out of the blue in 1982 – and it is almost certain that it is still evolving. It is probably descended from an ordinary *E coli* that picked up genes for virulence factors from other bacteria.[6] Other serotypes have done this as well – like *E coli* O111. Are strains like these, which cause problems in Europe and Australia, going to affect Scotland as well? This is an important question because these strains are much more difficult to detect in the routine diagnostic laboratory than *E coli* O157.

In summary, therefore, *E coli* O157 is a new and evolving pathogen. Consequently, our scientific knowledge about it is imperfect. This deficiency is great enough to significantly impede our ability to predict its behaviour and develop rational specific control measures. Infection with the organism is much commoner in the UK than elsewhere in Europe. *E coli* O157 shares these properties with another infectious agent which has also emerged to become a public health problem over the last decade. It causes bovine spongiform encephalopathy, BSE.

This new disease was first identified in November 1986 following the examination of the brains of two cows that had been sent to the main government Veterinary Laboratory from locations in south east and south west England.[7] Pathologically the changes in these brains resembled those seen in scrapie, a transmissible disease in sheep characterised by the appearance of vacuoles – empty sherical regions – in certain brain cells. These changes and the clinical features of the disease indicated that it belongs to the class of conditions known as transmissible spongiform encephalopathies – neurodegenerative diseases affecting a wide range of species, from mink to man.[8] In contradistinction to the characteristic and well-described histopathological and clinical features of these diseases, the precise nature of the infective agent that causes them remains a subject for research. It is a field currently far from closure.[9] There is little doubt that a central role in the disease is played by a naturally occurring protein found in cells in the brains and other organs of unaffected animals. Termed the prion protein (PrP) it becomes altered in animals with spongiform encephalopathies. In them its molecules fold up in a new and abnormal way. They build up in brain cells where they exert a toxic and lethal effect on them. The dominant scientific view is that this altered protein is in itself infectious and can transmit the disease from individual to individual – when it is eaten, for example. Others believe that this hypothesis cannot explain the occurrence of large numbers of different sub-types of agent found in diseases like scrapie and postulate that another molecule – probably a small nucleic acid – is essential. If this exists it is clear that it is not a conventional virus, because it has long been known that, unlike agents of this type, the transmissible agents of spongi-form encephalopathies are extremely resistant to heat, X-rays and reactive disinfectant chemicals like formaldehyde. Experimentation on spongiform encephalopathies is very difficult. The prion protein, for example, is very sticky, making it almost impossible to purify. Another very significant impediment to progress via experimentation is the very long incubation period that occurs between inoculation and the onset of disease. For cattle this ranges from three to six years, averaging five years.

After its initial diagnosis and description in Britain, the number of cases of BSE rose rapidly (Table 1).[10]

Table 1. *Confirmed cases of BSE in UK Cattle*

Year	No. of confirmed cases
1988	2,184
1989	7,136
1990	14,181
1991	25,027
1992	36,681
1993	34,360
1994	23,944
1995	14,076
1996	7,751

It is generally agreed the most probable aetiological hypothesis is that BSE was caused by an agent contained in meat-and-bone meal (MBM). This was prepared from ruminant carcasses and was included in cattle rations as a source of protein. It has been calculated that effective exposure of the cattle population to the agent started in 1981/82, a time coinciding with a significant reduction in the use of hydrocarbon solvents for the extraction of fat during MBM production. Strong epidemiological evidence favouring meat-and-bone meal as a vehicle for the agent was the large difference in the incidence of affected dairy herds compared with beef suckler herds. About 60 per cent of British dairy herds have been affected compared with 15.3 per cent of beef suckler herds, with an even greater proportional difference in Northern Ireland. Beef suckler herds receive much less concentrate rations in their overall diet. The occurrence of spongiform encephalopathies in exotic antelopes and other related animals in zoos that had been fed MBM also supported the hypothesis.

The actions taken by the UK Government action in response to BSE have been based on this hypothesis. In essence they have been:

a) to exclude from cattle feed all ruminant material which could convey BSE to cattle

b) to exclude from the human food chain parts of the bovine carcase which, laboratory experiments show, could convey BSE infectivity, if the animal were infected, and which could convey BSE to man, if it were transmissible to man.

A large body of rules to achieve these twin aims has been introduced by legislation since June 1988, in total amounting to more than 50 legal instruments. Three key features of this legislation have been:

a) progressive steps towards the complete exclusion of mammalian meat – and bonemeal – from all farm animal feed

b) a requirement that all cattle which are suspected of having BSE are slaughtered and destroyed

c) a requirement to remove Specified Bovine Offals (SBO; now called Specified Bovine Material – SBM: parts of the carcase known to contain the BSE agent in infected animals) from healthy cattle carcases at the time of slaughter, and to destroy them under strict controls.

Key policy decisions and actions taken by the UK Government between 1988 and 1994 are summarised in Table 2.

Table 2. *Key policy decisions and actions taken by the UK Government between 1988 and 1995.*

1988	February	Ban of beef offal in baby food
	June	BSE made a notifiable disease
	July	Sale or supply of ruminant animal protein banned
	August	All clinically suspect animals slaughtered and carcases to be destroyed. 50 per cent compensation (approx £400/cow) to be paid
	December	Milk from suspect animals to be destroyed
1989	July	EU ban on trade of live cattle born before 1988
	November	Specified bovine offals (SBOs) from all cattle over 6 months banned for human consumption
	February	100 per cent compensation for slaughter of infected cattle introduced
	April	BSE made notifiable throughout EU
	September	Specified bovine offal prohibited in all animal feeds
1994	June	Gillian Shephard, Minister of Agriculture: 'I should repeat that the Chief Medical Officer continues to advise that there is no evidence whatsoever that BSE causes CJD and, similarly, not the slightest evidence that eating beef or hamburgers causes CJD'.

On 20 March 1996 the Minister of Health announced to the House of Commons that:

The ten cases of a new variant of Creutzfeld-Jakob disease (CJD) identified in people aged under 42 which have been studied by the CJD Surveillance Unit in Edinburgh University were considered by SEAC (the Government's advisory committee on Spongiform Encephalopathies). SEAC concluded that the most likely explanation at present is that these cases are linked to exposure to BSE before the specified offal ban in 1989.

The response to this announcement was:

i)   a total ban on use of MBM in all farm animal feed to ensure that no cross-contamination of cattle feed is possible

ii) the whole head of bovine animals now proscribed as SBM

iii) a ban on sale for human consumption of meat from cattle over 30 months old

iv) the slaughter, rendering and incineration of all bovine animals over 30 months.

So far more than 70 cases of new variant CJD have been definitively diagnosed. It is too early to say whether they stand at the beginning or the middle of an epidemic, and, if the former, what its eventual size will be. Only time will tell. This uncertainty comes, of course, from our incomplete understanding of the relationship between BSE and new variant CJD. While it is certain that many individuals must have eaten infected material from cattle infected with the BSE agent,[11] it is not known how transmissible the agent is to man by this route or what incubation period intervenes between ingestion and the development of disease.

The agents of BSE and O157 are new pathogens which first appeared in the 1980s and which caused dramatic public health crises in the late 1990s. Their impact as public health problems has been very great. BSE has been a particularly British disease and Scotland currently has the highest incidence of infection in the world with *E coli* O157. Whatever the reasons for this – and it would be rash to reject stochastic explanations at least for the latter – their occurrence and spread has shown that the current British system for protecting the public from unsafe food has significant deficiencies. These however, are highly unlikely to be UK-specific. This is not the only lesson that these diseases have taught us. They have also forcefully reminded us that the evolution of pathogens is an active process which proceeds in real time and is one that for all practical purposes is impossible to predict. So as a microbiologist it gave me no happiness to suffer schadenfreude when recalling the misguided 1967 statement by the US Surgeon General 'the time has come to close the books on infectious disease'!

POSTSCRIPT

Notable developments have occurred since the symposium. The incidence of human infections with *E coli* O157 in the United Kingdom has continued to increase, particularly in England and Northern Ireland. While the number of cases of BSE in cattle continues to fall in line with predictions, showing that control measures are working satisfactorily, the evidence linking the disease with new variant CJD in man has been significantly strengthened by strain type studies.[12] No differences could be found between the agent present in brain tissue from BSE-infected cattle and from individuals with new variant CJD.

The award of the 1997 Nobel Prize for Medicine or Physiology to Stanley Prusiner has been controversial. He is a leading proponent of the infectious protein hypothesis. A not untypical comment refers to remaining uncertainties about the nature of the transmissible agent in spongiform encephalopathies:[13]

> It would be tragic if the recent Nobel Prize award were to lead to complacency regarding the obstacles still remaining. It is not more detail, but rather the central core of the problem, that remains to be solved.

The Food Standards Agency – largely organised along the lines proposed by Philip James – started work in April 2000. Evidence of benefits from it are eagerly awaited – as are the imminent findings of the BSE Inquiry set up in December 1997 and chaired by the judge, Sir Nicolas Phillips.[14]

BIBLIOGRAPHY

Advisory Committee on the Microbial Safety of Food. Report on Verocytotoxin-producing *Escherichia coli* (HMSO), London, 1995.

Almond, J and Pattison, J. Human BSE, *Nature*, 389 (1997), 437.

Anderson, R M et al. Transmission dynamics and epidemiology of BSE in British cattle, *Nature*, 382 (1996), 779.

Bruce, M E et al. Transmissions to mice indicate that 'new variant' CJD is caused by the BSE agent, *Nature*, 389 (1997), 498.

Chesebro, B. BSE and prions: uncertainties about the agent, *Science*, 279 (1998), 42.

Hill, A F et al. The same prion strain causes vCJD and BSE, *Nature*, 389 (1997), 448.

Izumiya, H et al. Molecular typing of Enterhaemorrhagic *Escherichia coli* O157: H7 isolates in Japan using pulsed-field gel electrophoresis, *Journal of Clinical Microbiology*, 35 (1997), 1675.

James, W P T. *Food Standards Agency. An interim proposal*, 1997.

Prevention and Control of Enterohaemorrhagic Eschericia coli (EHEC) infections. *Report of a WHO Consultation, Geneva, Switzerland 28 April–1 May 1994* (World Health Organization), 1997.

Spongiform Encephalopathy Advisory Committee. *Transmissible Spongiform Encephalopathies: A summary of present knowledge and research*, (HMSO), 1994.

The Pennington Group. *Report on the Circumstances Leading to the 1996 Outbreak of infection with E coli O157 in Central Scotland, with Implications for*

Food Safety and the Lessons to be Learned, (The Stationery Office) Edinburgh, 1997.
Wells, G A H et al. A novel progressive spongiform encephalopathy in cattle, *Veterinary Record*, 121 (1987), 419

NOTES

1 The Pennington Group.
2 James, 1997.
3 Advisory Committee on the Microbial Safety of Food.
4 Prevention and Control of Enterohaemorrhagic (EHEC) Infections.
5 Izumiya et al, 1997.
6 Advisory Committee on the Microbial Safety of Food.
7 Wells et al, 1987.
8 Spongiform Encephalopathy Committee.
9 Chesebro, 1998.
10 Anderson et al, 1996.
11 ibid.
12 Bruce et al, 1997; Hill et al, 1997; Almond and Pattison, 1997.
13 Chesebro, 1998.
14. www.bse.org.uk

Part 1

Nutrition, the Carnegie Survey
and Sir John Boyd Orr

2 Glasgow Corporation and the food of the poor, 1918–24: a context for John Boyd Orr

John E Burnett

INTRODUCTION

'Poverty, bad housing, poor food, were sectors in a vicious circle'[1] – a vicious circle which resulted in ill health. Thus wrote Archibald Kerr Chalmers, Medical Officer of Health (MOH) to the City of Glasgow, suggesting the connections which John Boyd Orr was later to demonstrate unanswerably in *Food, Health and Income* (1936).

By 1920, when Chalmers penned these words, public health workers in the larger cities of Britain were aware of the link between poverty and diet on one hand, and on the other, infant mortality, retarded growth and susceptibility to disease. Indeed, some had perceived such a link in the first half of the nineteenth century. The rejection of a disturbing proportion of potential army recruits for the Boer War because they were small, malnourished or diseased, had made the problem quite clear. The public health profession, used to dealing with issues which affected people in the mass rather than individually, and also seeking new areas of activity as the incidence of infectious diseases declined, began to take an interest in diet. Yet the causal links between restricted diet and ill-health were not proven: was it lack of money which forced the poor to eat badly, or lack of common sense in selecting their food? What really constituted an adequate and healthy diet?

Glasgow was one of the first industrial cities. In the eighteenth century it grew to become the second largest city in Scotland; by 1901 it was the second city of the British Empire with a population of 760,000. It grew on the basis of cheap labour, and people there lived cheaply because they endured poor food and cheap accommodation. In the 1840s Chadwick said that 'the structural arrangements and the condition of the population of Glasgow were the worst of any we had seen in any part of Great Britain.'[2] In the language of social historians there was a poor wage–rent relationship in Glasgow.[3] It was a centre not just of manufacturing but of heavy industry, and it depended on the work of coal and ironstone miners in and around the city. In the shipyards and locomotive works there were many skilled trades but ironworks and chemical factories required a large pool of unskilled labour and even the engineering works needed unskilled hands: many men were forced to accept low wages.

It is recognised that by 1900 working people in and around Glasgow had a poor diet, containing insufficient energy and lacking variety: malnourished children grew into stunted adults, smaller than their grandparents.[4] The same pattern of the decrease of the mean height of a population of an industrialising society can be seen in the United States and in Austro-Hungary in the middle of the nineteenth century.[5] The decline in maternal and infant mortality in the years before World War I was partly due to a diet which was improving in the train of slowly increasing wealth. Nevertheless, means and averages conceal the fact that the very poor and weak were never sure of an adequate supply of food.

The purpose of this essay is to describe some of the issues relating to food and diet faced by the Glasgow Corporation Public Health Department between 1918 and 1924, and the difficulties they had in taking intelligent action. In particular the food of the very poor is considered because some of them, particularly pregnant women, mothers and children, came close to the *restricted diet famine* in Oddy's typology of famine.[6] Those who had a little more money were able to maintain a satisfactory diet. They were typically artisans living in a room and kitchen, who were members of a provident society or trade union, and had their own savings.[7] But the poor did not have this financial ballast, and their diet became a matter of civic concern.

As Simon Szreter has emphasised, the improvements in health brought about by public health professionals have first to be understood at the local level, in terms of 'fallible, blundering, but purposive human agency.'[8] It is necessary, therefore, to say a little more about Glasgow. The city's political character was unusual. Before World War I it was dominated by *municipal socialism*. The Corporation was controlled by men who were already successful in business rather than by professional politicians. The 'municipal socialists' wanted effective local government and they were prepared to work for it: they attended meetings including those of committees, and did not regard membership of the Corporation as a sinecure. They were not afraid to invest if they could see resulting benefits. They knew that social and political stability was good for business, and sought to minimise the possibly disruptive influence of the Catholic Irish.[9] Their Protestant morality made them dislike poverty, but they also feared it as a possible cause of unrest. 'Bolshevism, like tuberculosis, is a disease of poverty', said their mouthpiece, the *Glasgow Herald*. On the basis of the ideology of municipal socialism, Glasgow had developed a high level of municipal ownership of its infrastructure. Water and gas supply, and electric power, tramways and lodging houses were all owned by the Corporation.

The municipal socialists lost their power during World War I and in the subsequent collapse of the economy. The social and political divisions which they had sought to suppress were revealed. The Independent Labour Party (ILP) became prominent: Clydeside went red. Men who were later to become famous at Westminster joined the Corporation, including Mannie Shinwell and Jimmy Maxton, perhaps the most principled of them all. Though their politics were different from their predecessors', their concern for the poor and support for the Public Health Department were unwavering. In the Labour landslide at the General Election of November 1922 Glasgow's leading socialists were elected to Parliament. After the departure of these firebrands to London the membership of Glasgow Corporation was less vividly radical, though the Public Health professionals were no less active.

Glasgow had a record of taking vigorous action in matters of public health.[10] In 1857 the city had opened the greatest of Victorian water supply works, bringing water from Loch Katrine in the Trossachs. Fifty years after it opened, it was still seen as the finest water supply scheme in Britain.[11] James B Russell (1837–1904) had from 1872 to 1898 been the City's MOH, a campaigner and administrator of schemes which tackled many difficulties. Glasgow had a particularly good record of establishing effective institutions to promote change, of which the City of Glasgow Improvement Trust and the City's own Sanitary Department were the most important.

Russell was succeeded by Archibald Kerr Chalmers (1857–1942).[12] He was born in Greenock and took his degree in medicine at Glasgow and Diploma in Public Health at Cambridge. He joined Glasgow's Public Health Department in 1891 and took over from Russell as MOH eight years later. Chalmers held the post for 26 years, a significant period during which public health moved from being purely concerned with removing disease to monitoring health and taking measures such as education and providing food for the newborn. Working in parallel with Chalmers was the vigorous and lively Alexander M Trotter, Glasgow's first Veterinary Officer. He was appointed in 1899.

Chalmers saw his Department standing 'between the citizen and disease', serving the public by saving them from 'chronic invalidism and dependence' which were caused by disease.[13] There was a pragmatic side to this view, which it shared with Lloyd George's National Insurance Act of 1911. This legislation aimed to support not the whole population, but the breadwinner in each family: a sick man who returned to work quickly could continue to support his family.

Chalmers may in one sense have been atypical of MOHs. Anna Davin has shown that public health professionals at the beginning of the twentieth century stressed maternal ignorance as the prime cause of infant mortality, rather than environmental factors, infection, or an insufficient number of doctors.[14] Chalmers always emphasised the environment as a cause – even in the surprising instance of *alcoholism*. Chalmers used the term to mean excessive drinking which resulted in death following *delirium tremens*, or from cirrhosis, or from other direct results of consuming alcohol. Chalm-

ers believed that alcoholism was caused by 'the essentially unhealthy conditions of social and industrial life',[15] 'the nerve-racking strain of incessant
noise from machinery and traffic.'[16] In other words, it corresponded to the
traditional view of the public health professional that infectious diseases
derive from physical surroundings, whatever the causal mechanism. However, by 'social' conditions he meant aspects of life which had deteriorated
since the war years when factory canteens had fed people properly and
there had been an understanding that national efficiency depended on the
efficiency of the individual.[17]

This is not so say that Chalmers imagined that individuals had no role
in promoting health. In 1922 the Corporation published a pamphlet which
gave guidance to mothers on the care of their newborn children. The first
piece of advice was that the mother should have a plain diet, and that:

> Above all things she should avoid whisky or alcohol in any form. For a mother
> to drink whisky is almost as bad as to give it to the child directly, which would
> be to poison it.[18]

This is shocking. Yet it was appropriate, for there is anecdotal evidence that
drunken women were a common sight on the streets of Glasgow.[19] Chalmers did not advocate abstinence from alcohol, for he was not a moralist and
his concern was not with the way in which the poor used their money. His
distant goal was to see a healthy people with an adequate income, living
in sound housing. To Chalmers it was the environment, as much as the individual's behaviour, which raised the level of disease.

FOOD IN POSTWAR BRITAIN

Britain went through a period of social instability after World War I. It
was not the kind of ferment which Germany and Austria experienced at the
same time; nevertheless, it was probably as acute as anything Britain had
undergone since the 1820s. Government expenditure, distended during the
War, fell under the Geddes axe in 1922. Agricultural prices, at first artificially high, collapsed. Unemployment rose rapidly during 1921–2 and there
was a miners' strike. The Irish war of independence of 1919–22 affected the
west of Scotland because there were family ties with both the Unionist and
Nationalist communities.[20]

The government's control of the distribution of food had grown during
the War. A Food Department at the Board of Trade was created in August
1916, the Ministry of Food four months later, and rationing and control
of the food supply began on 1 January 1918.[21] Control ensured that the
peoples' diet did not deteriorate, and full employment meant that the whole
of the working population was able to afford the food they needed.[22] The
Ministry of Food was abolished in 1921. Despite the improvement in the
health of most sections of the community, except the elderly, during World
War I,[23] food again posed acute problems in the early 1920s.

The end of the War brought a rapid reduction in the government's demand for food, both locally and generally. There were many government-funded organisations throughout the country, including war hospitals, and canteens had been added to munitions works to ensure that the workers were properly fed. For the supply of some forms of food, such as fresh milk, this change was sudden.[24]

When Lloyd George introduced the slogan 'Homes fit for heroes' he was doing more than committing himself to a housing policy. He was also indicating a vision – an ill-defined vision – of postwar Britain as being something which was worth fighting for, something which would justify sacrifice. An editorial in the *Glasgow Herald* in February 1919 took up the theme. It argued that the better world which had been earned included physical wellbeing for all. It recognised that this would be 'the fruit of sys-tematic instruction, thorough organisation, long views, and the calculated expenditure of considerable funds.' An adequate diet was part of this con-ception of the future for:

> There is a longing that the energy of man and the resources of science, which have been bent to the destruction of wealth and human life, should be concen-trated on conserving and building up the race and on relieving its lot . . .[25]

This idealism was to be made irrelevant when in 1922 it became clear that the State was incapable of the calculated expenditure of considerable funds. After Geddes had slashed government expenditure, what remained was the idea that government was responsible for the well-being of the nation and that it could take legislative action to exercise this responsibil-ity. Similar thinking appeared in industry, where the concept of *welfare* had been developed during the War. It covered not only the provision of facili-ties such as canteens which sold nutritious food, but also 'welfare supervi-sion' whose aim was to control the behaviour of individuals.[26] There was thus a climate of ideas in which it was possible for a local authority like Glasgow Corporation to intervene in the feeding of the poor to an extent which had not been possible before 1914.

INSTITUTIONS AND INDIVIDUALS

The legislative situation of food in Britain was by 1920 extraordinarily complex.[27] In the second half of the nineteenth century the number of local government bodies had increased rapidly, and in many cases each func-tion – policing, or road repair – had its own authority with a particular geo-graphical area of operation and its own relationships with other authorities. Before the Local Government (Scotland) Act 1929 there were 204 burgh councils in Scotland, 107 of their rural equivalent, district committees, 876 parish councils and 947 school boards.[28] Many also operated on the motto *that government governs best that governs least*, and did not make full use of their powers. Much of the legislation was permissive: it gave powers but did not require them to be exercised. The elected members who controlled these bodies always hoped to minimise expenditure.

During the Great War the situation changed. Central government took upon itself many new powers, affecting a wide range of life: it passed Acts, changed them by Miscellaneous Clauses at the end of other Acts, and issued Orders and Circulars. It also issued powers to local government, and expected them to be active in implementing and acting upon these powers. At the same time, some existing powers were dropped – *de facto* if not *de jure*. Before 1914 the Glasgow Public Health Department could inspect a farm outside its boundaries if it were supplying diseased milk, but it could not find the staff to do this in the later years of the War. When food was short during the War, tuberculous meat was not destroyed by the meat inspectors in Glasgow: it was eaten. After the Armistice, the level of complexity increased further. Some, but by no means all of the wartime legislation was dropped, or changed.

Which official bodies had rôles which affected the food eaten in Glasgow? The Corporation, through its Medical Officer of Health and Veterinary Officer, was able to comment on the nature and quality of the food consumed, and the City Chemist sought adulteration. When it came to feeding the poorest Glaswegians, several other parties were involved. Chalmers said:

> One Authority is charged with the relief of destitution, another with feeding the children whose education is handicapped by inadequate feeding, and a third with the feeding of nursing or expectant mothers and of children under five, where more adequate feeding is medically certified to be necessary and the circumstances necessitous.[29]

These three authorities were the Parish – there were two in Glasgow – the Local Education Authority, whose concern was with children over five, and the Corporation. Their relationships were often strained. When in 1923 it was suggested that these three Glasgow authorities should co-operate with one another, nothing happened.[30] The Parish Councils were less powerful than the Corporation, and their membership was not made up of civic leaders but of minor capitalists, particularly shopkeepers. Thus they were notoriously reluctant to pay for relief, which they continued to insist would be given to able-bodied men only if they took the humiliating step of entering the workhouse.[31]

Whatever the views of the health professionals, they had to be aware of those of the elected members of the Corporation who in turn were both trying to find solutions to Glasgow's problems and to manipulate public opinion. For example, Manny Shinwell, before leaving for a long career at Westminster, protested about the need for local supply of milk to nursing mothers, rather than requiring them all to travel to the centre of the city.[32] Glasgow's socialist MPs raised in parliament the need for milk for mothers and children among their constituents.[33]

Local authorities had to report both to arms of government in London such as the Ministry of Health, and also parts of the Scottish Office in Edinburgh, the Boards of Education and Health. The rôle of the Boards was complex in that although their permission had to be sought to take certain action – such as supplying free milk to the poor – they would also bear half of the cost if approval were given.

The institutions and individuals mentioned above had formal rôles which affected the food eaten by the poor in Glasgow. Others acted informally, including academic nutritionists such as Dairmid Noel Paton and Annabel Tully, both at Glasgow University. It is probably impossible to know how much influence they had. Some local charities, such as the Cowcaddens Soup Kitchen, supplied food; and national charities such as the Babies of the Empire Society agitated on a broader front.

Local Authorities other than those in Glasgow could affect the quality of food supplied to the city. When cases of 'sore throat' – diphtheria – in the city were traced to a dairy in Dunbartonshire, Glasgow could take no more action than to say that no more of its milk should be sold in the city.[34] Dunbartonshire was solely responsible for the health of the cattle. Glasgow was, however, able to insist that milk cows which were being tended in the city were slaughtered if they were suffering from tuberculosis.

A similar situation was discovered in 1923. Much of Glasgow's milk came from Ayrshire, and the County Clerk of Ayrshire suggested that in order to implement new legislation, Glasgow should either provide staff to inspect cattle in Ayrshire, or bear part of the cost. In raising the issue, the County Clerk revealed that Ayrshire had never implemented the Dairies, Cowsheds and Milk Order (1899). This had included some of the most basic precautions against tuberculosis, including the requirement that milk from a tuberculous cow should not be mixed with that from other cattle. Ayrshire had, quite simply, ignored the Order. The officials in Glasgow wrote angry minutes to one another about their irresponsible colleagues and the proposed financial burden on Glasgow, but Trotter, the Veterinary Officer, was clear about the priorities:

> It is not a matter of money. It is a matter of health and ... it is imperative that we be in the position of safe-guarding the health of the citizens of this City.[35]

The idea emerged of creating a 'Milk Board' for the West of Scotland, not as a device for marketing in the manner of the Milk Marketing Boards of the 1930s, but as a way of supervising the quality of milk.[36] Chalmers felt that Ayrshire should bear the whole cost, but acidly observed that a Milk Board 'might avert what appeared to be an impending arrest of administrative effort' in Ayrshire.[37] But were local authorities empowered to co-operate in this way? After some prodding the Scottish Board of Health gave its opinion that there was no legislation to support 'the combination of local authorities' in matters of milk supply – but the Board agreed in principle with the closest co-operation.[38] Whatever fine sentiments the Board of Health might express, absence of legal power meant that the idea of a Milk Board could not be carried forward.[39] Yet correspondence must have had one effect: Ayrshire now knew that the Board of Health was aware of the absence of veterinary inspection of dairy cattle in the county.

The smaller authorities exhibited varying degrees of energy and competence, and most of them did not employ full-time professionals to act for them and advise them: many Medical Officers of Health were in general practice, and a few scientists in the cities acted as Public Analysts for a dozen or so authorities each, as well as having their own consulting practice.

In the midst of this administrative maze the most powerful figure commenting on the diet of the poor was Glasgow's Medical Officer of Health. Chalmers was a leader in a profession which had attracted great respect because of its apparent ability to solve one problem after another. The ideas of Public Health had dealt with one disease after another. It had developed methods for quantifying problems, usually by finding a way to use local legislation as a way of recording the incidence of a problem. Chalmers and his staff were not only professionals but also Glaswegians with an understanding of the people of the city. Nevertheless, action was limited by the complexity of local government.

FOOD SHORTAGES AND HUNGER

Food became a crucial issue at the end of the War, when there were acute shortages and rationing had to be applied rigorously. In the winter of 1918–19 there was an inadequate supply of milk in some areas of the city.[40] The following summer the Scottish Board of Health asked the city to circulate a card which explained to housewives that they should take steps to stop milk from souring and so being wasted; the Corporation preferred to place notices in the newspapers.[41]

The food shortage raised the issue of food wastage. Trotter observed that in the slaughterhouse the blood of pigs, calves and sheep was being allowed to run into the sewers when it could be used as food or at least for animal feeding or as a component in manure. He also pointed out that fat was being wasted by the carelessness of the men who rendered the cattle, such as the 'gut drawers' who removed the fat attached to the guts. He was also concerned that tripe, ox feet and sheep trotters were being sent to the North of England,[42] where there was a stronger tradition of eating offal, rather than being consumed in Glasgow.

In the winter of 1919–20, the Ministry of Food raised the price of milk over the whole country. In the poorest areas of Glasgow, such as Milend, the consumption immediately fell by a third despite there being a surplus of milk on the market in the city. A Welfare Nurse who worked in the Calton said 'the very poor here never use milk in the quantity they should, but give the infants tea with toast soaked in it.' Porridge made with milk, and milk puddings had been given up, and rice with milk at midday had been

replaced by cocoa. Nurses reported that mothers understood the importance of milk for babies, and tried to make up for the lack of cows' milk
by breast feeding as much as possible.[43] At the beginning of 1920 the great
influenza epidemic of 1918–19 was still a vivid memory and Chambers
pointed out that babies needed milk to grow up strong enough to resist
infectious diseases.[44]

The rapid rise in unemployment between the summers of 1920 and 1921
brought the threat of starvation back to Glasgow. Under the organisation
of the Independent Labour Party demonstrators carried banners reading
'1914 – Fighting, 1920 – Starving'.[45] John Maclean, the communist leader,
said that if people could not afford the food they needed, they should take
it, and was jailed for sedition.[46]

The miners' strike of 1921 posed new problems. The Corporation began
to supply meals to expectant and nursing mothers and to children under
five in 'necessitous' cases. It had already been supplying some school meals
through the Local Education Authority, but during the strike the demand
for meals exceeded the LEA's ability to organise them, and the Corporation
contracted the United Co-operative Baking Society to do so.[47]

During the period of high unemployment the Corporation itself paid for
the feeding of mothers and children: in the year to June 1922 they spent
£133,221: in March the figure peaked at 10,166 mothers and their children.[48] Since each meal cost about 3½d, each mother brought on average
three children to be fed. The meals supplied were organised on a weekly
pattern:

Monday	Mince, bread and margarine, tea
Tuesday	Steak pie, potatoes, sago pudding
Wednesday	Vegetable broth, bread and margarine, plum pudding
Thursday	Mince, potatoes, Creamola pudding and milk
Friday	Lentil soup, bread and margarine, sago pudding and milk
Saturday	Steak pie, bread and margarine, tea

The first aim in shaping this dietary plan was to provide energy. Chalmers
used the Royal Society's figure of 3390 calories for a man doing an average day's work, and concluded that a woman should have 2700 and a child
under 5, 1350. He was also aware that the diet of the poor was usually
protein- and fat-deficient, and he tried to remedy this. The dinners were
designed on the assumption that families would continue to take 'tea' in the
morning and evening – 'tea' meaning tea with milk and sugar accompanied
by bread and margarine.[49]

The most important evidence of the famine conditions which were being
experienced by the poor in the summer of 1922 was an examination of the
diet and health of twelve families from the 'labouring class', a total of 97
people. The fathers of these families were either unemployed or working
short time or irregularly.[50] They were making every attempt to apply their
relief from the Parish or from National Insurance to their food, by borrow-

ing money, by delaying the payment of rent until legal action was taken
against them, and by obtaining credit from shopkeepers. The collapse of
agricultural prices had lowered the cost, compared with a year earlier,
of bread, margarine, sausages, potatoes and corned beef. The amount of
energy content which they were able to buy with each penny had risen by
a third in the year. Despite this, the energy intake per man had fallen from
2500 to 2200 calories per day in the same period, and the weight of boys
and girls in poor families fell by 7.5 per cent and 7.0 per cent respectively
between 1919–21 and 1923. This report did not examine the way in which
food was distributed within the family, though in one case it commented
that the children looked surprisingly well, but the mother seemed severely
undernourished. The diet of all the families was based on bread, and mothers were making money go as far as possible by buying 'end loaves', or
loaves which were burnt or misshapen and so cheaper.

The authors of this study were two women, one medically qualified,
working in Glasgow University. Chalmers made further observations on
their data. He emphasised that milk was almost absent from their diet, that
margarine had been substituted for butter, that bread was the staple, and
that although fresh oranges were cheap, neither they nor any other fruit
formed any part of the food intake. He also considered 'vitamines'. The
existence of 'accessory food factors' had been emerging in the scientific
world since the 1880s and in 1912–13 three of them were defined as vitamines A, B and C.[51] The lack of milk caused deficiencies in all three vitamins, and the cheapest margarine (unlike butter) contained no vitamin A.
Chalmers also pointed out that vitamin A – in fact the component of it
which we would now call vitamin D – could have been gained from oranges
and vitamin C from apples. His conclusion was that relief was essential.

THE QUALITY OF FOOD

So far we have been discussing the quantity and nature of the food which
the poor were able to consume. The quality of the food was also an important issue. It relates to quantity because the poor were forced to buy the
cheapest food, which was often of low quality.

Glasgow had solved its water-supply problem by vast capital expenditure.
Milk supply was a similar problem in that it involved bringing a large quantity of liquid to the city from the surrounding country. It was different in
that the production of milk could not be concentrated in one place and
piped into the city: there was no opportunity for a capital project like the
Loch Katrine water supply scheme which would deliver a corporate solution. Milk production was in the hands of dairy farmers most of whom
operated on a small scale, and its supply was controlled by middle men.[52]

In the first decade of the twentieth century milk became central to ideas
about child care. It was seen as essential for the growth of the babies who
would become the healthy adults who would improve Britain's industrial

competitiveness and who would be a fighting resource in time of war. Yet at the same time milk was a highly effective communicator of disease, particularly tuberculosis, and an ideal environment for the rapid multiplication of bacteria.

Glasgow's interest in its milk supply began in 1888 when James B Russell was asked by the Town Council (the predecessor of the Corporation) to write a pamphlet to explain how a dairy farm should be managed in order to produce clean milk. It was a fine demonstration of his ability to write plain prose for the layman, but its significance is that it was the only means by which the City could put pressure on farmers outside its boundaries: no legal powers were available. In New York, Public Health Inspectors were in 1902 sent into the surrounding countryside to encourage farmers to improve the hygiene of milk production, and in 1910 all drinking milk in the city was required to be pasteurised.[53] Such legal powers were not available in Britain, and milk remained a potent transmitter of tuberculosis to Glasgow children.[54] Chalmers estimated in 1906 that only 221 of the 312 local authorities in Scotland had implemented Dairy Regulations under the Dairies, Cowsheds and Milk Order (1899).[55]

Tuberculosis had become a major issue, if an unresolved one, before World War I. The Milk and Dairies Act (Scotland) (1914) was passed and the Tuberculosis Order (1914) issued, but the declaration of war meant that neither came into force. The tuberculosis question took some time to re-emerge. Chalmers and Buchanan saw the Second Conference of the International Union Against Tuberculosis, held in London in July 1921, as an important step in reawakening interest.[56] It was not until 1923 that Glasgow Corporation began to agitate for the implementation of the 1914 legislation and the strengthening of the Order so that it applied not only to cows which were suffering from tuberculosis with emaciation of the udder, but to all cows with TB. The Corporation felt so strongly that it sent a deputation to call on the Minister of Agriculture in London.[57]

Milk carried not only tuberculosis but also other infectious diseases, and milk with a high bacterial count, even if it did not contain disease, went sour quickly. Consequently the Corporation resolved in March 1920 to examine 'the desirability of securing a pure milk supply for the citizens of Glasgow'.[58] They had in mind the example of Sheffield which under a left-wing council had taken powers to municipalise its milk supply.[59] Glasgow's aim was not to supply the whole population with milk, but to make available a supply of milk of assured quality which could be given to, or bought cheaply by, impoverished mothers and their children. The supply would also be used in hospitals and childrens' homes. This move was not the new beginning which it might seem to be in contemporary rhetoric (probably encouraged by the ILP), for the Corporation had been supplying some infants with milk by 1907. Their first step in 1921 was to contract supply to a co-operative group, the Scottish Farmers' Dairy Association Ltd, and this reduced the price by 2½d per gallon.[60] They also set up a sub-committee to examine the whole question of milk supply, and they focused on the idea of the Corporation owning a herd on a farm to the south-west of the city.[61] The wholesale reduction of the quantity of milk containing tuberculosis did not begin, however, until the 1930s.[62]

One of the tasks of the city's Veterinary Surgeon was the detection of tuberculous cows. He also had a more general role in inspecting animals which were slaughtered and carcasses which were offered for sale. Indeed, this was Trotter's principal task. His office was in the Cattle Market, whereas Chambers' office was beside the City Chambers.

The number of animals slaughtered in 1913, and of diseased carcasses condemned, was:

Cattle	91,525	3,123	3.4%
Sheep	300,097	366	0.1%
Pigs	35,793	249	0.7%
Goats	34	1	2.9%

Based on the breakdown of the number of condemned carcasses ten years later, almost half of the cattle had been suffering from tuberculosis, and another ten–fifteen per cent were actually decomposing by the time they were offered for sale.[63]

Glasgow relied on imports for much of its supply, and much of it came from Ireland and was landed on the Clyde. It was made up by other imports which came, under the control of the Ministry of Food, through Birkenhead. The city's Veterinary Surgeon complained that in the week of 17 August 1919, of 949 sides of beef which had arrived from Birkenhead, 94 sides and seven quarters were completely unfit for human consumption, and many more had to be trimmed. He complained 'Glasgow has always been the "dumping" ground of inferior cattle but . . . that is no reason why the Ministry of Food should continue this dumping process.'[64] Shortly afterwards, 126 carcases from the same source were condemned out of a consignment of 212.[65]

The Ministry of Food responded to Trotter by saying that supplying poor quality meat was the only way of meeting public demand.[66] There was some justification in this, for the people of Glasgow were used to eating cheaply by eating badly. A speciality of the meat trade in Glasgow and Liverpool was the import of boneless meat in bags. This was used to make sausages, and was an inexpensive form of protein. The use of sulphur dioxide to give meat the appearance of freshness was common and in Glasgow the gas was called *Madam Rachel* after an adventuress who had claimed to restore youth to women – for a fee.[67]

CONCLUSIONS: PUBLIC HEALTH AND JOHN BOYD ORR

John Boyd Orr (1880–1971) was not trained in public health administration and never practised it. Yet his attitudes and ideals were those of an effective MOH in an industrial city: in effect, he placed himself in the public health tradition. He was brought up in rural Ayrshire. When he went to Glasgow as a student he was shocked by the slums and later said that they, the poorest parts of Edinburgh and 'some other cities in the north of England were the worst housing in western Europe'. On Saturday nights he walked around Glasgow, building up his hatred of poverty and drunkenness.[68] Sydney Checkland has said that Boyd Orr was 'radicalised by his inquiries', meaning his studies of diet in the 1930s, but he had radical views on poverty before World War I.[69] In June 1923 Jimmy Maxton, the Independent Labour Party MP for Bridgeton, angered by the government's proposal to withdraw the provision of free meals to severely under-nourished schoolchildren, called the Conservative party 'murderers': he was suspended from the House of Commons.[70] Boyd Orr, who regarded himself as a Conservative, later wrote in praise of Maxton's intervention.[71]

There was a separate tradition of regarding the health problems of the poor as being caused, at least in part, by their own failings. Paton and his colleagues writing on diet in Edinburgh regarded them as feckless or irresponsible.[72] As late as 1922 he rejected the idea that rickets was a deficiency disease, instead seeing its cause in poor housing and the large size of families which prevented mothers giving as much attention as they should to individual children.[73] Many believed that the health problems of unskilled workers and their families were of their own making, and often related to drink.[74] A report of the Medical Research Council on the diet of miners said that their ill-health was caused by their wives' inability to choose and cook suitable food. A similar wish to see fault in working class behaviour lay behind the attempt to suppress Boyd Orr's *Food, Health and Income* (1936).[75]

The public health profession regarded itself as the protector of the people, and particularly of the disadvantaged. This was not an altruistic view. If the poor were more likely to suffer from say, typhus, they were more likely to be responsible for its communication to the middle classes. The professionals thus believed that action could result in change for the better: indeed, it was their role to ensure that it did so. They sought environmental causes which could be quantified and localised, such as overcrowded housing. In the early twentieth century environmental explanations were expanded into what might be called circumstantial ones, including family incomes. Income was a central factor in Annabel Tully's paper and in other dietary research in the same period. One of the reasons for the clarity of the argument of *Food, Health and Income* was Boyd Orr's simple method of handling the financial side of the problem.

Boyd Orr's approach differed from the public health tradition in that he was comparatively independent. He did not have the support of a powerful local authority, and at the same time he was not hamstrung by having to consider how to implement his ideas. Many who held the post of MOH believed that poverty and ill-health were closely linked, but were reluctant to say so and thus fall foul of the Ministry of Health and so jeopardise their careers.[76] An MOH had, in the end, to be pragmatic and to accept that there were political and economic limitations, whereas Boyd Orr could afford to reveal his idealistic streak. Yet, at the same time, the most effective MOHs were driven by their ideals. Chalmers certainly was. His last words to his Department, written after his retirement, were, 'There can be no armistice with disease.'[77]

ACKNOWLEDGEMENTS

For their help in locating the source material for this paper, I am grateful to the staff of Glasgow City Archives and in particular to Robert M Urquhart.

REFERENCES

The printed *Minutes of the Corporation of the City of Glasgow* are abbreviated as *MCCG*, and Glasgow City Archives as GCA.

NOTES

1 Chalmers, A K. 'A complete health service', typescript of a lecture, 1920, GCA D-HE 1/2/1, 5.
2 Quoted by Comrie, John D. *History of Scottish Medicine*, 2nd edn, 2 vols, London, 1932, ii, 647.
3 Daunton, Martin. Housing. In Thompson, F M L, ed, *The Cambridge Social History of Britain 1750–1950*, 3 vols, Cambridge, 1990, ii, 195–250, especially 198–206.
4 See, for example, Kitchin, A H and Passmore, R. *The Scotsman's Food*, Edinburgh, 1949, 36–49; Steven, Maisie. *The Good Scots Diet*, Aberdeen, 1985, 100–1; Fraser, W Hamish and Maver, Irene. The social problems of the city. In Fraser and Maver, eds, *Glasgow: volume II: 1830 to 1912*, Manchester, 1996, 352–93, 361–2.
5 Komolos, John. Stature and health. In Kiple, Kenneth D, ed, *The Cambridge World History of Human Disease*, Cambridge, 1993, 238–43, 239.
6 Oddy, D J. Urban famine in nineteenth-century Britain: the effect of the Lancashire cotton famine on working-class diet and health, *Economic History Review*, 2nd series, 36 (1983), 68-86, 71.
7 Tully, Annabel M T. A study of the diet and economic conditions of artisan families in Glasgow in May 1923, *Glasgow Medical Journal*, 101 (1924), 1–11.
8 Szreter, Simon. The importance of social invention in Britain's mortality decline, c1850–1914: a reinterpretation of the role of public health, *Social History of Medicine*, 1 (1988), 1–37, 35.
9 Aspinwall, Bernard. *Portable Utopia: Glasgow and the United States*, Aberdeen, 1984, 151–84.

10 Checkland, Olive. Local government and the health environment. In Checkland, Olive and Lamb, M, eds, *Health Care as Social History: the Glasgow case*, Aberdeen, 1982, 1–15.

11 *Encyclopedia Britannica* 11th ed, 29 vols, Cambridge, 1910–11, s v Glasgow.

12 For the careers of Russell and Chalmers, see Comrie, *op cit*, ii, 645-9; for Russell, Chalmers, A K, Biographical note, in Russell, J B. *Public Health Administration in Glasgow*, Glasgow, 1905, xiii–xxviii; and Robertson, Edna. *Glasgow's Doctor: James Burn Russell MOH 1837–1904*, East Linton, 1998; for Chalmers, *Glasgow Herald*, 26 January 1942, 6d.

13 Chalmers, A K. Printed letter to the staff of the Glasgow Public Health Department, 31 October 1925, GCA LP 1/90.

14 Davin, Anna. Imperialism and motherhood, *History Workshop*, 7 (1978) 9–65.

15 Chalmers, A K. Some recent instances of the history of alcoholism in Glasgow, typescript of a lecture c1924, City of Glasgow Archives LP1/90/53, 6.

16 Chalmers, 'A complete health service' (ref. 1), 5.

17 *ibid*, 4–5, *Glasgow Herald*, 28 November 1919, 6g.

18 Chalmers, A K. *Hints About the Management of Children*, pamphlet dated in MS 22/5/22, GCA LP1/90/50, 1. The pamphlet does not bear an author's name, but is almost certainly by Chalmers himself.

19 Aspinwall, *op cit*, 164; Orr, John Boyd. *As I Recall*, London, 1966, 42–3.

20 For a description of the atmosphere in Glasgow, see O'Hagan, Andrew. *The Missing*, London, 1995, 14–38.

21 Burnett, John. *Plenty and Want: a social history of diet from 1815 to the present day*, London, 1966, 218.

22 *ibid*, 223.

23 Winter, J M. *The Great War and the British People*, London, 1986, 103–53.

24 *Glasgow Herald*, 28 November 1919, 6g.

25 *Glasgow Herald*, 21 February 1919, 6d–e.

26 Jones, Helen. *Health and Society in Twentieth-Century Britain*, London, 1994, 43–4.

27 On the administrative complexity of medical care at this period, see Brotherston, John. The development of public medical care 1900–1948. In McLachlan, Gordon, ed, *Improving the Common Weal: aspects of Scottish health services 1900–1984*, Edinburgh, 1987, 35–102, especially 60–2.

28 Hamilton, David. *The Healers*, Edinburgh, 1981, 266.

29 Chalmers, A K. MCCG, 1922, 1695.

30 MCCG, 1922–3, 788. On the medical side of the Poor Law in Scotland, see Brotherston, *op cit*, 42–7.

31 McShane, Harry. *No Mean Fighter*, London, 1978, 121. The Parish Workhouse disappeared as a consequence of the Local Government (Scotland) Act 1929.

32 *Glasgow Herald*, 12 December 1919, 6c.

33 *Glasgow Herald*, 11 December 1919, 10h.

34 MCCG, 1918–19, 355, 509.

35 Letter from Alexander M Trotter to Sir James Lindsay, 1 February 1923, GCA D-TC 8/66.

36 Fenton, Alexander. Milk and milk products in Scotland: the role of the Milk Marketing Boards. In den Hartog, Adel P, ed, *Food Technology, Science*

and Marketing: European diet in the twentieth century, East Linton, 1995, 89–102.

37 Chalmers, A K. Control of Milk Supply, paper dated 5 May 1923, in GCA D-TC 8/66.

38 Bain, A J S (Assistant Secretary, Scottish Board of Health), to Lindsay, 15 May 1923.

39 Letter from Lindsay to Shaw, J E. 29 May 1923, in GCA D-TC 8/66.

40 *MCCG*, 1918–19, 355.

41 *MCCG*, 1919, 1908.

42 *MCCG*, 1919, 2381.

43 *MCCG*, 1919–20, 480–1.

44 *MCCG*, 1919–20, 482.

45 McShane, *op cit*, 121.

46 Aldred, Guy. *John Maclean*, Glasgow, 1940, 47–8.

47 *MCCG*, 1921, 1452.

48 *MCCG*, 1921–2, 1683, 1040.

49 Chalmers, A K. The food values and diets supplied under the Maternity and Child Welfare Scheme, *MCCG*, 1922, 1687–97.

50 Tully, Annabel M T and Urie, Elizabeth M. A study of the diets and economic conditions of labouring-class families in Glasgow in June, 1922, *Glasgow Medical Journal*, 98 (1922), 353–68.

51 Singer, Charles. *A Short History of Medicine*, 2nd edn, Oxford, 1962, 611–18.

52 For general comments on milk and health in Scotland in this period, see Wilson, Scott. The public health services, in McLachlan, *op cit*, 277–321, especially 292–4.

53 Rosen, George. *A History of Public Health*, New edn, Baltimore, 1993, 335–6.

54 Pennington, Caroline. Tuberculosis. In Checkland and Lamb, *op cit*, 86–99.

55 Chalmers, A K. *Increase of the Powers of Local Authorities with Regard to Milk Supply*, London, 1906, 5; GCA, LP 1/90/21.

56 *MCCG*, 1921, 2485.

57 *MCCG*, 1923, 1542.

58 *MCCG*, 1919–20, 1249.

59 Sheffield Corporation Act 1920; *MCCG*, 1921, 1715.

60 *MCCG*, 1921, 1724.

61 *MCCG*, 1921, 1712.

62 Fenton, *op cit*.

63 Report of the Glasgow Corporation Subcommittee on Meat Inspection, D-TC 8/66.

64 *MCCG*, 1919, 2036, 2381–5.

65 *MCCG*, 1919, 2205.

66 *MCCG*, 1919, 2383.

67 Burnett, John. Madam Rachel and the meat trade, *Review of Scottish Culture*, 12 (1999), 123.

68 Orr, Boyd, *op cit*, 29, 42–3, 118.

69 Checkland, Sydney. British urban health in general and in a single city. In Checkland and Lamb, 170–90, 178.

70 Brown, Gordon. *Maxton*, Edinburgh, 1986, 130–4.

71 Orr, Boyd, *op cit*, 148–9.
72 Smout, T S. *A Century of the Scottish People*, London, 1986, 128–9.
73 Paton, D. Noel. Rickets: the part played by unhygienic social conditions in predisposing to the disease, *Glasgow Medical Journal*, 97 (1922), 120–44.
74 Brotherston, *op cit*, 38–9.
75 Jones, *op cit*, 59-60; Orr, Boyd, *op cit*, 116–17.
76 Webster, Charles. Healthy or hungry thirties?, *History Workshop*, 13 (1982), 110–29.
77 Chalmers, letter of 31 October 1925 (ref 13).

Epidemiological follow-up of the
Carnegie (Boyd Orr) Survey of diet
and health in pre-war Britain

David Gunnell

INTRODUCTION

In January 1937 a family of seven living in the Woodside district of Aberdeen was visited by a researcher from the Rowett Research Institute. Over the next seven days a record was made of their food consumption. The age and sex of family members, their occupations, food expenditure and quality of housing were also recorded. Two months later the family's children underwent a medical examination to assess their health and nutritional status.

This household was the first of some 40 similar families living in Aberdeen to undergo detailed assessment of their diet, social circumstances and children's health in the early months of 1937. These assessments were pilots for the largest national study of children's diet and health up to that time in Great Britain – the Carnegie Survey of Diet and Health in Pre-war Britain. By April 1939, over thirteen hundred families consisting of around 8,000 individuals living in sixteen districts of England and Scotland had undergone detailed dietary assessments (Figure 1 and Table 1). In addition, some 3,800 children from these families were examined by a team consisting of two doctors and their assistants. The study was planned by Sir John Boyd Orr, and David Lubbock was in charge of the direction and administration of the project.

Although some elements of the research were written up shortly after completion of the field work, the outbreak of war interrupted the main analyses and these were not completed and published until 1955.[1] 'Interim conclusions' were, however, made available to the government at the outbreak of war and were reported to have influenced war-time food policy.[2] Detailed analysis of many aspects of the survey was never undertaken.

In 1988 the original survey material and correspondence relating to the survey was obtained on loan from the Rowett Research Institute by a research team from Bristol University. The records included the one week dietary diaries for the survey families, full medical examination records

Hopeman
Barthol Chapel
Methlick
Tarves
Aberdeen
Kintore
Dundee
West Wemyss
Coaltown of Wemyss
Edinburgh
Barrow
Yorkshire
Liverpool
Wisbech
Fulham
Bethnal Green

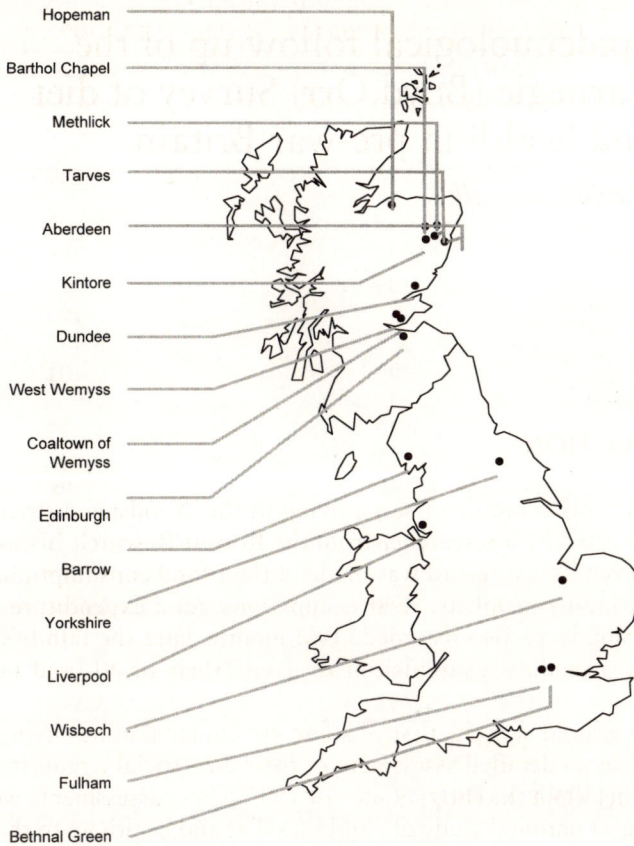

Fig. 1. *Survey centres used in the Carnegie Survey 1937–9*

(including anthropometry) for the children who were examined and corre-spondence relating to the design, conduct and analysis of the survey.[3] The records also contained detailed information on household structure, type of housing, family food expenditure and living conditions. These records have been entered into a computer database. The names, ages and addresses of the children surveyed have been used to trace the individuals who took part in the original study. Additional details about the design and conduct of the survey have been obtained from interviews conducted with some of the surviving researchers (the late Mr D Lubbock (Survey Administrator), Professor J Pemberton (Clinical Survey Team) and Mrs I Crichton (Diet Survey Team)).

This paper describes the design of the Carnegie Survey and summarises a selection of the early findings from a follow-up study based on this survey – the Boyd Orr Cohort. The cohort is currently being used to investigate rela-tionships of childhood nutrition and nutritional status with adult health.

Table 1. *Centres involved in the Survey of Family
Diet and Health in Pre-War Britain (1937–9)**

Centre	Total number of participating families (recorded in original report[1])	Number of families whose records were found in the Rowett Archive
English Centres		
Barrow-in-Furness	100	100
Bethnal Green	286	286
Fulham	103	103
Liverpool	103	103
Wisbech	162	163
Yorkshire	103	101
Scottish centres		
Aberdeen	37	35
Barthol Chapel	35	35
Coaltown and West Wemyss	98	98
Dundee	99	94
Edinburgh	50	49
Hopeman	27	27
Kintore	6	6
Methlick	38	38
Tarves	105	105
TOTAL	1,352	1,343

*Modified from Gunnell et al, 1996[3]

BACKGROUND TO SURVEY

Survey centres

The sixteen survey centres were selected to represent the range of living conditions and diet in Britain's rural and urban areas. Many of the districts surveyed in Scotland were close to the Rowett Research Institute. Centres were chosen because their Medical Officer of Health and the Local Authority and School Medical Officer agreed to co-operate following contacts made by Boyd Orr and the survey administration. Families were then selected using a number of techniques in order to obtain a range of families in different income groups within each centre. A greater proportion of families surveyed were working-class and thus middle- and upper-class families are relatively under-represented.

Measurement of family diet

In the dietary survey the weighed food consumption of an entire family over a period of one week was recorded in standardised notebooks. All food on hand in the house at the beginning of the survey was itemised. Over the survey week each acquisition of food (whether purchased or otherwise) and its cost was recorded. At the end of the survey week another inventory of food present in the home was taken. Notes were made of which family members were present for each meal and on the methods of preparation and cooking of the meals. In addition, household refuse was measured and details of family income, occupations, and housing quality were recorded. Members of the dietary survey team visited participating families on a regular basis to encourage full recording of food bought and consumed during the week of study. At the end of the survey week the diet records were sent to the Rowett Research Institute for analysis. From these per capita daily consumption of calories, fat, protein, carbohydrate, iron, calcium, phosphorus, and vitamins A, B1 and C were calculated for each household.

Physical examination of children

Children from all districts except Edinburgh and Kintore were examined by the medical examination team. These examinations took place either at their school or in halls booked in advance. Pre-school children were collected from their homes and brought to the examination centres in the survey car. A draft report of the Carnegie survey describes the examination process:

> As each batch of children arrived their names, ages, home address etc. were checked, then they undressed, were weighed, measured and photographed and, in earlier survey areas, prints of the soles of their feet were taken. They were then examined clinically by the doctors and their teeth condition recorded at the same time. They then dressed again and in some survey areas their eyes were tested for dark adaption and their ears for hearing loss . . .
>   . . . To minimise subjective influences, it was arranged so that it was not known by the doctors what expenditure group any child came from. Periodically the doctors examined the same children and the results of their examinations were compared. (Source: Rowett Archive)

A 'portable measuring stand'[1] was used to measure height to the nearest millimetre. 'All children were measured in bare feet against a vertical scale with feet together, ankles touching and head horizontal (Source: Rowett Archive). Cristal height ('leg length') was also recorded as 'the distance between the summit of the iliac crest and the floor.'[1] This was measured using a steel measuring tape to the nearest millimetre. Weight was measured using a W&T Avery standard model 'calibrated level balance and recorded to the nearest ounce.' Children under the age of eleven years were weighed naked, those aged eleven years or over 'wore only trousers or knickers for which standard reductions were made.'[1]

As well as anthropometry physical examination of the children included:

> Assessment of nutritional deficiency: signs of rickets and anaemia.
> Signs of chronic disease: enlarged lymph glands, bronchitis, evidence of TB, otitis media.

A dental examination.
Audiometry.
Haemoglobin assay on a capillary blood sample.

Dietary intervention study

In eight of the Carnegie Survey centres a diet supplementation study was conducted (Table 2). Food supplements were given to selected children to determine whether the effects on growth and health of undernourishment could be ameliorated. In three of these centres (Tarves, Wisbech and West Wemyss) supplements were given to children attending particular schools. Other children from these districts as well as children from three of the other survey centres (Methlick, Coaltown of Wemyss and Barthol Chapel) acted as controls. In the other two centres (Bethnal Green and Dundee) supplemental foods were sent to families for consumption at home ('home feeding') and children from other families in these areas acted as their controls. The supplements given in particular areas were 'planned to make good the main deficiencies revealed by the diet survey in that area'.[1]

To determine whether the provision of supplements resulted in relative increases in height and weight serial measures of growth and health were made on over a thousand children in the intervention and control groups. Such experimental methods had previously been used by Orr and others to assess the effect of milk supplements on children's growth.[4-6]

CONTEMPORARY ANALYSES BASED ON THE BOYD ORR COHORT

Tracing of subjects

The National Health Service Central Register has been used to trace children whose families took part in the original study. To date (July 1997) 85 per cent of survey members have been identified on the NHS central register and over 800 members of the cohort are known to have died.

Analyses of recreated dataset

Early analyses of the survey data have examined three broad areas. First, we have examined associations of childhood stature with diet and living conditions. These analyses are based on the 2,990 children who were aged between two years and fourteen years nine months when they were examined.[7] Few study members were aged over fifteen and anthropometric measurements in younger children are prone to inaccuracy. Second, we have examined relationships between childhood stature (a marker of nutritional status) and adult mortality.[8] These analyses are based on 2,324 study members who have been traced and who have complete records of their medical

Table 2. *Survey centres used in the nutritional supplementation trial*

Survey centre (number of children aged 2–14 given supplements according to survey report)	Supplements given to children
Tarves (151) Children from Methlick and Barthol Chapel districts acted as controls	Soup and 1/3 pint of milk daily; 16,000 international units of Vitamin A weekly (halibut oil capsules). Some pre-school children also given 1 pint of milk daily 24,000 IU Vit A and 3 oranges per week. These were given over 220 school days between 22/11/37 and 9/12/38.
Wisbech (96) Children from Parson's Drove school in Wisbech acted as controls	Soup and 2/3 pint of milk daily; 16,000 international units of Vitamin A (halibut oil capsules) and 1.3 oranges per week. These were given during term time between 02/08/38 to 16/06/39.
West Wemyss (63) Children from Coaltown of Wemyss acted as controls	1 pint of milk and 0.25 oz Marmite per day. These were given from 15/06/38 to 31/03/39.
Bethnal Green and Dundee (242) Other families in these areas were chosen to act as controls	Weekly food packages given to families. These contained milk, cheese, Bemax, Marmite, oranges, halibut liver and cod liver oil. Eggs were also included in Dundee and in Bethnal Green small amounts of blackcurrant puree and malt and cod liver oil suspension were also given.

examinations, childhood diet and living conditions. Third we have examined the associations between childhood calorie intake and adult cancer mortality in all traced subjects with records of family diet.[42]

Statistical methods used in analyses

To enable height comparisons to be made between children of different ages and gender all anthropometric measures have been converted to standard deviation scores (z-scores). The z-score expresses a child's measurement as the number of standard deviations their value is from the mean, given their age and sex. They provide a measure of relative height for age and sex. Positive z-scores indicate that the child is taller than expected for their age and sex; negative z-scores imply the opposite. Because representative British standards for height, cristal height and trunk length in the 1930s and 1940s do not exist we used the study members themselves as the reference population to calculate the z-scores. Regression models were used to estimate expected values for height, cristal height and trunk length and their standard deviations. Boys and girls were analysed separately.

Childhood calorie consumption was estimated by dividing total household consumption by the number of consuming heads within the family, weighted for their age and sex using weightings for 'man value' calorie requirements modified from a BMA Report of Committee of Nutrition, 1933.[9] Per capita family food expenditure was calculated in a similar way.

Cross-sectional associations of the z-scores for overall height, cristal height and trunk length with childhood living conditions and diet have been examined using correlation and regression techniques. Mortality analyses to examine associations between nutritional status, diet and mortality in traced cohort members have been carried out using Cox's proportional hazards models.[10]

SELECTION OF RESEARCH FINDINGS TO DATE

Cross-sectional analyses

Relatively strong associations have been found between a number of measures of childhood socio-economic circumstances and height (Table 3). These associations are similar in males and females and suggest that adverse childhood socio-economic circumstances and diet are associated with shorter stature. In particular these data suggest that the socio-economic differences in height are due in greater part to differences in leg length than differences in trunk length.[7] This is probably because legs are the component of stature which grow most in the period leading up to puberty. The existence of socio-economic differences in height is well established in the research literature.[11] These data confirm the presence of such differences in the Boyd Orr cohort.

The average height of children who were surveyed in the Bethnal Green and Fulham areas of London have been compared with heights recorded in a 1938 survey of London schoolchildren.[12] The Carnegie children examined in these areas were generally shorter than the average child of that age living in London in 1938.[3] This is in keeping with the fact that children were predominantly drawn from working-class families.

Longitudinal mortality analyses

Figure 2 shows the age-standardised hazard ratios and their 95 per cent confidence intervals for coronary heart disease (CHD) mortality in relation to stature in males and females. These are based on 103 coronary heart disease deaths among survey members with height measurements. The hazard ratios were derived from Cox's proportional hazards models and represent the increase (or decrease) in the risk of death associated with a one standard deviation increase in height, leg length or trunk length. Thus hazard ratios greater than one indicate increased mortality rates associated with increasing stature, hazard ratios less than one indicate decreasing mortality rates in relation to stature. In both men and women greater stature is associated

Table 3. *Pearson's correlation coefficients between anthropometry and childhood dietary and socio-economic variables*

Anthropometric, dietary or socio-economic index (n)	'z' score for height	'z' score for leg length	'z' score for trunk length
Males			
Weighted per capita food expenditure[1]	0.28*	0.28*	0.15*
Number of people per room[2]	-0.19*	-0.20*	-0.08*
Relative family per capita calorie consumption	0.23*	0.26*	0.08*
Females			
Weighted per capita food expenditure	0.25*	0.23*	0.15*
Number of people per room[2]	-0.15*	-0.17*	-0.05
Relative family per capita calorie consumption	0.20*	0.25*	0.05*

1 Weighted according to the age and sex of family members
2 High = overcrowded; low = not overcrowded
*$p < 0.05$

with a decreased risk of CHD, although this difference only reaches statistical significance in women ($p = 0.007$ for overall height and $p = 0.003$ for leg length). In both sexes leg length was the component of height associated with reduced CHD mortality risk.

Figure 3 shows the mortality rate ratios for all-cause, all cancers, smoking and non-smoking related cancers associated with an increase in energy intake of 1,000Kcal/day in men and women. These hazard ratios are based on 206 cancer deaths among subjects who were aged up to 16 when their families took part in the survey. There is an increased risk of cancer mortality associated with increased childhood energy consumption, and this risk appears to be greatest in relation to non-smoking related cancers.

DISCUSSION OF EPIDEMIOLOGICAL ANALYSES

Over the last 60 years epidemiological analyses have shown that poverty, undernutrition and disease in childhood may have important long term effects on adult health and life expectancy.[13] In more recent years the possibility of such influences have been the subject of intense epidemiological research[14, 15] and debate.[16, 17] Research to date in this area has generally been confined to the analysis of associations between birth measurements and cardiovascular risk factors and mortality in later life, although more recently, interactions have also been demonstrated between birthweight and adult weight in determining cardiovascular risk.[18, 19] These suggest that adversity in early infancy may influence disease risk only if coupled with being overweight in adulthood.

CHD mortality rate ratios (95% CI) for males in relation to 1 SD increase in stature

CHD mortality rate ratios (95% CI) for females in relation to 1 SD increase in stature

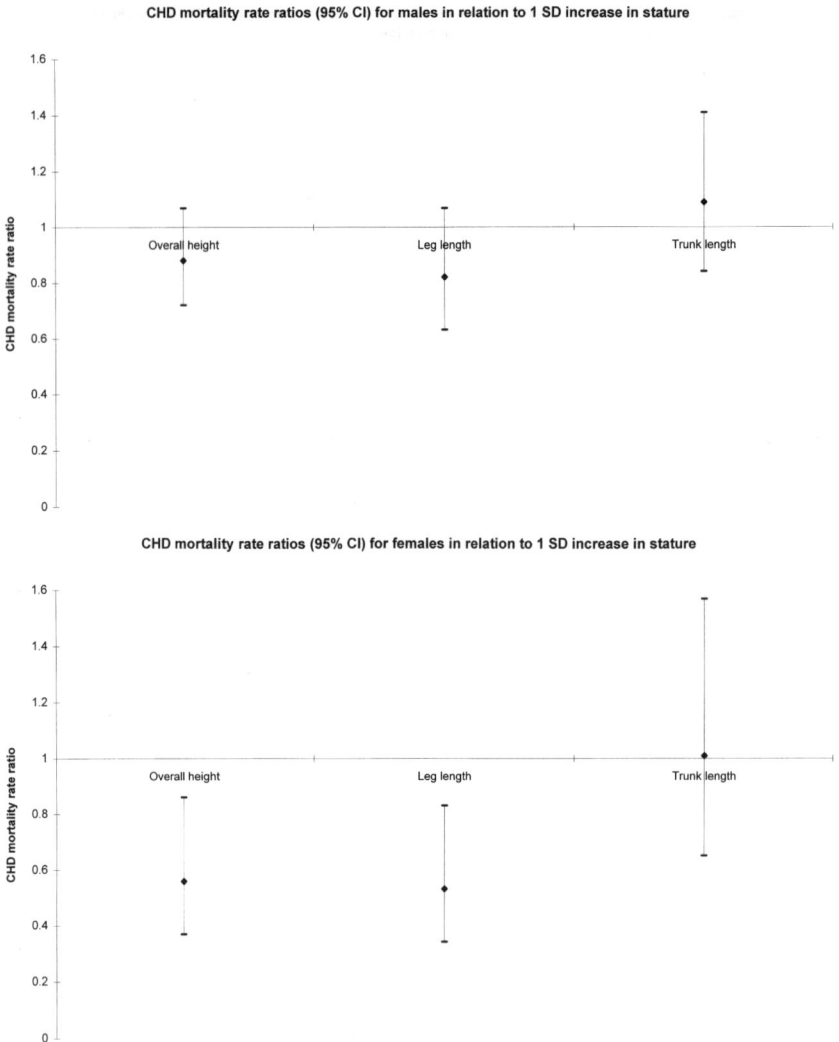

Fig. 2. *Association of childhood height, leg length and trunk length with adult coronary heart disease mortality in males and females.*

Height and coronary heart disease

Few epidemiological analyses have examined the influence of childhood diet and health after the first year of life on adult health. In part this is because few cohorts of individuals currently at risk from coronary heart disease and cancer have detailed records of their childhood diet and nutritional status. Adult height is sometimes used as an indicator of past nutritional status – although final height is limited by genotype, environmental

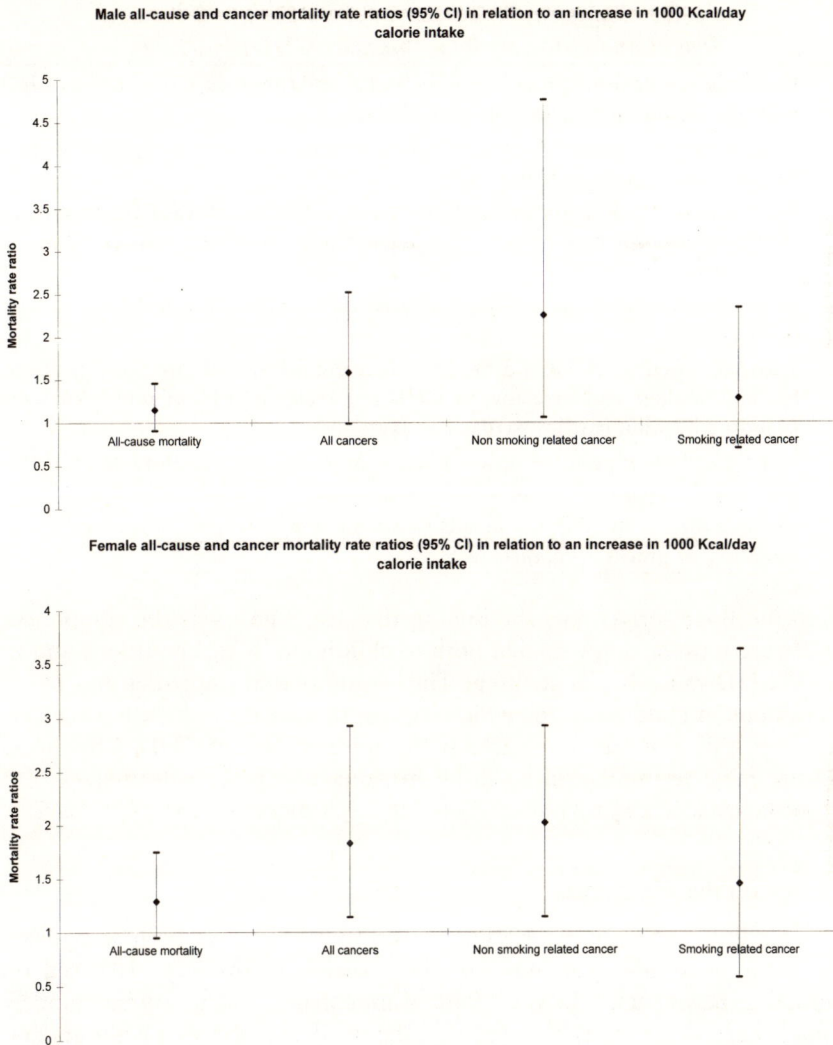

Fig. 3. Association of childhood energy intake with adult all-cause and cancer mortality in males and females.

influences may restrict attainment of full growth potential.[11] Inverse relationships between *adult* stature and coronary heart disease (CHD) are generally found in adult cohort studies.[20-25] These are in keeping with the relationships found in relation to *childhood* height in the Boyd Orr cohort. Biological mechanisms underlying the observed associations are uncertain (Table 4).

Table 4. *Possible explanations for the association between*
height and coronary heart disease (CHD) mortality

1. Height is a marker for socio-economic status and this in turn is related to CHD mortality (confounding by adult social class)

2. Height is related to birthweight, which in turn is associated with CHD mortality (confounding by early life factors)[15, 23]

3. Factors that effect height in childhood (diet, infectious disease exposure, psychological health) may in turn be related to adult mortality (confounding by these factors).[26, 28-30, 39]

4. Taller people have larger coronary arteries and are therefore at decreased mortality risk.[21]

5. Those exposed to childhood factors which retard growth are more likely to become smokers and have adverse CHD risk factor profiles in adulthood (confounding by adult cardiovascular risk factors).[40]

6. Taller children experience upward social mobility and therefore enjoy better adult socio-economic circumstances (confounding by adult social class).[41]

7. Chronic disease in adulthood leads to a reduction in height ('shrinkage') (confounding by pre-existing disease.[22]

In the Boyd Orr cohort the finding that leg length was the component of stature most strongly related both to childhood living conditions and to adult CHD mortality is striking. This suggests that poor diet and living conditions in childhood, for which leg length appears to be a particularly sensitive indicator, are associated with increased risk of CHD. Childhood stature may be influenced by ill-health, diet and psychosocial stress.[26-28] These factors have in turn been linked to adult mortality risk.[29, 30]

Energy intake and cancer

Possible links between calorie intake and mortality have been recognised for many years although most of the research in this area is based on animal experiments.[31] In the 1940s Tannenbaum, using animal models, found that calorie restriction reduced the incidence of breast tumours and carcinogen induced skin cancer and sarcoma.[32, 33] Several mechanisms for the association between caloric intake and cancer risk have been suggested. Albanes and Winnick hypothesise that higher calorie intake results in a greater number of dividing stem cells, each at risk of undergoing malignant change.[34] Caloric intake may also reflect total dietary carcinogen load, and in addition reduced calorie intake is thought to be associated with diminished oncogene expression.[35, 36]

A large number of epidemiological studies have investigated possible links between diet and cancer in humans. The findings from these are often conflicting. A recent review of fat intake and studies of breast cancer concluded that there appears to be little or no relationship with dietary fat in adulthood, however, dietary influences and in particular energy intake, during *early life* may be important.[37] The Boyd Orr cohort thus provides an opportunity to examine the influence on adult health of an array of dietary exposures, measured in childhood, and cancer development in later life. Findings to date support a role for early diet in relation to later adult cancer risk.

FUTURE AND CURRENT RESEARCH BASED ON THE BOYD ORR COHORT

Postal questionnaires are currently being sent to all surviving survey members to obtain information concerning their adult diet, health, occupations and other disease risk factors (ie smoking, exercise, weight). These factors may confound associations between adult health and childhood exposures and information on these will provide a more complete picture of the life-courses of these individuals. Contacts already made with respondents to this questionnaire demonstrate the striking ability of many to recall details of the original study. The dietary intervention study is being re-analysed using modern statistical techniques. The purpose of this re-analysis is to determine whether the effects of food supplementation on children's height has differential effects on leg length growth and whether childhood supplementation has long term effects on adult health. Birth records for around 500 survey children have recently been retrieved from maternity hospital archives and these will be used to investigate the relative influences of early life and childhood exposures on adult health.[43]

In addition, detailed interviews are being conducted with a sample of 300 surviving survey members both to reconstruct more fully their life-course exposure to adverse environments and to investigate the role of such exposures in the well recognised socio-economic variations in adult health.[38] Funding is being sought to examine and clinically investigate a sample of survey members and obtain fuller information regarding their adult health and cardiovascular risk factors.

FUNDING

This work was funded by grants from the World Cancer Research Fund, the British Heart Foundation and the Medical Research Council

ACKNOWLEDGEMENTS

This research was initiated and has been continually supported and developed by Professors Stephen Frankel and George Davey Smith. Professor Philip James, director of the Rowett Research Institute has allowed us the use of the Boyd Orr archive and this has been supported by Walter Duncan, honorary archivist to the Rowett who has helped us with access to the survey records. Dr David Smith, University of Aberdeen, has given us access to his interviews with surviving members of the survey research team. Sara

Seavill, Sue Williams, Andrea Wilson, Jenny Eachus and Sarah Pike have helped with data entry. Tim Peters, Kiran Nanchahal, Martin Kemp, Fiona Braddon, Sara Brookes, and Phil Chan have provided statistical and technical assistance. We also wish to acknowledge all the research workers and subjects who participated in the original survey in 1937–9. In particular we thank Professor J Pemberton, Mrs I Crichton and the late David Lubbock for information concerning the design and conduct of the original survey.

NOTES

1 Rowett Research Institute. *Family Diet and Health in Pre-war Britain* (Carnegie United Kingdom Trust), Dunfermline, 1955.

2 Baines, A H J, Hollingsworth, D F, Leitch, I. Diets of working-class families with children before and after the Second World War. With a section on height and weight of children, *Nutrition Abstracts and Reviews*, 33 (1963), 653–69.

3 Gunnell, D J, Frankel, S, Nanchahal, K, Braddon, F E M, Davey, Smith, G. Lifecourse exposure and later disease: a follow-up study based on a survey of family diet and health in pre-war Britain (1937-9), *Public Health*, 110 (1996), 85–94.

4 Leighton, G, McKinlay, P L. *Milk Consumption and the Growth of School Children. Report on an investigation in Lanarkshire schools* (HMSO), Edinburgh, 1930.

5 Orr, J B. Milk consumption and the growth of school-children, *Lancet*, i (1928), 202–3.

6 Leighton, G, Clark, M L. Milk consumption and the growth of school-children. Second preliminary report on tests to the Scottish board of health, *Lancet*, i (1929), 40–3.

7 Gunnell, D J, Davey Smith, G, Frankel, S J, Kemp, M, Peters, T J. Socioeconomic and dietary influences on leg length and trunk length in childhood: a re-analysis of the Carnegie survey of diet and health in pre-war Britain (1937–9), *Paediatric and Perinatal Epidemiology*, (1997), in press.

8 Gunnell, D J, Davey Smith, G, Frankel, S J, Nanchahal, K, Braddon, F E M, Pemberton, J, Peters, T J. Childhood leg length and adult mortality – follow up of the Carnegie survey of diet and growth in prewar Britain, *Journal of Epidemiology and Community Health*, 52 (1998), 142–152

9 *Report of Committee on Nutrition* (British Medical Association), London, 1933.

10 *SAS Technical Report P-217, SAS/STAT Software: The PHREG Procedure.* Version 6 ed, (SAS Institute Inc), Cary, NC, USA, 1991.

11 Rona, R J, Chinn, S. Genetic and environmental influences on growth, *Journal of Medical Screening*, 2 (1995), 133–9.

12 Daley, A. *Report on the Heights and Weights of School Pupils in the County of London in 1949* (London County Council), London, 1950.

13 Kuh, D, Davey Smith, G. When is mortality risk determined? Historical insights into a current debate, *Social History of Medicine*, 6 (1993), 101–23.

14 Barker, D J P. *Mothers, Babies, and Disease in Later Life* (BMJ Publishing Group), London, 1994.

15 Barker, D J P. *Fetal and Infant Origins of Adult Disease* (BMJ Publishing Group), London, 1992.

16 Paneth, N, Susser, M. Early origin of coronary heart disease (the 'Barker hypothesis'), *BMJ*, 310 (1995), 411–12.

17 Elford, J, Whincup, P, Shaper, A G. Early life experience and adult cardio-vascular disease: longitudinal and case-control studies, *Int J Epidemiol*, 20 (1991), 833–44.

18 Leon, D A, Koupilova, I, Lithell, H O, et al. Failure to realise growth potential in utero and adult obesity in relation to blood pressure in 50 year old Swedish men, *BMJ*, 312 (1996), 401–6.

19 Frankel, S, Elwood, P, Sweetnam, P, Yarnell, J, Davey Smith, G. Birthweight, body mass index in middle age, and incident coronary heart disease, *Lancet*, 348 (1996), 1478–80.

20 Rich-Edwards, J W, Manson, J E, Stampfer, M J, et al. Height and the risk of cardiovascular disease in women, *Am J Epidemiol*, 142 (1995), 909–17.

21 Hebert, P R, Rich-Edwards, J W, Manson, J E, et al. Height and incidence of cardiovascular disease in male physicians. *Circulation*, 88 part 1 (1993), 1437-43.

22 Leon, D, Davey Smith, G, Shipley, M, Strachan, D. Adult height and mortality in London: early life, socioeconomic confounding or shrinkage? *J Epidemiol Community Health*, 49 (1995), 5–9.

23 Yarnell, J G W, Limb, E S, Layzell, J M, Baker, I A. Height: a risk marker for ischaemic heart disease, *Eur Heart J*, 13 (1992), 1602–5.

24 Walker, M, Shaper, A G, Phillips, A N, Cook, D G. Short stature, lung function and risk of a heart attack, *Int J Epidemiol*, 18 (1989), 602–6.

25 Watt, G C M, Hart, C L, Hole, D J, Davey Smith, G, Gillis, C R, Hawthorne, V M. Risk factors for cardiorespiratory and all-cause mortality in men and women in urban Scotland: 15 year follow up, *Scottish Medical Journal*, 40 (1995), 108–12.

26 Martorell, R, Habicht, J-P. Growth in early childhood in developing countries, in Falkner, F, Tanner, J M, eds. *Human Growth. A Comprehensive Treatise.* Second edn, vol 3, New York, 1986, 241–62.

27 Widdowson, E M. Mental contentment and physical growth, *Lancet*, i (1951), 1316–8.

28 Peck, M N, Lundberg, O. Short stature as an effect of economic and social conditions in childhood, *Soc Sci Med*, 41 (5) (1995), 733–8.

29 Patel, P, Mendall, M A, Carrington, D, et al. Association of Helicobacter pylori and Chlamydia pneumoniae infections with coronary heart disease and cardiovascular risk factors, *BMJ*, 311 (1995), 711–4.

30 Schwartz, J E, Friedman, H S, Tucker, J S, Tomlinson-Keasey, C, Wingard, D L, Criqui, M H. Sociodemographic and psychosocial factors in childhood as predictors of adult mortality, *Am J Public Health*, 85 (1995), 1237–45.

31 McCay, C M, Maynard, L A, Sperling, G, Barnes, L L. Retarded growth, life span, ultimate body size and age changes in the albino rat after feeding diets restricted in calories, *J Nutr*, 18 (1939), 1–13.

32 Tannenbaum, A. Effects of varying caloric intake upon tumor incidence and tumor growth, *Ann NY Acad Sci*, 49 (1947), 5–19.

33 Tannenbaum, A. Relationship of body weight to cancer incidence, *Arch Pathol*, 30 (1940), 509–17.

34 Albanes, D, Winick, M. Are cell number and cell proliferation risk factors for cancer? *J Natl Cancer Inst*, 80 (1988), 772–5.
35 Weindruch, R. Effect of caloric restriction on age-associated cancers, *Experimental Gerontology*, 27 (1992), 575–81.
36 Kritchevsky, D. The effect of over- and undernutrition on cancer, *European Journal of Cancer Prevention*, 4 (1995), 445–51.
37 Hunter, D J, Willett, W C. Diet, body size and breast cancer, *Epidemiol Rev*, 15 (1993), 110–32.
38 Blane, D. Collecting retrospective data: development of a reliable method and a pilot study of its use, *Soc Sci Med*, 42 (1996), 751–7.
39 Thomson, A M. Fourth Boyd Orr memorial lecture. Problems and politics in nutritional surveillance, *Proc Nutr Soc*, 37 (1978), 317–33.
40 Notkola, V. Living conditions in childhood and coronary heart disease in adulthood, *Commentationes Scientiarum Socialium*, 29 (1985), 1–119.
41 Power, C, Fogelman, K, Fox, A J. Health and social mobility during the early years of life, *Quarterly Journal of Social Affairs*, 2 (1986), 397–413.
42 Frankel, S, Gunnell, D, Peters, T, Maynard, M, Davey Smith, G. Childhood energy intake and adult cancer: the Boyd Orr cohort, *BMJ*, 316 (1998), 499–504.
43 Kemp, M, Gunnell, D, Davey Smith, G, Frankel, S. Finding and using inter-war maternity records, *Social History of Medicine*, 10 (1997), 305–29.

4 The paradox of diet and health: England and Scotland in the nineteenth and twentieth centuries

Derek J Oddy

The displacement of traditional foods from the diet and the alteration of food patterns is an essential part of the process of social change that accompanies the spread of industrialization and urbanization. In Britain this process began in the eighteenth century and was largely completed by the inter-war years of the twentieth century, though its extent and pace varied in different parts of the United Kingdom. Nowhere was the switch away from traditional foods more obvious than in Scotland. From the late eighteenth century, when Robert Burns could write 'The healsome *Porritch*, chief of SCOTIA's food',[1] dietary change was described by Professor Roy Campbell in *Our Changing Fare*[2] as: 'the modern history of diet in Scotland is fundamentally that of the rejection of oatmeal as its leading item.' The result was obvious: 'a decline in the standards of nutrition of the people . . . The history of diet in Scotland is, therefore, the story of an exercise in choice that must be regretted by the nutritionist.' Roy Campbell believed these changes to have occurred, broadly speaking, in the timespan bounded by the *Old Statistical Account* (which described Scotland in the 1790s[3] – only a few years after Burns's poem appeared in the Kilmarnock edition of 1786) and the outbreak of war in 1914. After World War I, Roy Campbell thought, 'differences between diets of the varying parts of Great Britain are relatively slight.'

During the first half of the nineteenth century, there was no great evidence of change. The patterns of food consumption for the early 1840s revealed by the *New Statistical Account* and the *Report of the Royal Commission on the Poor Law (Scotland)*[4] showed only limited variety across the country. Oatmeal was the most widely consumed cereal, though where oats grew less well, as in the Hebrides, its usage was less common. In general, though, other cereals, such as wheat or barley, were little used, except where oats did not grow as well as wheat. Thus oats were replaced by barley in the north and west, and wheat around the Firth of Forth. The other principal foodstuff widely used was potatoes. Consumption varied inversely with income, being greatest in the north and west of Scotland so that crop failure in 1846 brought famine to the western straths, where the potato was of fundamental importance. Fish, particularly herrings, was commonly eaten in coastal districts but vegetable consumption was often confined to what went into broth. Kailyards were common but usually too small for vegetables to be a regular part of the diet.[5] Some regional variation was evident: whilst all areas relied to a greater or lesser extent upon oatmeal and potatoes, the presence or absence of additional foods reflected differences in agricultural production. Diets in Caithness and the Northern Isles, where meat, fish, oatmeal, barleymeal and green vegetables were eaten, differed markedly from the Hebrides and western Highlands, which had little oatmeal and relied on fish and milk as additions to the ever-present potato. In the north-east, oatmeal was universal, supplemented by milk and some green vegetables while potatoes were less important. Further south, in Argyll, the lowland areas of Perth and the eastern coastal counties, meat and milk appeared in the diet alongside the basic foods. Across central Scotland, there was clear distinction between west and east but, even in urban areas, oatmeal and potatoes remained the mainstay of the diet. In the industrializing west, cheese, butter and meat were added to the diet, while around the Firth of Forth basic foodstuffs were augmented by tea and wheaten bread. In the south-west and the Borders, dairy produce and fish were the principal supplementary foods. Lastly, in the south-east, the presence of barleymeal, pease-meal, meat and tea gave the diet a quite distinctive character from other regions.[6]

Within the second half of the nineteenth century, as dietary change began, the domestic economy of Scotland could be categorized by three distinct types. There were the rural workers of the south-west and the eastern coastal counties, the city-dwellers of Dundee, Edinburgh and Glasgow, and the Highlands and Islands. As might be expected, dietary change was slowest in the countryside; here oatmeal held its ground best though, by the last quarter of the nineteenth century, tea, bread and meat were all entering the diet as additional foods to the traditional oatmeal, milk and, in coastal districts, at least, herrings. In the towns, by the same time, bread, butter, jam and tea had largely displaced traditional foodstuffs. To the north and west in the Highlands, the potato remained the staple food. Roy Campbell provided two additional points of information on dietary change which we should note. First, that dietary change in the nineteenth century took place initially through the male wage earner's food consumption, before later – and in some cases quite a long time later – becoming the pattern for the whole family. An illustration of this can be found in Hutchison's 'Report on the Dietaries of Scotch Agricultural Labourers' at the end of the 1860s:[7]

A field worker in Newton Stewart, Wigtownshire:

Breakfast – tea with oatcake and butter; family sometimes porridge and milk, and frequently tea, oatcake and butter.

Dinner – husband, a penny loaf of wheatflour and cheese or butter to it, and milk or cold tea as 'sap'; family, tea and oatcake.

Supper – with family, tea with oatcake and butter or porridge and milk.

This pattern, where 'the husband wins the bread, and must have the best food', to quote the observations constantly made to Dr Edward Smith in 1863,[8] was to be found throughout Britain during the nineteenth century: it meant, as Charles Booth put it in the context of the domestic economy of English towns: 'a good deal of bread is eaten and tea drunk by the women and children'.[9] Here, it is necessary to remember that the patterns of dietary change in England were different from those in Scotland: in England bread occupied a lower status as food than animal flesh; in Scotland it had a higher status than traditional foods, so that men ate bread while women and children still ate porridge or oatcake. Thus Hutchinson's example is from a stage when bread was beginning to enter the rural diet. Much the same pattern can be distinguished for meat, bacon, and fish. Since these are foods which need cooking – unless eaten cold as left-overs from the dinner cooked on Sunday – what is implied is that most cooking – at least in England – was done 'only for the father' as one witness explained to the Interdepartmental Committee on Physical Deterioration in 1904.[10] In Scotland, the difference was that when the wife did not work outside the home, the pot for broth or porridge was constantly at the fire.

The second point, perhaps made only indirectly by Roy Campbell, is that by the end of the nineteenth century when there was already in Scotland a group of physiologists concerned with dietary studies, observations of dietary patterns were closely combined with a moral judgement on the working classes. It is in the writings of Professor D. N. Paton, at Edinburgh, that this is clearest.[11] In short, the physiologists' thesis was this: food from animal sources is more expensive than food from vegetable sources; it is therefore wrong for the poorer classes to buy expensive foods when they can get as much or more energy per penny from cheaper foods. Whilst this view commended itself to the moral economy school of thought, it ignored the complementarity of foods, the importance of palatable foods in the diet and was in direct contradiction with the high protein requirements currently being specified by nutritionists and physiologists.[12] Later on, though they could not know it before World War I, their advice was in direct contradiction to the new theories on Accessory Food Factors, as vitamins were originally known in Britain. It may be unnecessary to labour this point but care is needed in using the contemporary evaluations of diets at the turn of the century by Scottish physiologists. This was not merely a passing phase: it may be that set attitudes unbalanced Paton's judgement. In the inter-war years he refused to accept the new vitamin theory and thus his last major work, *Poverty, Nutrition and Growth*[13] was not as successful as he might have hoped.

There is a need, therefore, to re-examine the material from the early part of the twentieth century and to make a fresh quantitative assessment of diet in Scotland. Before World War I, the Royal College of Physicians in Edinburgh attempted to make a rigorous investigation of the relationship between people's income, diet and health. Paton undertook this investigation on the College's behalf. He investigated only sixteen families in Edinburgh in 1900 but, although this was a very small sample, the painstaking recording and analysis was unsurpassed at a time when all calculations had to be made by hand and, moreover, there were no standard food analysis tables yet available in Britain. A similarly detailed survey of 60 families in Glasgow, which drew on Paton's earlier study for its methodology, was made by Dorothy Lindsay in 1912. Between these dates were two other surveys carried out by different means. The Dundee Social Union's investigation of 1906 is interesting because although its principal concern was with housing improvement, sixteen budgets were also taken, of which fourteen gave sufficient detail of food consumption for an analysis to be made. Finally, the Board of Trade's large-scale investigation of urban workmen's budgets by Hubert Llewellyn Smith in 1904, contained 455 returns from Scotland.[14] These returns, said to refer to 'a week in summer', were obtained through trade unions and co-operative societies, and reflected conditions amongst the better-off groups of town-dwellers.

In the same year, 1904, Mr Wilson Fox of the Board of Agriculture carried out an inquiry into wages, earnings and conditions of employment of agricultural labourers in Scotland and Ireland,[15] which was intended to complement his 1902 rural inquiry in England. This produced 97 returns but no more precise regional breakdown of distribution than 'Highlands and Islands' and 'Midlands and Lowlands'. It seems probable that this inquiry was not a true family budget survey. Wilson Fox seems to have used the system of farm correspondents who reported to the Board. After that the information obtained appears to have been standardized for an hypothetical family of a man, wife and four children.[16]

This pre-1914 material is shown in Table 1. The mean family incomes shown require two comments: first, that these returns all suggest families above Booth and Rowntree's 'poverty line' in England. Rowntree's figure for income at the poverty line was 21s.8d. [£1.08] and, excepting the rural survey in 1904, only the lowest income group of the 1904 urban survey is anywhere near that level. The second point is that a very high proportion of income in Scotland was spent on food. The 1904 urban survey produced an overall mean of 60 per cent from its 1,944 returns and so this became the weighting for food expenditure used in the 1913 Board of Trade Cost of Living Index. Thus, while in England some 50–60 per cent of income went on food, in Scotland it was common amongst the poorer classes to spend 70 per cent or more of family income on food. In the countryside, as Wilson Fox's *Report* noted, there was still some payment in kind to farm servants,[17] although the tendency was growing for farm servants to be paid in money; none the less, there was still some sale of allowances (oatmeal and pota-

Table 1.1. *Income and food expenditure*

| Survey | Families | Income | | Food Expenditure | | Expenditure |
| | | per family | per head | per family | per head | as % of family income |
	(number)	(sh/wk)	(sh/wk)	(sh/wk)	(sh/wk)	(%)
Urban						
Edinburgh 1900	16	25	4.2	18.1	3.1	72.6
Urban 1904	455	36.5	6.4	23.4	4.1	64.1
Dundee 1906	14	22.3	4.2	13.6	2.6	61
Glasgow 1912	60	28.1	4.2	20.8	3.1	73.9
Rural (1904)						
Highlands & Islands		16.5	2.8	13.8	2.3	83.4
Midlands & Lowlands		20	3.3	16.2	2.7	81
Mean	97	18.3	3	15.2	2.5	83.3
1904 Urban by Income Groups						
< 25s	48	21.7	4.3	15.9	3.2	73.4
25-30s.	77	26.9	5.4	18.9	3.8	70.3
30-35s.	117	31.8	6.4	20.9	4.2	65.7
35-40s.	83	36.4	7.3	21.9	4.4	60.1
> 40s.	130	51.9	7.4	32.1	4.6	61.7

toes) or even the bartering of them with fish-wives. The lower income levels shown for rural districts conceal these transactions and the 81–3 per cent of income going on food expenditure is an artificial figure.

Table 1.2 shows the food consumption per head per week. On this evidence, it is tempting to conclude that the diet in Scotland was still in a transitionary stage and not to have progressed as far towards the English urban pattern as Roy Campbell thought it had. Oatmeal, potatoes and milk arc prcscnt in sizcablc amounts but bread, sugar and butcher's meat (the heading 'meat' does not distinguish fresh from cured meat) are eaten universally. Even in the countryside, it was notable that agricultural labourers were buying: 'Bread, groceries, tinned meat (of which, especially in bothies, a good deal is used) jams, cake, etc., from the tradesmen's carts and vans which now frequently call at their houses'.[18] Not all the foods consumed are shown in this table but, except for vegetables (11–18 ozs [312–510 g] per head per week in town surveys) and fish (5–8 ozs [142–227 g] per head per week) other items were insignificant. Tea is not shown because it has no nutritive value but it was used, and even in rural districts families bought about ½ lb [227 g] per week. The question of oatmeal needs some special comment because of Roy Campbell's assessment that it had all but disappeared from the Scottish diet after 1914. In the countryside, it was still the basis of the diet – menus given in 1904 are very little different from those given by Hutchinson in 1868. In Argyll, for example, it was still:

Breakfast – Porridge, tea, bread and butter, scones, oatmeal cake (on Sundays fish);

Table 1.2. *Weekly Food Consumption per head*

Survey	Bread (lb)	Potatoes (lb)	Cereals (oz)	Sugar (oz)	Fats (oz)	Meat (lb(	Milk (pt)
Urban							
Edinburgh 1900	4.7	1.2	6.4	13	4.2	1.2	1.6
Urban 1904	6.2	3.7	17	17	7.3	1.1	2.8
Dundee 1906	5.4	2.8	10.1	13	4.9	0.5	2.9
Glasgow 1912	5.1	2.8	6.2	15	5.7	1.5	2.0
Rural (1904)							
Highlands-Islands	2.8	5.5	47.1	12	4.4	0.5	4.0
Midlands-Lowlands	5.2	4.2	25.6	14	5.2	0.7	3.5
Mean	4.2	4.7	35.7	13	4.9	0.7	3.7
1904 Urban by Income Groups							
< 25s	5.5	3.8	22.7	17	5.4	0.7	2.4
25-30s.	6.0	3.6	15.3	17	6.9	0.9	2.6
30-35s.	6.3	3.6	17	17	7.1	1.1	2.9
35-40s.	6.1	3.1	17	18	7.1	1.1	3.2
>40s.	6.7	4.1	16	18	8.4	1.2	2.7

Dinner – Broth, fish, potatoes (Butcher's meat occasionally and on Sundays);

Tea – Bread, scones, oatmeal cake, tea, butter and jam;

Supper – Porridge and milk, bread, butter and jam.[19]

The improvement lay in the variety of foods which now complemented the oatmeal, milk, broth and potatoes that remained the staples. Greater variety means that people will usually be able to eat more of a monotonous staple and so there is little chance that in rural districts, at least, people in Scotland were underfed. Nevertheless, there was always the risk of those in most need getting least, as the following diet sent in by a farm servant in Clackmannan shows vividly:

Breakfast – Children: Porridge and milk or syrup.

Father and mother: tea, bread and butter, an egg or a small bit of ham or a sausage (On Sundays something better for the children at breakfast and dinner);

Dinner – Soup (Potato, lentil or pea – usually enough made at once for two days) or broth with meat (the parents have the meat).

Supper – Bread, scones, butter, jam, tea. The children have rice boiled in water with sugar or with some milk if available (On Sundays a bit of cake or some biscuits as well).

In this instance, the children probably did not feel particularly hungry but they may well have been smaller than those in many other families. In towns, the consumption of oatmeal had largely given way to bread and other products based on wheat flour. In Scottish towns fat consumption was lower than in England (where it ranged between 5–10 ozs [142–284 g] per head per week) at this time, perhaps because of less use of margarine. Sugar consumption was very high and roughly on a par with English urban diets of the same period. Milk consumption was higher than England in every case except Paton's Edinburgh survey of 1900, while meat consumption was lower than in England in every case except Miss Lindsay's Glasgow survey in 1912. In one sense, the high cereal consumption and low fat and meat figure are reminiscent of the English diets of a generation or so earlier, such as Dr Edward Smith recorded in the 1860s.[20]

Something of this comparison can also be seen in the results of the daily nutrient analysis shown in Table 1.3. The high carbohydrate content of the diet is clearly visible in this table and the other feature which has a nineteenth-century look about it is the way in which the amount of protein is usually greater than that of fat, even if the difference is only measured by a few grams. In twentieth-century diets it is usual to find that fat intake is larger than protein intake. Energy levels are not as high as one might expect from a diet which has such a high carbohydrate content and in which such a high proportion of family income is devoted to food expenditure. Although the proportional figures for the sources of energy are not shown in Table 1.3, it is worth noting that in all these diets 62–70 per cent of energy came from carbohydrates and only 19–26 per cent from fats. Energy values of 1800–2100 kcals/day [7531–8786 kj/day] were too low for nineteenth-century families to maintain themselves in good health – comments in the Paton and Lindsay inquiries bear this out. What seems to be happening in this period is that the switch from oatmeal to bread had not been as wholehearted as was necessary to make up the deficit in energy value due to the reduction in oatmeal consumption. Families in England depending principally on wheaten bread with low fat and meat intakes had often eaten 9–10 lbs [4.08–4.54 kg] of bread per head per week in the nineteenth century. In England, as bread consumption fell between the 1860s and the 1930s, energy values were maintained and even increased by the introduction of additional foods to the diet. More fats, which had a high energy content, were the major component of this change. In Scotland, additional

Table 1.3. *Daily Nutrient Intake per head*

Survey	Energy value (kcal)	(kJ)	Protein (g)	Fat (g)	Carbo-hydrate (g)	Iron (mg)	Calcium (g)
Urban							
Edinburgh 1900	1,784	7,464	54	52	276	10.1	0.38
Urban 1904	2,691	11,259	74	75	430	14.2	0.61
Dundee 1906	1,968	8,234	54	41	345	10.2	0.58
Glasgow 1912	2,131	8,916	64	62	330	11.2	0.58
Rural (1904)							
Highlands-Islands	2,342	9,799	69	58	387	14.8	0.63
Midlands-Lowlands	2,402	10,050	66	60	397	12.3	0.61
Mean	2,365	9,895	67	59	391	13.3	0.62
1904 Urban by Income Groups							
< 25s.	2,444	10,226	66	60	411	13.3	0.54
25-30s.	2,523	10,556	68	68	409	13	0.56
30-35s.	2,693	11,268	75	75	429	14.3	0.62
35-40s.	2,720	11,380	76	78	427	14.4	0.65
> 40s.	2,862	11,975	79	82	452	15	0.62

foods did not compensate for low bread consumption in the years before 1914. On the other hand, the level of milk consumption did produce adequate calcium levels in excess of 0.5 g/head which few diets in England (where milk consumption was significantly lower) achieved. Iron intakes appear adequate from the mean figures in excess of 10 mg/head/day but, given the probable distribution of food in families, would not have met the requirements of teenage children. Of course, there were inadequate diets amongst the poorer classes in towns on both sides of the border but, in the countryside, and amongst the better-off townsfolk, Scottish diets were no worse than those in England and with regard to mineral salts, in many cases, a good deal better.

In the inter-war years, several significant surveys were undertaken in Scotland. In fact, Scotland was the only part of the United Kingdom in which coherent attempts were made to monitor the population's food consumption. At the Rowett Research Institute, near Aberdeen, the Director, Dr J. B. Orr, undertook these surveys for a variety of reasons: first, in clarifying its role, the new Ministry of Health in London had forced a 'concordat' on the Medical Research Council (MRC) in 1925, which reserved the right to carry out surveys relating to epidemiological problems to the Ministry rather than the MRC. However, George Newman, the Chief Medical Officer at the ministry, was unwilling to involve himself or his staff in this work and did not wish work undertaken by the MRC to be used to embarrass the Ministry's official policies. Since the MRC had a very limited budget and was committed to expenditure on vitamin research by its Accessory Food Factors Committee, it was anyway restricted as to what it could achieve. Its only attempt at a dietary survey in the 1920s, carried out by Professor E. P. Cathcart (Glasgow) on the nutritional status of miners and their families, left the MRC dissatisfied with both the results and the expense involved. Despite this, the Secretary of the MRC, Sir Walter Fletcher, was highly critical of what he saw as the failure of the Ministry of Health to implement the new knowledge which the nutritionists had recently acquired through the discovery of vitamins. He was eager to encourage research into the nutritional status of the population of Britain. The dislike of the Ministry of Health's inactivity by the MRC led Professor Edward Mellanby to propose to the Cabinet Committee on Civil Research in 1927 that a Board of Nutrition should be established as a government department independent of the Ministry of Health.

Fortunately, no such concordat had been imposed by the Board of Health for Scotland, and its Parliamentary Under-Secretary, Walter Elliot became a key figure in promoting dietary surveys in Scotland. After 1926, when Elliot was moved from the Board of Health to be Parliamentary Under-Secretary of State for Scotland, he also acquired a seat on the Empire Marketing Board which had grown out of the Imperial Exhibition at Wembley. As chairman of the Empire Marketing Board's Research Sub-Committee, Elliot had a budget of £1m to spend and had long-standing personal links with the Rowett's Director, Dr J. B. Orr.[21] The Empire Marketing Board, which was hopeful of stimulating agriculture in Britain as well as in overseas territories, found common cause with the nutritionists after the appearance of the MRC Report by Dr H. Corry Mann on the *Diets for Boys during the School Age*.[22] Corry Mann had demonstrated the growth potential of dietary supplements in children's homes and this idea was taken up by the Empire Marketing Board to show the nutritive value of milk. It was hoped that this knowledge would increase consumption and in turn would stimulate British dairy farming. The Board's Research Sub-Committee was therefore eager to provide funds for research which would show what existing levels of milk consumption were. To Orr, who had been invited to become a member of the MRC's Nutrition Committee and was therefore party to its decision to give up plans for a national survey of diets[23] under the Ministry of Health's pressure, the Empire Marketing Board's proposal was second best. Orr accepted milk promotion as the means which justified the end of getting into working-class homes and carrying out dietary surveys. He was granted funds of approximately £25,000 in 1926 for an inquiry into seven Scottish towns after an MRC pilot study had been carried out in St Andrews. By April 1928, the Empire Marketing Board was running full-page advertisements in the *Daily Mail*, the Glasgow *Sunday Mail* and the national Sunday newspapers, based on the Corry Mann Report, headed 'What Milk Can Do' – 'Results that "Startled" the Medical Research Council'. The MRC was less than enthusiastic about this coverage and the quotations from the Corry Mann Report that accompanied the trade advertising campaign that followed. But they could not deny the slogan 'Take Fresh Milk – and Plenty of it' and Neville Chamberlain's broadcast on the subject in May 1928, in his role of Minister of Health, eased their discomfort. However, Orr never received cash so freely again and by April 1931 the Research Committee of the Empire Marketing Board was reviewing its financial commitments 'in view of reduced financial resources'.

The analysis of the surveys in Scotland during the inter-war years shown in Tables 2.1 and 2.2 result from the use of the original returns which have survived at the Rowett Research Institute. To date, there seems to be little, if any, surviving evidence for the planning and execution of these surveys, so that the process by which the families in the surveys were chosen is unclear. However, it is necessary to take note of the scale of the inquiry which Orr undertook. To have completed surveys of over 100 families in several of the towns required a major effort from a large team and, at the same time that records of food intake were being accumulated, children's health was being assessed by clinical examination at their schools. The second section in Table 2 resulted from John Boyd Orr's attempt to measure the impact of the depression upon food consumption in Scottish families. Unfortunately, this was on a smaller scale and concentrated only on Aberdeen and Peterhead in the north-east.[24] The third section of Table 2 shows

Table 2.1. *Weekly Food Consumption per head*

Survey	Number of families	Bread (lb)	Potatoes (lb)	Sugar (oz)	Fats (oz)	Meat (lb)	Milk (pt)
Seven Towns (1928)							
Glasgow	57	5.7	3.8	14	8.8	1.1	2.6
Greenock	132	5.3	3.3	16	8.6	1.0	2.2
Paisley	31	7.0	3.3	15	8.1	1.3	2.4
Edinburgh	112	5.4	3.2	14	8.1	1.1	1.7
Dundee	37	5.3	3.1	13	7.2	1.2	1.6
Aberdeen	150	4.1	3.6	17	7.6	1.2	3.3
Peterhead	104	4.1	4.5	17	5.9	0.8	2.6
Depression (1933)							
Aberdeen	66	3.6	2.2	16	4.2	1.0	2.6
Peterhead	49	4.4	2.9	15	4.0	0.8	1.9
Carnegie (1937)							
Scotland	70	4.6	2.9	16	8.6	1.1	3.2
England	140	5.1	3.2	17	11.6	1.4	2.8

Table 2.2. *Daily Nutrient Intake per head*

Survey	Energy value (kcal)	(kJ)	Protein (g)	Fat (g)	Carbo-hydrate (g)	Iron (mg)	Calcium (g)
Seven Towns (1928)							
Glasgow	2,669	11,167	80	74	414	15	0.62
Greenock	2,495	10,439	75	67	399	13.5	0.55
Paisley	2,900	12,134	87	77	464	16	0.61
Edinburgh	2,545	10,648	76	68	407	14	0.61
Dundee	2,409	10,079	72	67	379	13.1	0.53
Aberdeen	3,030	12,678	91	88	470	16	1.38
Peterhead	3,002	12,560	90	77	488	16.3	1.31
Depression (1933)							
Aberdeen	1,926	8,058	67	49	303	11.6	0.48
Peterhead	2,118	8,862	69	47	355	12.2	0.4
Carnegie (1937)							
Scotland	2,457	10,280	74	79	362	13.7	0.7
England	2,538	10,619	76	96	343	13.7	0.65

the results of the Carnegie Trust-financed inquiry of 1937–9 and is based upon a stratified sample of the surviving returns.[25] The use of such a sample has tried to deflect criticism that the Carnegie Survey concentrated upon poor families and also large families with young children. The results shown are based upon a ten per cent sample which is weighted towards smaller families rather than larger ones. It was impossible to include many families with no children at all as the whole Carnegie inquiry covering 1352 families contained only four families with no children. Taking into account the repeat surveys, there were 667 family budgets for Scotland (and 1046 for England) of which 70 were recalculated for Table 2.

Food consumption in Table 2.1 shows an interesting relationship to the pre-1914 diets. In the Seven Towns inquiry, fat and potato consumption had risen and even bread of which, though broadly unchanged, slightly more was eaten in some instances among families in Edinburgh and Glasgow. Sugar, meat and milk figures remained more or less unchanged: these were all 'expensive' foods – sugar becoming so as its price went up from 1903 onwards. The comparison between Aberdeen and Peterhead in 1928 and the later Depression inquiry figures is also interesting. Family-budget analysis shows that the 'Giffen-good' theory – that if a family's income is reduced severely, food consumption will be restricted to one food, such as bread, even if the price of that food should rise – is inappropriate for real life. In depressions, families do not eliminate some items from their diet altogether but instead it is more usual to see a proportional reduction all-round. In this case, some foods reveal greater proportional falls than others: potato consumption fell by 35–39 per cent, fats by 32–45 per cent and milk by 21–27 per cent. Potatoes, so often described as the food of poverty, show one of the two largest reductions. Sugar consumption dropped by only 6–12 per cent and meat was surprisingly resistant to falls in consumption. While bread consumption rose by 7 per cent at Peterhead, as Giffen would have predicted, it fell in Aberdeen along with all other foods. By the later 1930s, it seems possible that fat and milk consumption were rising, or had recovered to the pre-Depression levels, though bread and potatoes had not. Even if one was tempted to see further movement towards an English pattern of food consumption, it is necessary to note the various comments by the Carnegie Survey research team that the traditional diet of oatmeal, potatoes and milk was still strong in the north-east and that it was reinforced by the system of payment to farm labourers.

These figures are based on an analysis which was carried out some years ago and which omitted one useful indicator of change in diet in Scotland, namely a breakdown of cereal consumption. In consequence, Table 3, which is based on the Carnegie Report, attempts to show various features of inter-war diet in Scotland which deserve comment. Patterns of cereal consumption are shown in Table 3.1. The principal items were recorded by the Carnegie Survey in three categories: first, white bread, second, rolls, buns, and scones, and third, oatmeal and oatcake. In Table 3.1, each of these is set out by the expenditure groups used. The contrast is marked. In the rural north-east, as shown in columns 1–5, there were only about 2 lbs [0.9 kg] of bread eaten per head per week whereas in the Fife coalfield (columns 6–7) and in the towns of Dundee (column 9) and Edinburgh (column 10), 3 to 4 lbs [1.4-1.8 kg] was being eaten. Aberdeen (column 8) lay somewhere between the two. Perhaps unsurprisingly, bread consumption declined as expenditure on food rose but the picture would be incomplete without considering the consumption of rolls and buns. Here again, a pattern of low consumption in rural districts contrasted strongly with Fife and the urban centres. Aberdeen made up for its lower bread consumption with rolls and buns. Conversely, oatmeal consumption in rural areas at up to 2 lbs [0.9 kg] per head per week was still a major component of the diet which had almost

Table 3.1. *Differences in cereal consumption in Scotland, 1937*

Expenditure Group	Rural north-east					Mining Districts		Urban Areas		
	1 (oz)	2 (oz)	3 (oz)	4 (oz)	5 (oz)	6 (oz)	7 (oz)	8 (oz)	9 (oz)	10 (oz)
White Bread										
1 < 3s	—	—	—	—	—	—	—	—	33	61
2 3-5s	39	37	30	32	34	50	54	45	51	71
3 5-7s	34	32	31	35	33	50	64	40	50	64
4 7-9s	42	26	26	31	24	62	53	20	49	71
5 9-11s	—	—	32	21	24	58	44	23	36	—
6 > 11s			29	30	21	50	51	25	20	—
Rolls, Buns and Scones										
1 < 3s									6	4
2 3-5s	4	12	3	4	4	19	15	20	13	5
3 5-7s	4	12	5	7	8	19	15	25	17	14
4 7-9s	14	22	8	12	15	19	19	22	10	14
5 9-11s	—	—	8	16	10	28	17	13	11	—
6 > 11s	—	12	2	7		23	7	15	10	
Oatmeal and Oatcakes										
1 < 3s	—	—	—	—	—	—	—	—	2	3
2 3-5s	12	5	35	30	34	0.1	1	2	2	3
3 5-7s	14	3	30	30	31	1	2	6	1	5
4 7-9s	21	5	36	18	24	1	2	5	10	nil
5 9-11s	—	—	29	26	17	2	2	8	7	—
6 > 11s	—	—	36	30	16	3	3	10	3	—

Key (Columns 1–10):   **Rural N-E:** 1 Kintore; 2 Hopeman; 3 Barthol Chapel; 4 Methlick; 5 Tarves
Mining Districts: 6 West Wemyss; 7 Coaltown of Wemyss
Urban Areas: 8 Aberdeen; 9 Dundee; 10 Edinburgh

Table 3.2 *Differences in weekly food consumption
in Scotland and England, 1937*

Expenditure group	Vegetables				Potatoes		Fresh fruit		Rolls, buns and scones	
	Green		Root							
(shillings/head)	Scot (oz)	Eng (oz)	Scot (oz)	Eng (oz)	Scot (oz)	Eng (oz)	Scot (oz)	Eng (oz)	Scot (oz)	Eng (oz)
< 3s	0.3	5.8	6.4	1.8	32	45	1	3	5	0.5
3 to 5s	1.5	8.2	4.9	2	49	52	4	7	9	0.7
5 to 7s	1.9	8.9	6	2.6	62	59	7	12	13	1.5
7 to 9s	3.3	10.9	7.8	3.5	61	64	12	18	15	2.3
9 to 11s	5.7	18	7.7	2.9	63	56	22	29	16	2
>11s	4.4	21.5	9.4	7.3	59	54	29	47	11	3

disappeared from Fife and the towns.[26] Orr's team felt that there was still reluctance to accept margarine in Scotland, which probably contributed to a lower fat consumption by comparison with England but, that with the greater use of rolls, buns and scones, there had developed an increasing use of jams, marmalade and syrup. Table 3.2 extends the comparison of Scottish and English preferences for food to fruit and vegetables. Scottish consumption of fresh fruit and green vegetables, although showing an increase as food expenditure rose, was low and markedly different from that of English families surveyed by the Carnegie inquiry. By contrast, the consumption of root vegetables was greater than in England and increased as food expenditure rose. Potato consumption, in which there was little difference between the two countries, is also shown to complete the picture. In both countries potato consumption showed signs of decline above expenditure groups 4 or 5, that is over some figure around ten shillings [£0.50] per head per week on food. The last column reinforces the predilection towards cereal products in the Scottish diet; the consumption of rolls, buns and scones exceeded that in England significantly at every food expenditure level.

The nutrient analysis of inter-war diets is shown in Table 2.2. The bottom line, that of the English families in the Carnegie Survey, shows how far the average English diet had changed since the nineteenth century. Then, the 'typical' intake of the high carbohydrate English diet had an energy value of around 2,200 kcals per day [9205 kj]. The largest component providing this energy value was carbohydrate and an average intake of 380 g per day will be found when analyzing family budgets. By the end of the inter-war years, bread consumption in England had fallen, though potato and sugar consumption remained stable. The gradual rise in energy value to around 2,500 kcals/day [10,460 kj] was the result of increasing amounts of fats in the diet. By the 1930s, the proportional sources of the energy in the typical English diet were 12 per cent protein, 34 per cent fat and 54 per cent carbohydrate, very similar, as might be expected, to the figures which result from analyzing the diets in John Boyd Orr's *Food, Health and Income*. The English Carnegie diets confirmed the trend: fat intake exceeded protein and was approaching 100 g/day; carbohydrate intake had fallen from the nineteenth-century level of 380 to 340 g/day. Calcium levels – the target of the Empire Marketing Board's milk campaign – remained low.

Diets in Scotland in Table 2.2 show some general advance on the pre-1914 surveys analyzed in Table 1.3. Energy values, on the whole, are higher – in some cases significantly so – as are carbohydrate intakes. Some levelling up of iron and calcium intakes had occurred but the fat intake was still low and not much above those shown before 1914. In the Seven Towns inquiry, the sources of the energy value were, proportionally, 12 per cent from protein, 62–65 per cent from carbohydrate but only 23–26 per cent from fat. While these proportions were quite common in England in the nineteenth century, they had almost entirely disappeared by the 1930s. The two Depression surveys in Aberdeen and Peterhead show very clearly the effects of food restriction: very low fat intake and dangerously low levels of calcium in the diet. In proportion, the changes in the source of energy during the Depression were that carbohydrates provided 63–67 per cent and fat only 20–23 per cent. The Carnegie Survey in 1937 provided the real comparison of families in the two countries surveyed by the same methods. Scottish diets had lower energy values, fat intake was lower but carbohydrate intake higher.

What general conclusions might be drawn from this comparison and what questions remain unanswered? Scottish diet undoubtedly went through a period of modernization between the late nineteenth century and World War I. At a superficial level of analysis, there might be grounds for regarding these changes as adopting English patterns of eating but with a time lag of around a generation or so. A second generalization stems from the limited evidence of differences in diets between towns and the countryside. It seems likely that rural diets in Scotland were significantly better than many in the towns, particularly among the poorer town-dwellers. By contrast the general impression resulting from looking at English diets is that the reverse was true, namely, that town-dwellers – even among the poor – often ate better than those in the country.

However, it is important to modify that picture by recognizing that change in Scotland began from a different pattern of traditional foods. Thus, the process of modernization in Scotland was expressed by eating more bread and more fats, some of which was offset by a decline in traditional cereals and milk. This, in Roy Campbell's view, led to a decline in the standards of nutrition in Scotland. Assembling family budget evidence suggests that while such a statement may reflect changes in food consumption patterns, the nutritional analysis reveals that during the period 1900–39, families in Scotland maintained or even slightly improved their nutritional status in terms of the energy value, protein and fat intakes and the mineral content of their diets. In a wider sense, the changes shown by this study suggest that modifications were occurring in inter-war Scotland that had taken place in England 30 or 40 years earlier. However, Scottish diets in the inter-war years were not progressing towards the higher consumption of fat as rapidly as those in England. The Scots, of course, were still learning to eat more bread in the inter-war years, an accomplishment they perfected in the period from the end of World War II until about 1963.[27] From then on, a gradual decline in bread consumption set in. The fundamental aspect of dietary change in Scotland during the twentieth century, therefore, is that for those sectors of the Scottish population that began adding new foods to their traditional diet, the greater variety of foodstuffs consumed led to more energy and more fat in the diet. On the other hand, for those sectors of the population that gave up traditional cereals and milk to eat more bread, the result was the development of a restricted diet similar to the poorer English families of the late nineteenth and early twentieth centuries. By the inter-war period, this led to sub-clinical and even overt malnutrition in Scotland.

The historian, lacking clinical evidence to test any hypothesis based on the effect of these dietary changes, must make some arbitrary assessments. The new knowledge of vitamins, which stimulated scientists into much political activity in the inter-war years, is probably the key. In the absence of any fortification of foods during the inter-war years, low fat intakes probably restricted the vitamin D content of the diet. It is possible that deficiencies of vitamins A and C also occurred but were, on balance, unlikely. After all, potatoes provided the most significant source of vitamin C in British diets in the first half of the twentieth century rather than fresh fruit or green vegetables. On the other hand, low extraction white flour may have reduced the B vitamins in bread. In general, the deficiency diseases most likely to be present in Scotland were rickets and anaemia. Rickets was certainly of concern in Scottish towns before 1914. There is a reference to rickety children in Miss Lindsay's 1912 Glasgow survey but evidence for the extent of rickets in either Scotland or England in the inter-war period is much harder to find. By the inter-war period, it is possible that some deficiency diseases were not so pronounced and existed mainly in sub-clinical forms though, since the functions of vitamins are to facilitate growth, evidence of any restriction of growth might confirm dietary deficiencies.

The Carnegie Survey made the point that children in the families surveyed in Scotland were smaller than in other parts of the United Kingdom (see Table 4). Feeding experiments carried out in some of the Carnegie Survey populations accelerated children's growth by contrast to slower growth rates in the control groups. Unfortunately, the data were not disaggregated to show differences between Scottish and English children. In his appendix to the Carnegie Report, Professor A. F. Thomson said of the 1930s: 'We had a population in which frank deficiency disease was rare but in which generalized malnutrition was undoubtedly widespread, manifested by imponderable but evident impairment of health and vitality and by easily measured defects of growth and form.'[28] The confident ring of this assessment owes much to the experience of war-time rationing and full-employment in postwar Britain. At the time, in the 1930s, there was no political will to implement any solution to the problem of poor growth and health and, indeed, more energy was devoted to denying the existence of any problem than to its solution. After 1937, when the Ministry of Health's Second Nutrition Committee reported, government responsibility for 'feeding the nation' became a common figure of speech. Nevertheless, during

Table 4. *Heights and weights of children, 1937–39*

Survey	Age 5		Age 8		Age 12	
	Height (cm)	Weight (kg)	Height (cm)	Weight (kg)	Height (cm)	Weight (kg)
Boys						
Carnegie	106.9	17.9	124.5	24.4	141.5	34.3
English Urban	108	18.9	124.2	25.2	142	35.5
LCC	109.2	19.4	125.7	26.1	144.8	37.7
Girls						
Carnegie	106.6	17.5	123	23.3	143.3	35.2
LCC	108.5	18.9	124.7	25.5	146.8	37.7

Source: Baines, A. H. J. and Hollingsworth D. F., 'Diets of working-class families with children before and after the Second World War' *Nutrition Abstracts and Reviews*, 33 (1963), 666.

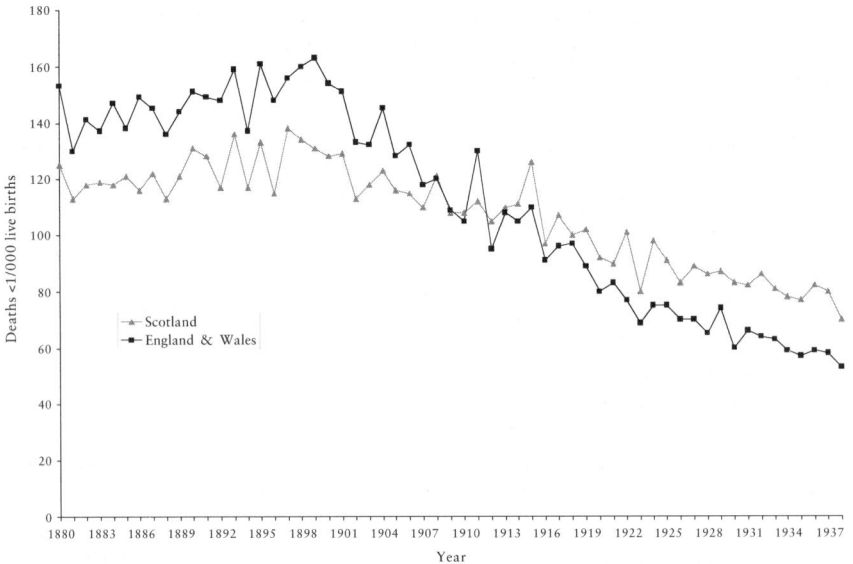

Fig. 1. *Infant mortality in Britain 1880–1938*

the 1930s, no one was prepared to discuss the implementation of large-scale supplementary feeding programmes for children. The introduction of the school-milk schemes in 1934, while satisfactory as an outcome of the Empire Marketing Board's campaigns, was no substitute for the failure of governments to integrate nutritional knowledge into social policy in the inter-war years.

Nutritional status is, of course, only part of the explanation of ill health and restricted growth. Levels of infant mortality are an indicator of the status of the most vulnerable group in the population, those in the first year of life. Nutritional status, and particularly maternal nutrition, is part of the explanation of infant mortality, but infection resulting from environmental hazards need to be considered and may outweigh nutritional status. Some indication of the environment's impact may be deduced by examining the differing levels of infant mortality in England and Scotland before World War II. Figure 1 shows that in the 1880s and 1890s, infant mortality rates were much higher in England than Scotland and remained so up to World War I. Between 1911 and 1931, however, infant mortality in England was halved, while in Scotland it fell only by a quarter. During the inter-war years, therefore, Scottish infant mortality was appreciably higher than in England and Wales.

Can the contrasting reduction of inter-war infant mortality rates in Scotland and England be explained by differences in the rate at which dietary patterns changed, or do they reflect other differences in the state of the economy and the quality of the urban environment? In the inter-war years, the strong growth of housing and new industries in the English midlands and

Table 5. *Exploring demographic data: constructing housing ratios for England and Scotland*

Census Year	Total Population		Crude Birth Rate		Housing Stock		Housing Ratio	
	England (000)	Scotland (000)	England (/000)	Scotland (/000)	England (000)	Scotland (000)	England (persons/ house)	Scotland (persons/ house)
(1)	(2)	(3)	(4)	(5)	(6)	(7)	(8)	(9)
1881	25,974	3,736	33.9	33.7	5,218	799	4.98	4.68
1891	29,003	4,026	31.4	31.2	5,824	869	4.98	4.63
1901	32,528	4,472	28.7	29.5	6,710	986	4.85	4.54
1911	36,070	4,761	24.5	25.8	7,550	1,102	4.78	4.32
1921	37,887	4,882	22.8	19.1	7,979	1,109	4.75	4.40
1931	39,952	4,843	15.8	19.1	9,400	1,197	4.25	4.05
1951	43,758	5,096	15.5	17.7	12,389	1,442	3.53	3.53

Housing ratio = column (2)/column(6) for England and Wales
and column (3)/column(7) for Scotland

Source: Central *Statistical Office, Annual Abstract of Statistics*, Vol 97, 1960, London, 1960; B. R. Mitchell and P. Deane, *An Abstract of British Historical Statistics*, Cambridge, 1962

south-east, compared with the structural problems in the Scottish industrial economy, meant that employment and levels of incomes were stronger influences on food consumption patterns and standards of living in England and Wales than tradition and culture. Spending power meant that diets in England and Wales were being modernized, except in the Special Areas where the depression prevailed. However, in Scotland, where dietary change was slower, restricting the use of traditional foods, when new foods were not substituted in sufficient quantities to make up for the loss of the old, compounded economic difficulties. Urban working-class families in Scotland experienced shrinking employment and overcrowded housing, which accentuated the impact of the inter-war depression.[29] The stress can be seen even at aggregate levels in Table 5, as Scotland's population fell in the 1920s and the progressive decline in the crude birth rate was halted. Under these circumstances, it is not surprising that the fall in the infant mortality rate in England and Wales between 1911 and 1931 was not mirrored in Scotland.

BIBLIOGRAPHY

Barker, Theo C., McKenzie, J. C. and Yudkin, J. *Our Changing Fare*, London, 1966.

Barker, Theo C., Oddy, D. J. and Yudkin, J. *The Dietary Surveys of Dr Edward Smith, 1862–3*, London, 1970.

Levitt, I. and Smout C. *The State of the Scottish Working Class in 1843*, Edinburgh, 1979.

Orr, John B. *Food, Health and Income*, London, 1936.

Paton, D. N., and Findlay, L. *Poverty Nutrition and Growth*, London, HMSO, 1926.

Report of the Royal Commission on the Distribution of the Industrial Population [the Barlow Commission], (Cmd 6153) London, 1940.

Rowett Research Institute. *Family Diet and Health in Pre-War Britain*, Dunfermline, 1955.

NOTES

1 Robert Burns, 'The Cotter's Saturday Night', verse XI.
2 Barker, McKenzie, and Yudkin, 1966, 60.
3 Though by the nature of the evidence available, he had to draw more from the *New Statistical Account*, Edinburgh, 1845, which described Scotland in the early 1840s.
4 *Report of the Royal Commission on the Poor Law (Scotland)*, Parliamentary Papers (P.P.), 1844, XX–XXV.
5 This account of diet in Scotland in the early 1840s depends on Levitt and Smout, 1979, ch 2.
6 Ibid, 28–9.
7 Hutchison, R. Report on the Dietaries of Scotch Agricultural Labourers, *Transactions of the Highland and Agricultural Society of Scotland*, II, 1868–9.
8 *Sixth Report of the Medical Officer of the Committee of Council on Health*, P.P., 1864, XXVIII, 249.
9 Booth, Charles. *Life and Labour of the People in London*, 2nd ser Vol 5, London, 1903, 327.
10 *Report of the Interdepartmental Committee on Physical Deterioration*, P.P. 1904 (Cd 2175) XXXII, para 290.
11 Paton (1859–928) left Edinburgh in 1906 to become Regius Professor of Physiology in Glasgow, where he remained until his death.
12 See *British Medical Journal*, 1903. R. H. Chittenden was the sole advocate of low protein intakes at the time.
13 Paton and Findlay, 1926.
14 *Second Series of Memoranda, Statistical Tables and Charts*, P.P. 1905 (Cd 2337) LXXXIV
15 *Second Report by Mr Wilson Fox on the Wages, Earnings and Conditions of Employment of Agricultural Labourers in the United Kingdom*, P.P. 1905 (Cd 2376) XCVII.
16 ibid. No original questionnaire returns relating to this inquiry have been traced in the Public Record Office.
17 *Second Series of Memoranda*, op cit, 242.
18 Ibid, 242.
19 Ibid, 243.
20 See Barker, Oddy and Yudkin, 1970.
21 Walter Elliot was MP for Kelvingrove, Glasgow. He met J. B. Orr when they were both medical students in Glasgow. After the War, Elliot spent his Parliamentary vacations as a research student at the Rowett Institute, being awarded a DSc in 1922 for a 'Study in mineral metabolism with special reference to rickets and similar bone lesions in other animals and in the human'.
22 MRC, *Special Report Series, No 105*, London, 1926.

23 A further study in St Andrews convinced the MRC that they had not the resources to carry out large-scale investigations of diet.

24 It should be noted that the apparent omission of any diets from Orr, 1936, is because all the budgets used in that publication were collected from England between 1932 and 1935. Orr left the Aberdeen and Peterhead families out of the 1152 studies which were the basis of *Food, Health and Income.*

25 World War II delayed the appearance of the Carnegie Report until 1955 but even then its appearance led to criticism from the Ministry of Agriculture, Food and Fisheries in 1963. This reflected the political embarrassment, to the Ministry of Health in particular, that Orr's work had caused in the 1930s.

26 The low consumption in column 2 is for Hopeman, Morayshire, a fishing village east of Burghead.

27 By 1956, Scotland was top of the regional league in the National Food Survey for cereal consumption with a total intake of 82 ozs/head/week [2.33 kg]: by 1975 Scotland had fallen to second place behind the North of England and total cereal intake in Scotland was down to 62 ozs/head/week [1.76 kg].

28 Rowett Research Institute, 1955, Appendix I, 70.

29 See *Royal Commission on the Distribution of the Industrial Population* [the Barlow Commission], 1940 (Cmd 6153) 70, 266.

The Carnegie Survey: background
and intended impact

David Smith

The Carnegie Nutritional and Dietary Survey was funded by the Carnegie
United Kingdom Trust, and conducted from the Rowett Research Institute
near Aberdeen, between 1937 and 1939. The results were not published
until 1955,[1] but an interim report was sent to the Minister of Health, Secretary of State for Scotland, and the Trust, soon after the outbreak of World
War II.[2] At this time John Boyd Orr, Director of the Institute, urged cau-
tion: 'As the Report shows the inadequacy of diet in nearly one-third of
the population . . . it is most inadvisable that it should be made public at
the present time'. He claimed, however, that 'the findings . . . have proved
of great value to the Minister of Health in connection with the influence
of proposed rationing schemes on public health'.[3] In 1950 this claim was
repeated by David Cuthbertson, Orr's successor at the Rowett,[4] and the
former Minister of Food, Lord Woolton, emphasised the value of the findings in the foreword to the 1955 publication. No doubt the data did play
an important wartime role, but this awaits detailed analysis.[5] This chapter
instead sets the investigation in the context of the careers of Orr and the
Rowett, and the wider scientific, social, and political background, and illu-
minates the intended, rather than actual, impact.

In order to understand the context of the investigation, it is necessary
to consider various long-term developments, as well as the immediate situation. In the former connection, Orr's interest in expanding the remit
of the Institute to cover human as well as animal nutrition must be mentioned.[6] Similarly, his increasing involvement with questions of agricultural
economics and marketing, particularly milk marketing, should be considered. During the early 1930s Orr was appointed to various committees
that sought solutions to the problems of agricultural over-production and
depressed prices.[7] In addition, he became a member of the Advisory Committee on Nutrition of the Minister of Health and the Secretary of State for
Scotland, which was charged with investigating the British diet and advis-
ing on whether changes were desirable.[8]

Orr was greatly helped in advancing his ambitions through his association with Walter Elliot, MP, who, like Orr, was a Glasgow medical graduate. Elliot worked voluntarily at the Institute during the early 1920s, and
later, as chair of the Research Grants Committee of the Empire Marketing

Board, proved a valuable supporter. As Minister of Agriculture from 1932, Elliot was responsible for several of Orr's appointments to government committees.[9]

As Orr's interests expanded, and his involvement with the practical problems of managing Britain's food supply increased, he began to emphasise the role of poverty as the main cause of nutritional problems, and argued for cheap food policies as the solution. His argument linking the dietary habits and financial means of families was most clearly expressed and vividly illustrated in *Food, Health and Income*, published in March 1936, the reception of which forms the immediate context for the Carnegie Survey.[10]

ORIGINS OF *FOOD, HEALTH AND INCOME*

The work published as *Food Health and Income* began in response to a request by the Millers Mutual Association to the Rowett Institute in January 1935, for data about the consumption of staple foodstuffs, and the effects on health of varying consumption. Orr suggested to the Institute's governing body that the task might be entrusted to the Market Supply Committee, an organisation responsible for collecting food statistics, created under Elliot's 1932 Agricultural Marketing Act. Orr was authorised to explore the matter,[11] leading to a conference of representatives of the millers, agricultural marketing boards, and other interests. It was agreed that the Imperial Bureau of Animal Nutrition, which was based at the Rowett, should assemble the information, with the costs contributed by the food trade organisations. Orr leased a room adjacent to the offices of the Market Supply Committee in London, and Lord Linlithgow, Director of the Committee, agreed that the secretary, E. M. H. Lloyd, and staff, could co-operate in the exercise.[12] Orr and Linlithgow had earlier collaborated as members of the Agricultural Committee of the Scottish National Development Council, an initiative of Scottish local authorities, which aimed to rejuvenate Scottish industry by publicity and research.[13]

Old Etonian David Lubbock, Orr's future son-in-law, and half-brother of the wife of Walter Elliot, was sent to London to work on the project. Lubbock, a biochemist, had worked at the Institute voluntarily since October 1934, and acted as Orr's personal assistant.[14]

In July 1935 a conference of representatives of the funding bodies was held. Each received a general report, and a specific report on the foodstuff with which they were concerned. The sources of data included about 1,500 family budgets which had been collected between 1932 and 1935, by seven different projects carried out by social scientists, medical officers of health, and the Women's Co-operative Guild. These, and other statistics, were used to work out the consumption and expenditure at different income levels.[15] The resulting figures were presented in tables and graphs. The examples in Figure 1 also appeared in a paper presented by Lloyd to the Agricultural Economics Society in December 1935, as well as *Food, Health and*

PER HEAD
PER WEEK FRESH MILK
PINTS

AVERAGE 3·1 PINTS PER HEAD
PER WEEK

PER HEAD
PER WEEK BUTTER
OZS

AVERAGE 7·8 OZS PER HEAD
PER WEEK

PER HEAD
PER WEEK CONDENSED MILK
PINTS

AVERAGE 0·5 PINTS PER HEAD
PER WEEK

PER HEAD
PER WEEK MARGARINE
OZS

AVERAGE 2·5 OZS PER HEAD
PER WEEK

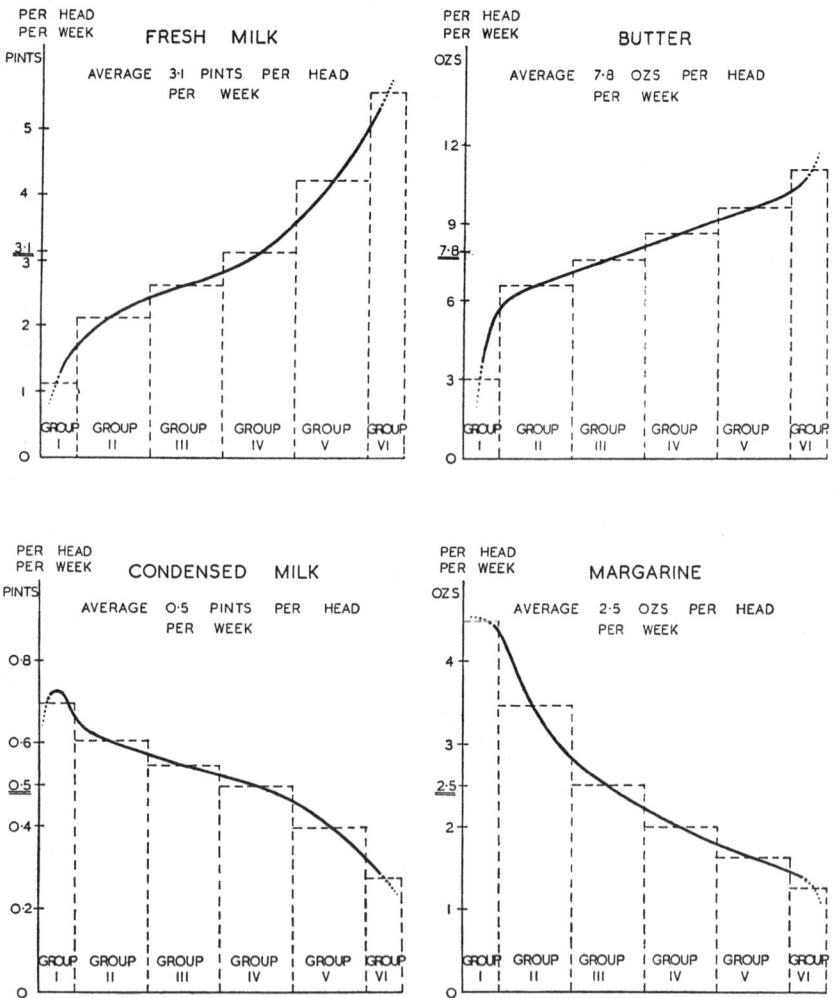

Fig. 1. *Estimated consumption per head of certain foodstuffs by income groups*

Income.[16] Another document based on these analyses was prepared for the Nutrition Committee of the League of Nations, which met in London at the end of November 1935.[17]

Food, Health and Income analysed consumption by income group in terms of nutrients, and incorporated a discussion of the variation in height and health with social group. It reproduced the graphs showing the consumption of individual foods, and also included the graphs shown in Figures 2 and 3. The report was ready in draft form by October 1935 and Orr obtained permission from Elliot to publish it, but they both came under pressure to delay from the Conservative Research Department (CRD). Henry Brooke was responsible for considering milk policy for the CRD,

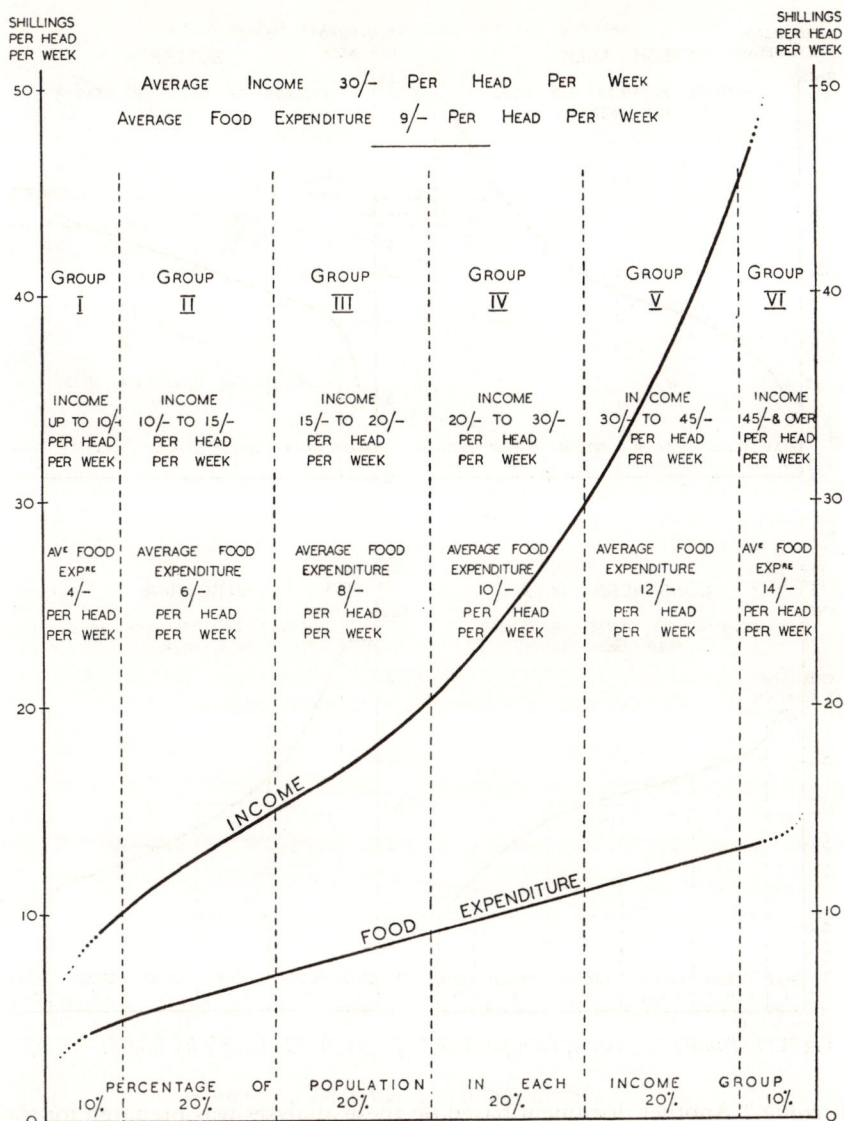

SHILLINGS PER HEAD PER WEEK

50 — 40 — 30 — 20 — 10 — 0

AVERAGE INCOME 30/- PER HEAD PER WEEK

AVERAGE FOOD EXPENDITURE 9/- PER HEAD PER WEEK

GROUP I	GROUP II	GROUP III	GROUP IV	GROUP V	GROUP VI
INCOME UP TO 10/- PER HEAD PER WEEK	INCOME 10/- TO 15/- PER HEAD PER WEEK	INCOME 15/- TO 20/- PER HEAD PER WEEK	INCOME 20/- TO 30/- PER HEAD PER WEEK	INCOME 30/- TO 45/- PER HEAD PER WEEK	INCOME 45/- & OVER PER HEAD PER WEEK
AVE FOOD EXPRE 4/- PER HEAD PER WEEK	AVERAGE FOOD EXPENDITURE 6/- PER HEAD PER WEEK	AVERAGE FOOD EXPENDITURE 8/- PER HEAD PER WEEK	AVERAGE FOOD EXPENDITURE 10/- PER HEAD PER WEEK	AVERAGE FOOD EXPENDITURE 12/- PER HEAD PER WEEK	AVE FOOD EXPRE 14/- PER HEAD PER WEEK

INCOME

FOOD EXPENDITURE

PERCENTAGE OF POPULATION IN EACH INCOME GROUP
10% | 20% | 20% | 20% | 20% | 10%

Fig. 2. *Estimated income and food expenditure by groups of the population*

and was introduced to Orr by E. M. H. Lloyd. After an interview in October 1935, Brooke advised the Director of the CRD that Orr intended publishing his book as soon as possible, which, in view of the general election in November, was an alarming prospect:

I view with some apprehension the prospect that an explosive booklet of this kind ... may quite likely appear in the middle of the election campaign. Neither he [Orr] nor Lloyd seems to have perceived in the least that it might have incal-

PERCENTAGE
OF STANDARD
REQUIREMENTS

EXPRESSED AS PERCENTAGE OF STANDARD REQUIREMENTS

140

120

CALCIUM
(STANDARD MINIMUM
OF 0·6 GRAM)

PHOSPHORUS

VITAMIN
C

LEVEL OF
ADEQUACY

100

IRON

80

VITAMIN
A

CALCIUM
(STANDARD REQUIREMENT OF 0·9 GRAM)

60

GROUP I | GROUP II | GROUP III | GROUP IV | GROUP V | GROUP VI

GROUPS OF THE POPULATION

AVERAGE INTAKE OF CALORIES PROTEIN & FAT

PERCENTAGE
OF STANDARD
REQUIREMENTS

EXPRESSED AS PERCENTAGE OF STANDARD REQUIREMENTS

140

120

PROTEIN

FAT

CALORIES

100

LEVEL OF
ADEQUACY

80

GROUP I | GROUP II | GROUP III | GROUP IV | GROUP V | GROUP VI

GROUPS OF THE POPULATION

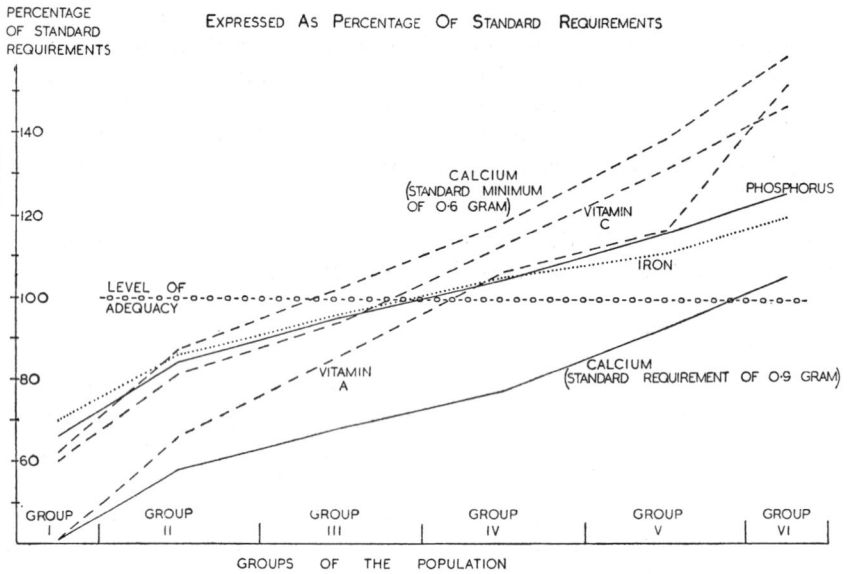

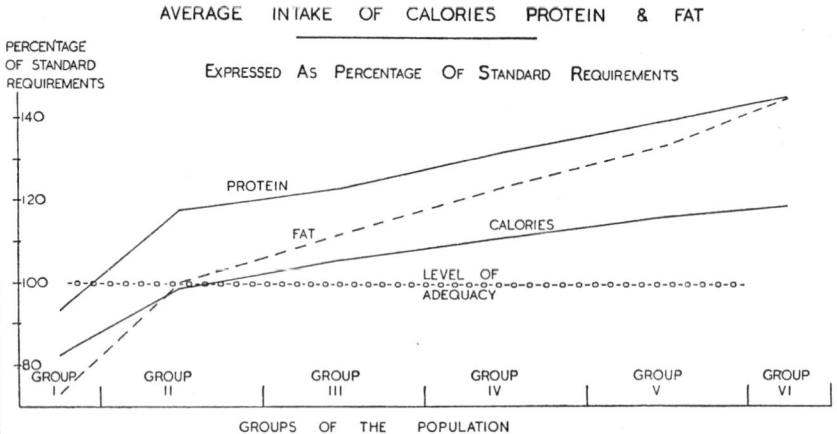

Fig. 3. *Average intake of minerals and vitamins*

culable political effects. If, therefore, you are seeing the Minister [Elliot] . . . I think it would be well to put to him that either he must restrain Sir John Orr from publishing until after the Election, or else he must be prepared to come out instantly on the day of its publication with a Government milk policy that is going to meet the implied criticism which the pamphlet will contain.[18]

A few days later a letter from Orr showed he had got the message. He told Brooke: 'We wish to avoid doing any damage to the party, and will probably hold back until after the Election'. Orr, however, clearly hoped that by being accommodating, some concessions might be forthcoming:

It would . . . be far better if the Party could make some general statement that so soon as they got back to power, the Government would immediately set up a commission to consider a National food policy which would take account of public health as well as agriculture. The setting up of such a commission before the Election would, to my mind, be an astute political move. You would have spiked the guns attacking the present Government on what is probably its only weak point. [19]

Brooke reported that 'the Minister's warning' to Orr 'not to publish his pamphlet until after the Election has taken effect'.[20]

MILK POLITICS

Orr told Brooke that he thought milk policy should aim to bring an adequate supply within reach of working-class mothers and children. He referred to a study initiated under the publicity provisions of Elliot's Milk Act of 1934,[21] and claimed that the improved health of children getting extra milk was already apparent even without clinical examination. Meanwhile, many households could not afford sufficient milk, while under the marketing schemes it was sold at 4d a gallon to manufacture plastic buttons.[22] Orr supplied a memorandum that he had prepared for the Milk Reorganisation Commission, of which he was a member, which was currently considering further reforms of milk marketing. Orr's memo argued that instead of the current Marketing Boards, which represented producers, a new Board of independent men should be created, with powers to acquire or construct wholesale milk depots, including pasteurisation plants.[23] Brooke was unconvinced. He replied that the economic case for converting the wholesale milk trade into a public utility had yet to be made.[24]

The CRD and the Reorganisation Commission were not the only bodies considering milk policy. A group of officials at the Ministry of Health held a series of discussions about how to head off political attacks concerning nutrition from September to December 1935, and agreed that the most promising course of action was to focus upon milk.[25] They established an interdepartmental committee to 'consider whether the consumption of milk can be increased and to advise upon the financial and other implications'. This committee reported at the end of January 1936, and concluded that the under-consumption of milk was largely a problem of indifference rather than poverty. A general reduction in price, which would have an appreciable effect upon consumption, was thought to be beyond the limits of state subvention, and therefore the committee concentrated upon mothers and children, costing possible schemes at between £1,530,000 and £12,000,000 per year.[26]

Earl de la Warr, parliamentary secretary to the Board of Education, prepared another document arguing for targeted milk schemes. He declared:

It is . . . becoming clear that we are in danger of public opinion getting ahead of us; indeed, had it not been for Abysinnia, the King's death, and armaments,

it might well have done so already. There is the further danger of the Labour
Party making it their platform and thereby gaining the credit for whatever is
ultimately done.[27]

De la Warr warned that nutrition was 'as explosive as housing' and could
not be 'damped down'. He argued that it was essential that the government
showed that it was prepared to make a 'serious start' by an extension of free
and cheap milk to mothers, infants and school children.

Meanwhile, the Ministry of Health drafted a bill to extend existing milk
schemes. This involved the removal of the need for malnutrition to be medically diagnosed in order for school children to receive free milk. For mothers and infants a scheme providing one pint per day was proposed with
the costs apportioned between local authorities and the Exchequer.[28] The
Minister, Kingsley Wood, asked for the opinion of the Chancellor, Neville
Chamberlain.[29] Chamberlain's advisers were not impressed. Their advice
was conflated with their concerns about the impending publication of *Food,
Health and Income*. One intimated:

> . . . Sir John Orr is publishing this week an alarmist book on nutrition. The
> Minister wishes to announce his scheme in advance of the book's publication.
> The scheme is half-baked, and only the vaguest guesses are possible of its prob-
> able effect.[30]

Another remarked:

> In general what I am afraid of is large and resounding generalisations over mal-
> nutrition and the production of ill-considered statistical material ... providing
> admirable material for opportunist propaganda and electioneering purposes;
> but this is the domain of Sir John Orr and his associates.[31]

Chamberlain told Wood that he felt that Ministry of Health's proposals
could not be adopted

> . . . even in principle without the closest examination . . . There are ideas about
> now on the subject of nutrition which give rise to serious misgivings in my mind
> and unless we are careful the development of these ideas may involve serious
> political risks and possibly unlimited expenditure. The ideas and their expo-
> nents are such, moreover, as to make me apprehensive lest a moderate govern-
> ment scheme should rather whet their appetite for more rather than satisfy their
> present demands.[32]

Elliot's suggestion was that when renewing his Milk Act, which was
to expire shortly, the limit on expenditure permissible under the publicity
clause (that paid for the Milk-in-Schools scheme) might be removed. Chamberlain objected to this. He argued that it would be inappropriate to take
any further action until the Milk Reorganisation Commission had reported,
and proposed extending the Act for a further period on more or less the
same basis as before.[33] This course of action was followed.[34]

FINAL PREPARATION OF *FOOD, HEALTH AND INCOME*

The CRD appears to have successfully delayed publication of *Food, Health and Income*, but by February 1936 Treasury officials thought that Ministers were again becoming anxious about the book.[35] The Chancellor wanted to avoid any large uncontrollable expenditure, but other Ministers wanted to be seen to be doing something about nutrition. Elliot even proposed to provide a foreword, and in early February 1935 sent a proof of the book to Chamberlain for his view of the matter. Elliot told Chamberlain that both he and Wood were both impressed by the desirability of keeping nutrition out of politics, and that Orr was also of this opinion. He had even offered to leave out 'anything which might be injudicious'.[36]

Sir Frederick Phillips, Under Secretary at the Treasury, remarked: 'This is an extraordinary case of the tail wagging the dog'. The Market Supply Committee had been set up to consider what to do with surplus food but had joined forces with Orr and busied itself in producing a new policy for the government. First a memorandum was prepared for the League of Nations Committee. Then Lloyd gave a paper to the Agricultural Economic Society, and now Orr had produced a book.[37] Phillips pointed out that economist Colin Clark, who had stood as Labour candidate in the 1935 election, was among those who had assisted Orr, and stated: 'There seems no reason why enthusiasts and people with axes to grind should be able to use Government machinery for advocating a policy in advance of Government approval'.[38] Chamberlain noted 'This is eminently an occasion to apply the brakes to our volatile Minister of Agriculture'.[39] He advised Elliot against writing the foreword and commented:

> It is unfortunate that a Government organisation, the Market Supply Committee, is already so closely connected with Sir John Orr's work. Unless we are careful the development of these ideas may involve serious political risks and there are almost unlimited possibilities of expenditure.[40]

Elliot took Chamberlain's advice. Orr signed the foreword.

PUBLICATION AND REFERRAL TO THE ADVISORY COMMITTEE ON NUTRITION

The publicity for *Food, Health and Income* was carefully managed. A talk by Orr on the wireless entitled 'Our Children's Scotland' at the end of February led to an article in the *Daily Herald* with the headline 'Third of the Population Half-Starved'. This referred to revelations that would appear in a report 'held up by anxious consultations in Government circles'.[41] On the date of publication detailed summaries appeared in the press under such headlines as 'Challenge to the Nation', 'Half of us Hungry' and 'Our Tallest Boys They come from Public Schools'.[42] *Food, Health and Income* compared estimates of the food consumed by six income groups with estimates of optimum food requirements and concluded:

The average diet of the poorest group, comprising 4½ million people, is . . . deficient in every constituent examined. The second group, comprising 9 million people is . . . deficient in all the vitamins and minerals considered. The third group, comprising another 9 million is deficient in several of the important vitamins and minerals.[43]

Orr's book immediately became the subject of questions in parliament, where it was announced that it would be referred to the Advisory Committee on Nutrition.[44] Orr explained to the Committee, which met at the end of March, his reasons for producing the publication:

For the last year or two . . . it was necessary to adopt drastic measures with regard to the food supply . . . Measures for limiting imports and raising prices and so on . . . but these measures had to be taken without considering . . . how it would affect the health of the poorer classes . . . there was no picture of any kind against which these very important measures could be considered.[45]

A long discussion followed and it was decided to refer those sections of the book dealing with 'medical aspects' to the Advisory Committee's Physiological Sub-Committee. The Statistical Sub-Committee, which had already considered the earlier Market Supply Committee documents, would also consider whether it had anything to add.

A month later a Physiological Sub-Committee meeting discussed Orr's book. The *verbatim* minutes indicate a remarkable contrast between the clear picture in *Food, Health and Income*, and the lack of agreement among Orr's colleagues. The following extract is taken from part of the meeting during which stature was under discussion:

Dr Buchan:[46]	Is there any greater value in height or weight? I cannot see any great advantage in it.
Professor Cathcart:[47]	Industrially, height is a drawback.
Dr Magee:[48]	Would you suggest that, as you know that food has to do with physique of the individual, we should feed people in accordance with the employment you think they ought to take part in?
Dr Buchan:	That was not my suggestion. My suggestion was that health was apart altogether from the question of height or weight. That was really my suggestion: if we want to feed people for good health or perfect health, the question of making them two or three inches taller does not to my mind necessarily arise.
Dr Magee:	You cannot make them two or three inches taller, you can satisfy, or you cannot satisfy, a growth impulse. That is what it amounts to.
Dr Mellanby:[49]	You can on average. It is a good thing to be taller and stronger.

Professor Cathcart: Industrially it is not.

Professor Mellanby: Quite apart from that, I would much rather see a fine Colonial people walking along the streets than the average person walking along our streets.

Professor Cathcart: Industrially, it is not an advantage. I see recruiting people, and they have a height of 5ft 8ins and that is all they want. They are more comfortable amongst machines.[50]

There was not a great deal that the Committee could agree on, but it was at least agreed that the average health of the community could be improved by means of preventative measures, and that it was desirable to increase milk consumption.[51]

When the Statistical Sub-Committee considered the Market Supply Committee's original analysis in October 1935, they had framed conclusions regarding the adequacy of the data. They also made recommendations about the new data collection exercises that were needed if a more accurate picture was to be obtained. It was agreed, however, that the variation in food consumption and expenditure was 'the best that can be made from the data at present available', and that the shapes of the curves showing food consumption by income group were broadly correct.[52] The Sub-Committee's verdict on *Food, Health and Income* was little different from their earlier conclusions.[53]

NUTRITION RESEARCH AND NUTRITION ACTION

Ministers were slow to grant authority for the investigations recommended by the Statistical Sub-Committee, and they were still largely at the planning stage when W. J. Peete, secretary to the Advisory Committee, sent out a draft interim report in September 1936. In response, Lloyd complained that Peete had over-emphasised the weaknesses of existing data, and ignored the Statistical Sub-Committee's conclusion about the shape of the curves showing consumption by income group.[54] Orr was also unimpressed. He told the Chair of the Advisory Committee that:

In my opinion, while there is need for further study of the position, there is abundant evidence to show that the health and physique of the people of this country could be greatly improved by improving the national dietary.[55]

Orr expressed this view to Edward Mellanby, Secretary of the Medical Research Council, and urged Mellanby to intervene at a meeting at which the draft was to be discussed.[56] As a result it was agreed to include the statement that health and physique could be improved by better food, and to emphasise the importance of milk.[57] Orr was pleased. He told Mellanby:

The publication of the Report as it stood would have been disastrous. I believe that the Government are now getting into the mood when they are really willing to do something big for nutrition, provided they got the necessary support and backing, and a luke-warm report . . . would have given the impression that all this talk about improving physique by better feeding is merely the exuberance of one or two fanatics . . .[58]

Subsequent events, however, showed that Orr's optimism, which was conditioned partly by his expectations of the report of the Milk Reorganisation Commission, was misplaced. The Interim Report of the Advisory Committee, as published, like the draft, placed most emphasis upon the need for new data.[59] The Reorganisation Commission did make some radical recommendations, but attempts to reform milk marketing were frustrated by the powerful Marketing Boards created under the earlier legislation.[60]

Meanwhile, by the end of 1936, the part of the Advisory Committee's investigations in which Orr was to be directly involved was finally about to get underway. It had been agreed that new dietary studies should be carried out, but the small sums allowed for the study covered only 300 families in England and 200 in Scotland. Of the latter Orr was allocated a study of 80 families in the Northeast.[61] At this time, however, Orr was also considering a possible career move. After the death of the Secretary of State for Scotland in October 1936, Chamberlain persuaded the Prime Minister to shift Elliot from the Ministry of Agriculture to the Scottish Office.[62] Elliot now offered Orr the post of Chief Medical Officer at the Department of Health for Scotland. Orr wanted to take the post for one year only, which he thought sufficient time to introduce the reforms he had in mind. He also wanted to remain director of the Institute, but Elliot rejected these conditions.[63] Having failed to seize this opportunity of working from within the civil service, Orr now sought to expand the modest survey that he had agreed to undertake for the Advisory Committee. He planned a much larger project, which, he hoped, would finally silence his critics and oblige serious government action. The larger project became possible with the help of funds from the Carnegie UK Trust.

ORIGINS OF THE CARNEGIE SURVEY

After Orr entered into discussions about the Advisory Committee's survey, it soon became clear that he was intent upon working according to his own agenda. In February 1936, he explained to the Department of Health for Scotland that he was linking the dietary study with an investigation into the clinical condition of families, with the assistance of members of the medical faculty of Aberdeen University.[64] However, at a meeting at the Department in early March, reservations were expressed about Orr's proposals. It was resolved that he should not combine dietary and clinical surveys because 'this might intensify the selection of the families in the northern area'.[65] By this time Orr was about to achieve a greater degree of independence, in view of the funding he was soon to receive from the Carnegie UK Trust.

The Trust's interest in supporting work supervised by Orr was stimulated by the publicity surrounding *Food, Health and Income*. At a meeting of the Trust in early March 1936, Lord Elgin, the Chairman, referred to Orr's recent wireless broadcast. Elgin, like Linlithgow, had worked with Orr on the Scottish National Development Council's Agricultural Committee. In connection with Orr's remarks about the co-existence of food surpluses and hungry people, Elgin asked 'Is it not possible that the impulse of an allocation from our resources might provide the spearhead of an attack to break through the vicious circle . . .?'[66] Elgin arranged for Orr's book to be sent to Trustees' Executive Committee members in preparation for their next meeting.[67] He asked them to consider what action they might take and the general consensus proved to be that

> . . . there had probably been sufficient investigation, and that what was now required was some practical step which might serve to confirm or correct the conclusions reached by the investigators.[68]

Orr subsequently met the Trustees' Policy Committee for a discussion at Elgin's home in London. He did not have a concrete proposal, but taking the Trust's previous work on land settlement as the starting point, suggested one important aspect that had been neglected was the need for a reorganisation of agriculture in order to increase the consumption of the more expensive foodstuffs.[69]

Orr was in no hurry to take advantage of the Trust's offer. It took additional prompting before he produced firmer proposals.[70] He suggested an experiment which aimed to create a 'new social grouping of unemployed under conditions which would keep them physically fit, give them a chance of part-time profitable employment on the land, and form a reservoir of reserve labour for urban industries'.[71] He suggested the establishment of an experimental fully mechanised farm close to an industrial centre, with nearby smallholdings, where unemployed workers could be settled. The smallholders would produce the foods they required for an improved diet, and would also provide seasonal labour for the large farm, and the nearby factories. A second proposal was for an 'investigation on the connection between economic and social factors and physical welfare' which would encourage co-ordinated government action for improving the condition of people.[72]

Orr was asked to elaborate his proposals but did not send another memorandum until mid-February 1937. He had dropped the land settlement experiment, but developed his other scheme, now entitled 'Suggested Inquiry on the connexion between economic factors and physical welfare'.[73] Orr noted that there was still much difference of opinion as to whether dietary deficiencies were due to poverty, ignorance or other causes. Furthermore, efforts to promote public health by improving nutrition were being frustrated by the attempts to re-organise agriculture by means of 'marketing schemes, subsidies, quotas, and tariffs'.[74] The enquiry described was similar to that eventually undertaken. It consisted of an economic, dietary, and clinical survey of 1,000 working class families and a demonstration of the effect on health and physique of bringing the diet of 200 families up to a 'Health Standard'. He explained:

> After spending the last three or four years on Government Committees and Commissions ... I have come to the conclusion that the kind of information which this investigation would give us is urgently needed ... getting out a report as early as possible would be more useful than sitting on rather futile committees which are working in the dark because they have not got the background of information against which the problems can be discussed.[75]

Orr proposed that Lubbock would be responsible for the supervision of the project, and suggested that two reports might be produced – one fully documented with scientific and statistical conclusions – the other shorter for the information of the public, MPs and others. The Policy Committee recommended that £10,000 should be granted for the investigation.[76] This would not be ratified until June, but Orr was told that there would be no risk in incurring expenditure meanwhile.[77]

Work on the project officially started in May 1937. Orr visited Edinburgh and London and explained the aims to the officials of the Department of Health for Scotland, and the Ministry of Health.[78] In July 1937 he spoke about the survey at a meeting of the Physiological Sub-Committee of the Advisory Committee on Nutrition. If there was 'anything in nutrition', he said, they should be able to show a

> . . . correlation between the diets and physical condition of the children, and if bringing up the diet to a higher standard will improve health, then it should show some difference within twelve months. If it shows that diet has such an effect on health, and health can be improved, then the whole agricultural policy, the policy of the Milk Board, and so on, will have to be reconsidered not only in the light of agricultural interests but in the light of the objectives of the Ministry of Health.[79]

Because the Carnegie investigation was much larger and more comprehensive than that being carried out under the Advisory Committee on Nutrition, it could not easily be ignored by the Ministry of Health and the Department of Health for Scotland. Furthermore, Orr was now able to effectively set the agenda. In September 1938 he reported to the Trustees, that the co-operation between the 'Government inquiry and the more extensive Carnegie inquiry has now become so close that the two inquiries have practically coalesced into one investigation'.[80]

CONCLUSION

Orr's hope that the results of the Carnegie Survey would settle many of the controversies of the 1930s and oblige the government to at last take nutrition seriously were frustrated by the outbreak of the World War II. The government was finally persuaded of the necessity for comprehensive intervention in managing the nation's food system, not because of the force of scientific results, but by the exigencies of war. After the war, dismantling of the wartime measures began within a few years, but some of the war-time machinery for the surveillance of British diet survived. The origins of the Committee on Medical Aspects of Food Policy and the National Food Survey, for example, may be traced to the war years. But since the war dis-cussion about Government responsibility for the application of nutritional knowledge has been more-or-less continuous, and, during the 1980s and early 1990s the relative importance of ignorance and poverty was debated in terms very similar to those used by Orr and others during the 1930s.[81]

There have been new areas for nutritional controversy, however, the most striking example being the question of the nutritional origins of heart dis-ease and other degenerative 'diseases of civilisation', which has been hotly debated since the 1950s. Ironically, it is in this new area that the Carnegie data may yet play a decisive role, in view of the new work under way at Bristol University, described by David Gunnell in Chapter 3.

ACKNOWLEDGEMENTS

Thanks are due to: the Wellcome Trust for financial support for the research upon which this chapter is based; Susan Williams for drawing the author's attention to the material in the archive of the Conservative Research Depart-ment; participants at the 5th ICREFH Symposium for their comments upon the spoken version of the Chapter; Walter Duncan, Honorary Archivist of the Rowett Research Institute for advice and support.

BIBLIOGRAPHY

Hammond, R J. *Food Vol. II Studies in Administration and Control*, London, 1956.

Lloyd, E M H. Food supplies at different income levels, *Journal of the Proceedings of the Agricultural Economics Society*, 4 (1936), 89–110.

Ministry of Agriculture and Fisheries, *Milk Report of Reorganisation Commission for Great Britain*, London, 1936.

Ministry of Health, *First Report of the Advisory Committee on Nutrition*, London, 1937.

Orr, J B. *Food, Health and Income*, London, 1936.

Orr, J B. *As I Recall*, London, 1966.

Rowett Research Institute, *Family Diet and Health in Pre-War Britain*, Dunferm-line, 1955.

Scottish National Development Council, *Report of the Committee on Agriculture*, Glasgow, 1934.

Smith, D F. The Rise and Fall of the Scientific Food Committee during the Second World War. In Smith, D F, and Philips, J, eds, *Food, Science Policy and Regula-tion in the Twentieth Century*, London, 2000.

Smith, D F. The early institutional and scientific development of the Rowett Research Institute. In Adam, A, Smith, D F and Watson, F, eds, *To the Greit Support and Advancement of Helth*, Aberdeen, 1996, 45–53.

Smith D F and Nicolson, M. Health and ignorance: past and present. In Platt, S, Thomas, H, Scott, S, and Williams, G, eds, *Locating Health Sociological and Historical Explanations*, Aldershot, 1993.
Taylor, E M M. 'The Politics of Walter Elliot', Ph D, Edinburgh University, 1979.

NOTES

1 Rowett Research Institute, 1955.
2 First Interim Report on Carnegie Dietary and Clinical Survey and Feeding Test, Rowett Research Institute Archive (hereafter RRI), DSC 14/13 pt 1/2.
3 J B Orr to Secretary, 20 November 1939, Scottish Records Office (hereafter SRO), GD 281/82/127.
4 D P Cuthbertson to J Wilkie, 20 February 1950, SRO GD 281/82/127.
5 For discussion of the roles of Orr and the Carnegie data in wartime food policy making see Smith 2000.
6 Smith, 1996.
7 For example, Scottish National Development Council, 1934.
8 Ministry of Health, 1937.
9 Orr, 1966, 90, 109–111.
10 Orr, J B. *Food, Health and Income*, London, 1936.
11 Special Meeting of the Finance Sub-Committee, 29 January 1935, Joint Committee Minute Books, RRI.
12 Lloyd, E M H. Secretary's Progress Report, 12 May 1935, PRO MAF 53/127; Note of meeting with contributing bodies, 29 July 1935, PRO MAF 38/23, PRO MAF 53/127.
13 Scottish National Development Council, 1934.
14 D Lubbock, interview with David Smith and George Davey Smith, 31 August 1992; Meeting of the Joint Committee, 8 October 1934, Joint Committee Minute Books, RRI.
15 Lloyd, E M H. Report of investigation into food consumption at different income levels, 4 July 1935, PRO MAF 53/127.
16 Lloyd, 1936.
17 Referred to in F Phillips, Memorandum, 7 February 1936, PRO T161/714/539490/01/1.
18 Mr Brooke to Director, 11 October 1935, Department of Western Manuscripts, Bodleian Library, Cambridge, Conservative Research Department Archive (hereafter CRD) 1/60/1.
19 J B Orr to H Brooke, 17 October 1935, CRD 1/60/1.
20 Mr Brooke to Director, 18 October 1935, CRD 1/60/1.
21 Ministry of Agriculture and Fisheries, 1936, 296.
22 J B Orr to H Brooke, 17 October 1935, CRD 1/60/1.
23 Memorandum by Sir John Orr on the Objectives of a Milk Marketing Scheme, CRD 1/33/8.
24 H Brooke to J B Orr, 25 October 1935, CRD 1/33/8.
25 Office Nutrition Conference Minutes, 25 November 1935, PRO MH 79/346.
26 Report of Inter-departmental committee on milk consumption, 30 January 1936, PRO T161/714/539490/01/1.

27 Earl de la Warr, Proposals for Nutrition Policy, paper sent with de la Warr to J Ball, 2 March 1936, CRD 1/33/7.
28 Outline of a Proposals for a Bill to Increase Consumption of Milk by Mothers and Infants and School Children, PRO T161/714/539490/01/1.
29 K Wood to N Chamberlain, 25 February 1936, PRO T161/714/539490/01/1.
30 Memorandum to F Phillips and R Hopkins, 9 March 1936, PRO T161/714/539490/01/1.
31 Memorandum to W Fisher and Mr Ferguson, 9 March 1936, PRO T/161/714/539490/01/1.
32 N Chamberlain to K Wood, 12 March 1936, PRO MH 79/347.
33 N Chamberlain to W Elliot, 11 February 1936, PRO T161/714/539490/01/1.
34 Ministry of Agriculture and Fisheries, 1936, 295.
35 Memorandum to Mr Barlow and F Phillips, 1 February 1936, PRO T161/714/539490/01/1.
36 W Elliot to N Chamberlain, 6 February 1936, PRO T/161/714/539490/01/1.
37 F Phillips, Memorandum, 7 February 1936, PRO T161/714/539490/01/1.
38 F Phillips, Memorandum, 7 February 1936, PRO T161/714/539490/01/1.
39 N Chamberlain, Annotation to Sir Warren Fisher or Mr Ferguson, 8 February 1936, PRO T161/714/539490/01/1.
40 N Chamberlain to W Elliot, 11 February 1936, PRO T161/714/539490/01/1.
41 Third of the Population Half-Starved, *Daily Herald*, 27 February 1936.
42 R Calder, Challenge to the Nation, *Daily Herald*, 12 March 1936; V. H. Mottram, Half of us Hungry, *The Star*, 12 March 1936; Special Correspondent, Our Tallest Boys They come from Public Schools, *Daily Mirror*, 12 March 1936, Press Cuttings Album, RRI.
43 Orr, 1936, 49.
44 *Parliamentary Debates (Commons)*, 1935–36, vol 310, 16 March 1936, col 23.
45 Minutes of Sixth Meeting of the Advisory Committee on Nutrition, 30 March 1936, PRO MH 56/49.
46 G F Buchan was medical officer of health for Willesden.
47 E P Cathcart was regius professor of physiology at Glasgow.
48 H E Magee was senior medical officer at the Ministry of Health, with responsibility for nutrition.
49 E Mellanby was secretary of the Medical Research Council
50 *Verbatim* minute of Physiological Sub-Committee Meeting, 28 April 1936, PRO MH 56/254.
51 Minutes of seventh meeting of the Advisory Committee on Nutrition, 28 April 1936, PRO MH 56/49.
52 Lloyd, E M H. Advisory Committee on Nutrition Food Consumption Statistics Sub-Committee Interim Report, 18 October 1935, PRO MH 56/50.
53 Minutes of Meeting of the Statistical Sub-Committee, 28 April 1936, PRO MH 56/50.
54 W J Peete to E M H Lloyd, 26 September 1936; Lloyd to Peete, 30 September 1936, PRO MH 56/258.
55 J B Orr to Lord Luke, 17 October 1936, PRO FD1/4429.
56 J B Orr to E Mellanby, 17 October 1936, PRO FD1/4429.

57 Minutes of Physiological Sub-Committee Meeting, 19 October 1936, PRO MH 56/254; E Mellanby to J B Orr, 27 October 1936, PRO FD1/4429.

58 J B Orr to E Mellanby, 29 October 1936, Contemporary Medical Archives Centre, Wellcome Institute, London (hereafter CMAC) B13/20.

59 Ministry of Health, 1937.

60 Hammond, 1956, 182–3.

61 Ministry of Health to Treasury, 16 September 1936, Department of Health for Scotland to Treasury, 5 September 1936, SRO HH 64/152/1.

62 Taylor, 1979, 190–1.

63 Minutes of Special Meetings of the Joint Committee, 11 December, 16 December 1936, Joint Committee Minutes Book, RRI.

64 J M Vallance, Minute on a meeting on 17 February 1937, 22 February 1937, SRO HH 64/152/1.

65 Note of meeting at Department of Health for Scotland, 1 March 1937, SRO HH 64/152/1.

66 Carnegie Trust Policy, *The Times*, 7 March 1936, 9 col a.

67 A T Heggie to Mitchell, 2 May 1936, Mitchell to Heggie, 4 May 1936; Annotation by Lord Elgin, 12 May 1936, added to J M Mitchell to Lord Elgin, 11 May 1936, SRO GD/281/82/126.

68 Extract of Minutes of Meeting, 5 June 1936, SRO GD/281/82/126.

69 Minute of Meeting of Policy Committee, 18 June 1936, SRO GD/281/82/126.

70 J M Mitchell to J B Orr, 23 November 1936, J B Orr to J M Mitchell, 30 November 1936, SRO GD/281/82/126.

71 Note on suggested experiment to create a new social grouping . . ., SRO GD/281/82/126.

72 Suggested investigation of the connection between economic and social factors and physical welfare, SRO GD/281/82/126.

73 J B Orr to J M Mitchell, 12 February 1936, SRO GD/281/82/126.

74 Memorandum by Sir John Orr, Appendix to Minutes of Special Meeting of the Policy Sub-Committee, 9 April 1937, SRO GD/281/82/126.

75 J B Orr to Lord Elgin, 24 February 1937, SRO GD/281/82/126.

76 Minutes of Special Meeting of the Policy Sub-Committee, 9 April 1937, SRO GD/281/82/126.

77 J M Mitchell to J B Orr, 24 April 1937, SRO GD/281/82/126.

78 Minute Sheet 93414/1/30, 2 June 1937; Meeting of representatives of the Departments of Health, Agriculture and Education with Sir John B Orr held at the Department of Health on 7 June 1937, PRO MH 56/220.

79 *Verbatim* Minutes of Physiological Sub-Committee meeting, 30 July 1936, PRO MH 57/254.

80 J B Orr, The Carnegie Trust Dietary Survey. Progress Report up to 31st August 1938, 1 September 1938, SRO GD281/82/127.

81 Smith and Nicolson, 1993.

Part 2
Food consumption and health

6 Milk Consumption and Tuberculosis in Britain, 1850-1950

PJ Atkins

INTRODUCTION

The 'cultural turn' which has swept through the Anglo-American social sciences in the 1990s has as one of its major themes the consumption of food and the various discourses which are deployed to understand it. This theme of consumption is particularly apposite because in recent times we have also seen a surge in consumer concern about the ethics of food production and the quality of foodstuffs at various stages in the food system. The sight of middle class English protesters blocking the export of live calves to the Continent in 1995 was symbolic of a growing resistance throughout society to intensive farming, and the declaration on 20 March 1996 that Mad Cow Disease (BSE) can be transferred from cattle to humans has confirmed our worst fears about consequences for health. The green and consumer lobbies are keen to present these issues as new but I wish to argue that the concern, in a fully mature form, about food quality is at least one hundred years old. In this chapter I will outline the history of bovine tuberculosis in Britain and argue that its study presents us with one possible way that food historians might approach the links between consumption and health.

THE DEBATE ABOUT BOVINE TUBERCULOSIS

Tuberculosis was the single greatest cause of death and disability in nineteenth century Britain. People in their 30s and 40s had a depressingly high chance of dying from it. It was a plague to match cancer or AIDS in our own time. Unfortunately, the World Health Organisation has just warned that respiratory tuberculosis is returning at present in a new form that is resistant to drug therapy and that deaths will exceed one hundred million world-wide in the next fifty years.[1]

The German microbiologist Robert Koch discovered the tubercle bacillus in 1882 and almost immediately it was realised that milk might be a powerful agent of its spread. Only four years later a survey by the Association of Municipal Corporations found that 85 per cent of English Medical Officers of Health believed that tuberculosis was communicable via raw milk and undercooked meat, a view endorsed subsequently by various parliamentary enquiries.[2] This was a remarkable sea-change in opinion, the medical and public health professions having previously been convinced that heredity and environment were the major factors. Scientific belief and public action are often lagged, however, and indeed very little was done to put into practical effect the new rhetoric that dominated the public health journals and local Medical Officer of Health Reports in the 1890s and 1900s.

There were two reasons for this. First, neither was there an administrative structure for inspecting cattle or collecting samples of milk, nor had technology for mass screening yet become readily available. These features appeared first in large cities such as Manchester at the turn of the century and gradually filtered down to smaller centres. Second, the belief in the transmissibility of the bovine strain of tuberculosis, *Mycobacterium bovis*, to humans was fiercely contested. Ironically it was Koch himself, at the International Congress on Tuberculosis held in London in 1901, who declared that he had found experimentally that the human version of the mycobacterium did not produce tuberculosis in cattle, the implication being that there was no danger of an infection in the other direction either. It is difficult to exaggerate the consternation this caused in the medical community but it did at least stimulate debate and there was a surge in tuberculosis-related laboratory research in Britain, Germany, France and the United States.[3]

In this country a Royal Commission was appointed with a brief to take evidence and conduct experiments. Several strains of bacilli were identified, with different pathogenicities.[4] Under laboratory conditions the most virulent was the *M bovis*, which in humans was shown conclusively to be principally responsible for non-pulmonary forms of tuberculosis.

TUBERCULOSIS IN THE CATTLE HERD AND LIVESTOCK PRODUCTS

A major reason for the prevalence of bovine tuberculosis in humans was the endemicity of the disease among the cattle herds that supplied Britain's liquid milk and much of its beef, especially those cows confined to cramped urban sheds where the probability of infection by airborne droplets was maximized.[5] From Table 1 it is clear that the cattle population in general, kept on the whole on open pastures, was infected to a far lesser extent.

The problem for farmers was that the early stages of tuberculosis in cattle are invisible. By the time there are symptoms, such as emaciation, a chronic cough or a diseased udder, both the carcase and milk are potentially dangerous for human consumption.[6] In the decade or so before World War I it was generally realised that tests were required to ensure detection at the earliest possible moment. There were several possibilities.

First, the veterinary inspection of cows was attempted. This was easiest among beasts tethered in urban settings but some local authorities also employed inspectors to tour the country areas supplying milk. The results

Table 1. *Tuberculosis discovered at slaughter*

	Cattle slaughtered	% TB
Belfast 1909–13, 1917, 1919, 1922–4	161,306*	15.00
Birkenhead 1892–8, 1915, 1920	225,228	0.53
Blackburn, 1920	*	9.69
Bradford 1918-21	56,659	2.74
Bury 1911–25	52,292*	1.33
Croydon 1920	757	1.72
Derby 1937	*	53.00
Edinburgh 1919–21, 1924–25	4,932*	42.19
Halifax 1915	9,185	0.05
Liverpool 1913–16, 1918, 1920	95,950	1.02
Liverpool 1921, 1925	4,674*	11.90
London (Metropolitan Cattle Market) 1881	*	90.00
London (Metropolitan Cattle Market) 1929	*	51.00
City of London abattoirs 1918–27	*	33.33
Newcastle 1917, 1919–25	158,700	0.68
Newcastle 1943	*	47.5
Salford 1920	1,365	2.05

Note: * cows only
Sources: Medical Officer of Health Annual Reports; Creighton (1881); Savage (1929), 41–2; Francis (1947), 22–24.

Table 2. *Evidence of udder tuberculosis in the early twentieth century*

	Cows inspected	% TB udder
Birmingham: 1900–5, 1917-19, 1923, 1925	14,445	0.14
Blackburn 1902–12, 1920	unknown	0.6-2.9
Bradford 1910–11, 1915, 1918–19	16,212	2.10
Cumberland 1927–30	39,641	0.10
Gloucestershire 1927–31	327,434	0.06
Lanarkshire 1926–9	141,285	0.12
Leeds 1914	2,000	0.85
Liverpool 1901–25	47,185 city cows	0.83
	29,325 country cows	0.79
Manchester 1900, 1903–11, 1921	92,073 city cows	0.02
	24,851 country cows	0.81
Newcastle 1908–25	9,223	0.54
Salford 1921	91	3.30
Sheffield 1901–14, 1921–29	unknown	country cows 0.59–4.84
		city cows 0.14–1.10
Yorkshire, West Riding 1928–30	256,988	0.13

Sources: Medical Officer of Health Annual Reports; Anon. (1932); Savage (1929).

were varied at first (Tables 2 and 3) but gradually farmers came to realise that diseased animals threatened their livelihoods and a 'slink' trade in 'wasters' developed as a hidden circuit in the livestock economy of some regions. In Cheshire, for instance, vets employed by the City of Manchester were well aware of the problem but were powerless to act:

Table 3. *Udder tuberculosis detected by Liverpool inspectors*

	City cowshed visits				Country cowshed visits			
	Cows examined	TB udders	%	Convictions	Cows examined	TB udders	%	Convictions
1901–5	1,156	184	15. 9	21	2,345	76	3. 2	12
1906–10	1,110	24	2. 2	0	3,445	29	0. 8	11
1911–15	12,526	73	0. 6	0	5,837	20	0. 3	4
1916–20	7,499	23	0. 3	0	4,278	29	0. 7	0
1921–25	24,894	89	0. 4	0	13,420	77	0. 6	0

Source: Medical Officer of Health Annual Reports

The number of cows suffering from tuberculosis of the udder found in this piece of inspection was comparatively small, but this is to a great extent accounted for by the fact that, as soon as it became known that the farms were being visited, large numbers of suspected animals were sent into the local auction market every week, and disposed of to individuals who evidently had no difficulty in disposing of this class of cattle.[7]

Second, the tuberculin test (TT) was available for detecting tuberculosis. A fold of the animal's skin was injected with dead mycobacteria and a reaction of swelling was taken as an indication that there was a problem of infection. This TT was adopted only slowly in Britain by comparison with countries such as Denmark, one possible reason being the alarming results. Cows supplying Birmingham's milk were the first to be tested on a large scale, and from 1907 to 1927 no fewer than 40.4 per cent were found to be reactors.[8]

Third, the microscopic detection of *M bovis* in milk allowed the sampling of a city's supply and the identification of infected herds. This was a cost-effective approach pioneered in the largest cities but it came to be used by many Medical Officers of Health around the country as a means of providing ammunition in their campaign about the dangers of the milk supply. Figure 1 is a compilation of data from Birmingham, Liverpool, London, Manchester, Newcastle, Salford and Sheffield. It shows that the proportion of samples found to be tuberculous was as high, if not higher, in 1930 as

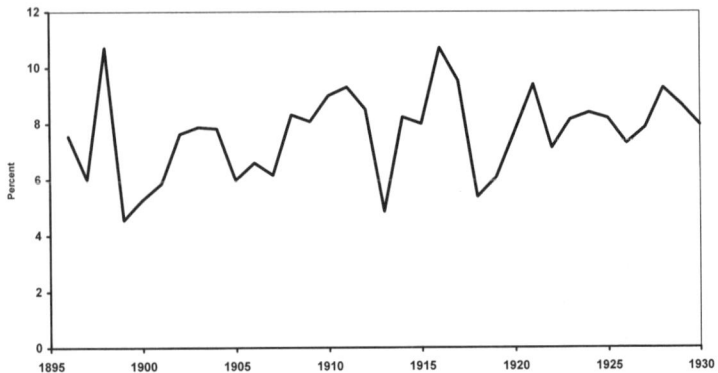

Fig. 1. *Tuberculous milk in selected cities, 1896–1930*

at the start of the series. This proved that government-sponsored remedial measures were necessary because the well-meaning efforts of local authorities had been ineffective.

This pooling of data from a number of cities hides the puzzling spatial variations of disease incidence shown in Table 4. Note the high figure for Manchester by comparison with other authorities. There are possible explanations in the differences in sampling methodology adopted and in the technicalities of testing, but these are insufficient reasons to account for the extremes of geographical variation.

THE IMPACT ON HUMANS

In some regions it seems likely that *all* of the milk drinking population would have been infected with bovine tuberculosis at one time or another. Thus 1,420 post mortems of children under 12 in the 1880s showed that 30 per cent had tuberculosis, no doubt mostly of bovine origin, and in 1930 58.3 per cent of a sample of London children reacted positively to the TT.[9] My estimates indicate that at least half a million (and possibly 800,000) human deaths in the period 1850–1950 are directly attributable to bovine TB, especially among young children who were the main milk drinkers.

One positive outcome of the Royal Commission on Tuberculosis was some detailed work on the typing of the mycobacteria found in human sputum, in surgical biopsies and in autopsy specimens. Stanley Griffith's work was the outstanding contribution, continuing through to the 1940s. As a result of his investigations we have a fair idea of the proportion of tuberculosis in each organ caused by bovine infection. From the data in Table 5 it seems that respiratory tuberculosis was rarely a consequence of milk consumption, but the non-pulmonary forms were.

Table 4. *Tuberculosis in milk samples*

	Dates	Samples	%		Dates	Samples	%
Aberdeen	1920–30	1,561	5.7	Leeds	1913, 20–30	1,080	4.4
Birmingham	1907–37	20,047	8.1	Liverpool	1896–1937	26,978	6.2
Blackburn	1915, 20–30	1,908	2.2	London	1908–37	53,195	8.1
Brighton	1915, 28–37	737	9.2	Manchester	1901–37	18,995	11.3
Bristol	1920–30	450	6.7	Monmouth	1927	213	1.4
Burton on Trent	1904–5	117	10.3	Newcastle	1913–37	6,819	4.4
Cambridgeshire	1927	46	0.0	Northumberland	1927	58	5.2
Cardiff	1920–30	682	4.6	Reading	1920–30	282	11.0
Coventry	1909–10	53	15.1	Salford	1904–6, 13–16, 20–30	4,401	8.0
Croydon	1900–21	547	8.0	Sheffield	1902–14, 20–37	20,580	8.0
Derby	1907, 09	94	8.5	Somerset	1926–8	683	2.2
Dorset	1926–7	243	4.9	Southport	1902–20	724	8.2
Edinburgh	1904, 6–7, 11–12, 26–37	3,541	8.5	East Suffolk	1927	33	6.1
Glasgow	1921–5, 28–37	4,647	6.7	Warwickshire	1927	85	3.5
Huddersfield	1926–30	237	6.3	Yorkshire, West Riding	1923–33	6,951	5.8
Hull	1925–30	449	6.7	Total	1896–1937	178,189	7.8
Lancashire	1924–7	1,753	10.2				

Sources: Medical Officer of Health Annual Reports; Anon. (1932); Savage (1929).

Table 5: *The estimated site-specific tuberculosis mortality of bovine origin*

Tuberculosis type	Savage (1929)		Griffith (1937, 1941) all ages	
	0–4 years (%)	>5 years (%)	England (%)	Scotland (%)
Respiratory	0	1	2	6
Abdominal	80	33	45	45
Nervous	20	20	25	30
Bones & joints	30	15	20	30
General	25	10	—	—
Other	20	5	34	36
Mean	29.5	3.2	27.8	34.2

Sources: Savage (1929), 27; Griffith (1937), 530–1; Griffith and Munro (1943).

The overall number of deaths from tuberculosis fell markedly between 1840 and 1920, but the proportion of this mortality attributable to non-pulmonary forms rose, peaking in the 1890s (Figure 2).[10] It seems likely that the respiratory disease was radically reduced in response to the environmental improvements of the late nineteenth century, especially in housing conditions, for the probability of catching 'phthisis' had been exacerbated by over-crowded and ill-ventilated accommodation. As the use of cows' milk increased in the second half of the century, *M bovis* infections became more common, especially amongst small children who had been taken from the breast. Unfortunately, the British taste for raw milk made this problem worse than it might have been had boiling been as common as on the continent.[11] Other dairy products were also sources of infection: *M bovis* can survive in butter for up to five months, and also for long periods in some types of cheese.[12]

In Scotland the non-respiratory tuberculosis death rate was consistently higher than in England, and there were also regional variations, the highest

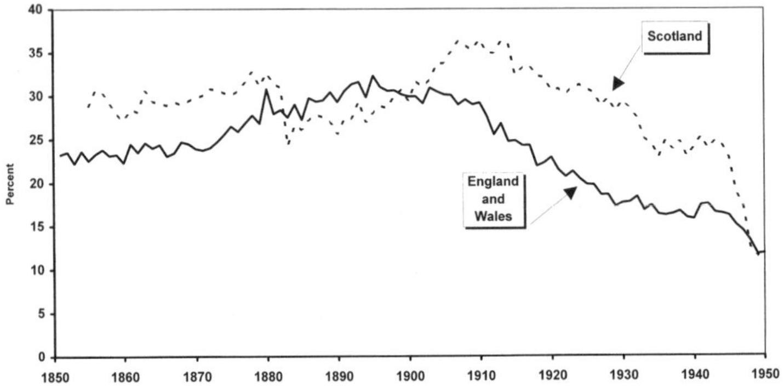

Fig. 2. *Non-respiratory tuberculosis as a percentage of all tuberculosis deaths, 1851–1950*

county figures lying in the northern half of the country. It seems likely that this distribution of human disease reflected that in cattle, but interestingly it was the inverse of the map of total tuberculosis mortality. It has been argued that this was due to an inoculation effect whereby regular low doses of *M bovis* induced a resistance to infection of the lungs by the respiratory route.[13]

THE LOCAL STATE AND THE REGULATION OF PRODUCTION AND DISTRIBUTION

It was generally recognised in the late nineteenth century that poor cattle housing was responsible for dirty and diseased milk.[14] The Dairies, Cowsheds and Milkshops Orders (1879, 1885) empowered local authorities to regulate the physical conditions in which animals were kept but improvements were gradual.[15] The crowding and lack of ventilation, which together created ideal circumstances for the spread of tuberculosis from animal to animal, remained common in rural areas into the 1920s and 1930s.[16]

Another hazard arose, ironically with technological progress in the 1920s. This was the mixing in 3,000 gallon tankers of the milk of 1,000 cows. If only one cow was diseased and excreting mycobacteria then the whole batch was contaminated because tuberculous milk can be diluted 10,000–1,000,000 times and still be infective.[17] Some forms of tuberculosis, such as that of the bones and joints, can be initiated by even small invasions of mycobacteria.

The dangers of tuberculous milk infected with tubercle bacilli may have been scientifically known from the 1880s, but policy reaction at the local level was slow. In 1885 the town council of Hull did enquire of the Privy Council about the possibility of using the Contagious Diseases (Animals) Acts to deal with the source of the disease, but nothing seems to have come of their initiative. Three years later a Departmental Committee even recommended compulsory slaughter of animals with tuberculosis, but this aspect of their report was ignored.[18]

Glasgow was the first city, under its Police (Amendment) Act of 1890, to take powers for its medical and sanitary officers to inspect any cowshed supplying the city and to prohibit the sale of any milk 'dangerous or injurious to health'.[19] Weak and permissive English law, however, was an obstacle to progress south of the border. Promisingly, Article 15 of the Dairies, Cowsheds and Milkshops Order of 1885 stated that 'If at any time disease exists among the cattle in a dairy or cowshed, the milk of a diseased cow therein shall not be mixed with other milk; and shall not be sold or used for human food', but the definition of 'disease' used was that of the 1878 Contagious Diseases (Animals) Act, which did not include tuberculosis.

Under the Infectious Diseases Prevention Act (1890) and The Public Health (London) Act (1891), sanitary authorities were given relevant powers.[20] A local authority's Medical Officer of Health had to obtain a magistrate's order to inspect a dairy and/or cows. Another order could then be made against the dairyman, forbidding the local sale of his milk. The procedure was cumbersome and there was nothing to prevent the dairy farmer or dairyman from switching milk to an area other than the one mentioned in the prohibition order. As a result few prosecutions were ever obtained.

In the absence of any real central government intervention it was left to a few pioneering local authorities to initiate measures against bovine tuberculosis. The so-called 'milk clauses' of the private Manchester Corporation (General Powers) Act of 1899, as amended in 1904, became a bench mark.[21] Officials were enabled to:

- prosecute anyone who knowingly sold milk from cows with tuberculosis of the udder;[22]
- demand the isolation of infected beasts;
- demand the notification of any cow exhibiting signs of tuberculosis of the udder;
- inspect the cows in, and take samples from, herds which supplied milk to the city.

By 1910, 67 boroughs and 24 urban districts had similar powers. Section 27 of the London County Council (General Powers) Act of 1904 allowed the compulsory slaughter, with compensation, of diseased animals, and Section 24 of the 1907 version of the same Act empowered the LCC to take samples at railway stations and to prevent tuberculous milk being sent to London. It was not until 1925 that central government measures advanced beyond this stage.

THE CENTRAL STATE AND THE RIGHTS OF THE CONSUMER

Faced with a mounting public outcry and with an overwhelming body of evidence, successive administrations felt the need to demonstrate, at the very least, a momentum in the direction of change. Concerted action was very slow in coming but there were experimental forays into enabling legislation.[23]

In 1909, after many years of discussion, it seemed likely that a Milk and Dairies Bill would receive the royal assent. This comprehensive legislation was meant, inter alia, to prohibit the supply and sale of milk likely to cause disease, including tuberculosis (Clauses 2 and 3). The Bill was not passed, however, and the Local Government Board was forced to withdraw its parallel Tuberculosis Order which would have given all local authorities powers of inspection and slaughter. A similar Order, made in 1913, was replaced in June 1914 by another, which in turn was revoked on the outbreak of hostilities.[24] The war also delayed the implementation of the Milk and Dairies Act (1914) and its replacement, the Milk and Dairies (Consolidation) Act of 1915. The Milk and Dairies (Amendment) Act (1922) further postponed any action until 1925, when at last the Tuberculosis

Order (1925) and the Public Health (Prevention of Tuberculosis) Regulations (1925) were made.[25]

Such a messy legislative process significantly delayed progress. One problem was that, although the problem of cattle disease was relatively well understood in the farming community, milk producers were on the whole small farmers who did not have the resources to clear out their own herds and start again with tuberculosis-free stock. There needed to be a policy of carrot (compensation for slaughter) and stick (legally binding regulation) but the politics of pragmatism meant that successive governments were content with steady, incremental change. Thus, the Tuberculosis Order of 1925 did establish the principle of slaughter with compensation, but the scheme was low key and not uniformly applied, and in practice it proved difficult to prevent tuberculous animals being recycled in the slink trade.[26] All of this contrasted with the United States where a more forceful slaughter policy was adopted, and most continental countries which settled for versions of Professor Bang's method of separating healthy from infected animals.

It was clear, to the veterinary and medical professions at least, that little improvement had been achieved by the early 1930s. Some consumers in urban areas had access to pasteurised milk, but not all of the equipment used was effective in killing the mycobacteria, and anyway it was merely treating the problem at an unacceptably late stage in the food chain. The People's League of Health in 1932 and the Gowland Hopkins Committee in 1934 both reported a major problem with the milk supply as a result of a minimum of 40 per cent of the dairy herds being infected with tuberculosis. This was difficult to ignore and the Milk Act of 1934 set aside a sum for upgrading milk quality. The notion of an 'attested herd' was introduced where cattle had passed the TT successfully, and milk guaranteed as disease-free attracted a premium. In 1937 the Ministry of Agriculture began moving towards an area eradication policy, an important advance that was interrupted by World War II.[27]

It was not until 1950 that bovine tuberculosis again came to the top of the political agenda. After decades of half measures the government finally decided on a stringent policy of area eradication which involved much disruption to the farming industry, through restrictions on the movement of cattle, and a considerable expenditure in compensation. The whole country was declared attested in 1960, and 'TT milk' as a category was abolished in 1964.[28]

Table 6 displays the geographical distribution of cattle taken for slaughter 1926–40 under the Tuberculosis Orders (1925, 1938). An alternative index would have been the proportion of positive reactors to the tuberculin test, but by 1938 only a small and unrepresentative sample of herds had been tested.[29] The most heavily infected areas were in north west and south east England, and in central and south west Scotland. Many of the worst affected counties were also the chief milk producing areas. Cheshire, for instance, in the mid 1940s still had 60–80 per cent of its cows infected,

Table 6. *The proportion of off-farm liquid milk sales in each Milk Marketing Board region in England and Wales, 1924/5–1938/9, compared with the percentage of cattle slaughtered under the Tuberculosis Order 1926–40*

Region	Milk sales (%)	Cattle slaughtered (%)
North	6.63	6.60
North West	28.01	38.44
East	5.36	6.98
East Midlands	7.70	6.57
West Midlands	8.44	7.47
North Wales	2.49	4.59
South Wales	3.83	2.73
South	7.49	3.41
Mid West	15.23	7.98
Far West	4.18	2.68
South East	10.65	12.56
Total	100.01	100.01

Sources: Francis (1947), 28-31; Barnes (1958).

when the estimated average for Britain was 30–35 per cent.[30] Large herds and older cows were especially susceptible.[31] Table 6 hints that people drinking milk produced in north west England were most at risk.[32] Much of that milk entered into the long distance supply of cities such as Manchester and may help to explain the high incidence of bovine tuberculosis among their citizens.

CONCLUSION

Recent public concern about Mad Cow Disease is by no means the first time that there has been a furore about cattle disease infecting humans. There have been many scares over the last one hundred years, and the reaction of politicians has been consistently reluctant and inadequate. On each occasion there appears to be a pattern of behaviour in the Ministry of Agriculture which suggests that public health is not, and never has been, at the top of its agenda.

By way of an overall conclusion we may assert that historians have a very important role to play in the analysis of food systems and food consumption. Examination of the temporal dimension can assist with a fuller understanding of structural and policy problems, many of which are not new. The ultimate aim is a theory of governance and food quality regulation that would act as context for analysing issues of food consumption and health.

BIBLIOGRAPHY

Anon. *Report of a Special Committee appointed by the People's League of Health Inc. to Make a Survey of Tuberculosis of Bovine Origin in Great Britain*, London, 1932.

Ashby, H T. *Infant Mortality*, 2nd edn, London, 1922.

Atkins, P J. The intra-urban milk supply of London, circa 1790–1914, *Transactions of the Institute of British Geographers*, new series 2 (1977), 383–99

Atkins, P J. White poison: the health consequences of milk consumption, 1850–1930, *Social History of Medicine*, 5 (1992), 207-27.

Barnes, F A. The evolution of the salient patterns of milk production and distribution in England and Wales, *Transactions of the Institute of British Geographers*, 25 (1958), 167–95.

Bryder, L. *Below the Magic Mountain: a social history of tuberculosis in twentieth-century Britain*, Oxford, 1989.

Cobbett, L. *The Causes of Tuberculosis*, Cambridge, 1917.

Creighton, C. Grounds for believing that the tubercular disease of animals which supply milk and meat for human use, is communicated by such food to man, *Transactions of the Seventh Session of the International Medical Congress*, London, 4 (1881), 481–6.

Cronjé, G. Tuberculosis and mortality in England and Wales, 1851–1910. In Woods, R. and Woodward, J, eds, *Urban Disease and Mortality in Nineteenth Century England*, London, 1984, 79–101.

Departmental Committee to Inquire into Pleuro-Pneumonia and Tuberculosis in the United Kingdom [Chairman: J. Wilson], 1888, C5461; C5461-I, xxxii.

Forrester, R B. *The Fluid Milk Market in England and Wales* (Ministry of Agriculture, Economic Series No16), London, 1927.

Francis, J. *Bovine Tuberculosis*, London, 1947.

Griffith, A S. Bovine tuberculosis in man, *Tubercle*, 18 (1937), 530-1.

Griffith, A S and Munro, W. T. Human pulmonary tuberculosis of bovine origin in Great Britain, *Journal of Hygiene*, 43 (1943), 229–40.

Hardy, A. Diagnosis, death and diet: the case of London, 1750–1909, *Journal of Interdisciplinary History*, 18 (1988), 387–401.

Kaplan, M M. Diseases transmitted through milk. In Abdussalam et al, eds, *Milk Hygiene: hygiene in milk production, processing and distribution*, (World Health Organization Monograph Series No 48), Geneva, 1962.

Ministry of Agriculture. *Animal Health: a centenary, 1865–1965*, London, 1965.

Myers, J A and Steele, J H. *Bovine Tuberculosis: control in man and animals*, St Louis, 1969.

Pennington, C. Tuberculosis. In Checkland, O and Lamb, M, eds, *Health Care as Social History: the Glasgow case*, Aberdeen, 1982.

Rich, A R. *The Pathogenesis of Tuberculosis*, Illinois, 1944.

Ritchie, J, Sir. The eradication of bovine tuberculosis and its importance to man and beast, *Conquest*, 52 (1964) 3–12.

Roberts, A E. 'Feeding and mortality in the early months of life; changes in medical opinion and popular feeding practice', PhD, University of Hull, 1973.

Rosenkrantz, B G. The Trouble with Bovine Tuberculosis, *Bulletin of the History of Medicine*, 59 (1985), 155–75.

Royal Commission to Inquire into Administrative Procedures for Controlling Danger to Man Through Use as Food of Meat and Milk of Tuberculous Animals [Chairman: H. Maxwell], British Parliamentary Papers, 1898, C8824; C8831, xlix.

Royal Commission to Inquire into Effect of Food Derived from Tuberculous Animals on Human Health, British Parliamentary Papers, 1895, C7703, xxxv; 1896, C7992, xlvi.

Savage, W G. *Milk and the Public Health*, London, 1912.

Savage, W G. *The Prevention of Human Tuberculosis of Bovine Origin*, London, 1929.

Smith, F B. *The Retreat of Tuberculosis, 1850–1950*, London, 1988.

Szreter, S. The importance of social intervention in Britain's mortality decline c1850–1914: a re-interpretation of the role of public health, *Social History of Medicine*, 1.

Thorne-Thorne, R. *The Administrative Control of Tuberculosis*, London, 1899.

Woodruff, H A. The Veterinary Inspection of Dairy Cows and Cowsheds, *Journal of the Royal Sanitary Institute*, 32 (1911) 87.

Youmans, G P. *Tuberculosis*, Philadelphia, 1979.

NOTES

1 *Guardian*, March 22 1996, 3.

2 Royal Commission, 1898, 155. Subsequently it transpired that meat was far less likely than milk to have been a source of infection. Savage, 1929, 1.

3 This was by no means the first time that Koch's work on tuberculosis had been found wanting. Cobbett, 1917, 132; Rosenkrantz, 1985.

4 There are 28 species of mycobacteria, nine of which can cause human disease. Youmans, 1979, 3–4.

5 Royal Commission 1896, qq 1508–9.

6 About four per cent of TT reactors excrete bacilli in their milk, but only 25 per cent of these show any udder lesions. Kaplan, 1962, 48.

7 *Annual Report*, Medical Officer of Health, Manchester, 1909, 134.

8 Savage, 1929, 38.

9 Cronje, 1984, 81; Smith, 1988, 12.

10 It should be noted that there are serious doubts about the accuracy of the mortality data on tuberculosis. The disease has complex manifestations and its diagnosis is very likely to have been confused with other causes of death. The term 'phthisis', for instance, was a general term for wasting diseases and would therefore have covered pulmonary tuberculosis, leukaemia and various internal cancers. Hardy 1988, 392. There are complex interactions between tuberculosis and other diseases which also need to be considered. Some deaths may, for instance, have been due to tubercular 'breakdown disease' in former sufferers initiated through a weakening of resistance by an unrelated infection. Szreter, 1988, 17; Rich, 1944.

11 Thorne-Thorne, 1899, 30; Ashby, 1922, 187; Smith, 1988, 190. Boiling reduces the nutritive value of milk and anyway was rejected as a practice by mothers in the 1880s as giving rise to constipation. Roberts, 1973, 86.

12 Savage, 1929, 2–6. The consumption of cream was also risky, but dried milk and condensed milk less so because of the heating process in their manufacture.

13 Savage, 1929, 137; 152; Ministry of Agriculture, 1965, 217; Cronje, 1984, 82; Bryder, 1989, 135.

14 Atkins, 1977; 1992.

15 The Dairies, Cowshed and Milkshops Order of 1899 amended Article 15 of the 1885 Order to include tuberculosis for the first time. The Order remained permissive, however, and even those local authorities which did make their own regulations were not necessarily conscientious in carrying them out.

16 Before World War I few rural authorities seem to have taken the problem of cattle welfare seriously. In many areas there was no veterinary inspection whatsoever. Woodruff, 1911, 87.

17 Individual cows may intermittently excrete five million bacilli per ml. Forrester, 1927, 17; Francis, 1947, 131; Kaplan, 1962, 48.

18 Departmental Committee, 1888, xxiii.

19 Royal Commission, 1898, 155; Pennington, 1982, 89–91.

20 Under these powers the London County Council kept a record of the number of instances of disease on milk retailing premises in their jurisdiction. The results were startling. In the short period 1895/6–1900/1, for instance, there were 680 cases of scarlet fever, 398 of diphtheria, 108 of enteric fever, and 23 of smallpox. *Annual Reports*, London County Council.

21 But one contemporary writer was sceptical that the Manchester Milk Clauses had any positive effect beyond their educational impact. Savage, 1912, 338; 1929, 104.

22 In practice it proved very difficult to track down the sources of tuberculous milk. Large dairy companies mixed their milk at rural depots before consignment. Savage, 1929, 107.

23 The farming lobby was politically strong enough to mobilise opposition in parliament to any anti-tuberculosis measure which might threaten the prosperity of dairying. Smith, 1988, 176–7.

24 Ministry of Agriculture, 1965, 216.

25 Grades of milk were established by the Milk (Special Designations) Order 1923 which guaranteed that the source herd had been tuberculin tested. The 1925 Tuberculosis Order was amended in 1938.

26 Notification and slaughter, with compensation, were compulsory for animals suffering from tuberculosis of the udder, emaciation, or chronic cough with clinical signs of the disease.

27 By 1947 only fifteen per cent of herds had qualified as 'attested'. Francis, 1947, 26.

28 Myers and Steele, 1969, 269-70.

29 The Milk and Dairies (Scotland) Act of 1914, which came into effect in 1925, was responsible for a rather different system of regular veterinary inspection north of the border.

30 Francis, 1947, 27; 32.

31 Ritchie, 1964, 4.

32 In Cheshire, Derbyshire, Lancashire, Staffordshire and the West Riding of Yorkshire.

7 Propagation of nutritional knowledge in Poland 1863–1939

Katarzyna Cwiertka

INTRODUCTION

After a century of political intrigue and instability, the vast territory of the Polish Commonwealth was finally annexed in 1795 and divided between the three neighbouring powers: the Russian, Prussian, and Austro-Hungarian Empires (Fig. 1). For more than a hundred and twenty years each annexed part was influenced by three different political bodies, and subjected to different social and economical policies. The country's reunion as the Polish Republic in 1918 meant a fresh start in all respects, including the state's involvement in issues concerning public health.

This paper investigates the dissemination of nutritional knowledge within the Polish population from the late nineteenth century until the outbreak of World War II in 1939. The basic sources are professional and popular magazines, and other related publications, which appeared in the Polish language in the period discussed. First, this paper will deal with the adoption, application, and promotion of Western nutritional science among the individuals professionally involved in dietary matters; and the dissemination of new ideas of healthy diet among the middle classes in partitioned Poland. Later, it will discuss efforts to propagate relevant knowledge among wider fractions of the population within the framework of the new state, concentrating on the government's involvement in this matter. The role of the Polish political situation in disseminating nutritional knowledge will stand at the centre of the investigation. Did the lack of central government influence the spread of nutritional knowledge in Poland?

There are two factors that need to be taken into consideration for this paper. First, the regional diversity of diet, already observed before partition, and increased as a result of the different economic, political, social, and cultural circumstances of Russian, Prussian, and Austrian Poland respectively. Moreover, living within one or other of three entirely different cultures marked the mentality and behaviour of every Pole, which in turn influenced attitudes toward nutritional knowledge and affected the reception of nutritional advice. Consequently, a uniform nutritional policy on Polish territory was lacking before 1918, and nutritional knowledge spread unevenly in different parts of the Polish Republic as well. Research on each region would be necessary to present an adequate picture of the entire territory. In this paper, I will focus on the situation of the Polish Kingdom, a semi-

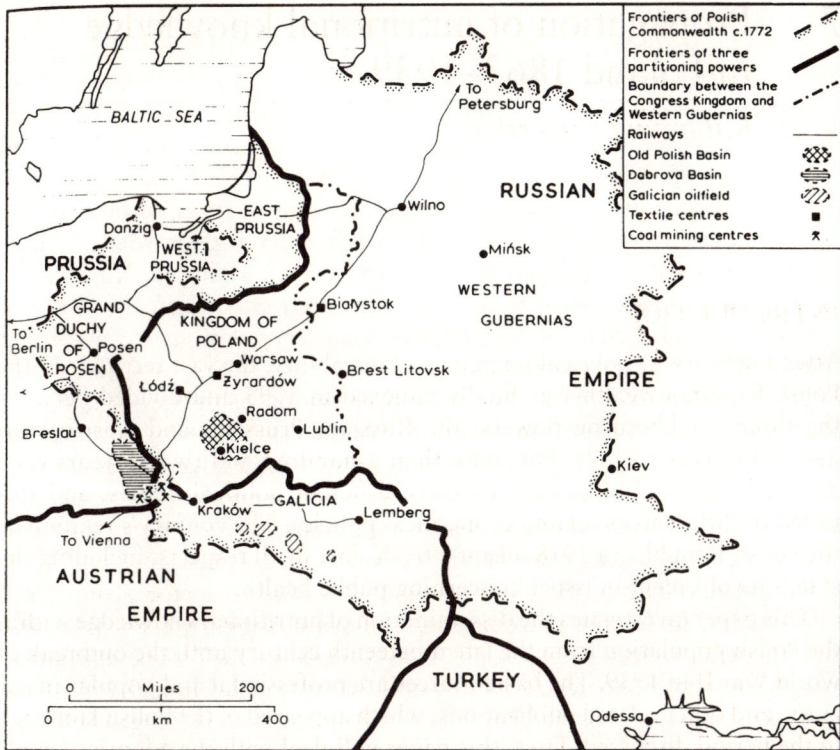

Fig. 1. *The lands of partitioned Poland, c1860 (after Zamoyski 1987, 303)*

autonomous unit belonging to Russia, and in particular its capital Warsaw, which from 1918 was also the capital of the Republic.

A second factor complicating the investigation of the spread of nutritional knowledge within the Polish population is the complex nature of the dynamics of the spread of knowledge itself. A balanced investigation should include the process of dissemination as well as of the reception of knowledge. However, the bulk of the historical data on which this paper is based concerns the propagation of knowledge rather than its diffusion. It is, therefore, impossible to indicate precisely the effect that the promotion of knowledge had on the daily lives of the people. Consequently, this paper merely reflects the efforts undertaken by various individuals, organisations, and institutions to propagate nutritional knowledge within the Polish population, and does not attempt to go further.

PROFESSIONALS c 1880

Numerous original editions in German and French of works by K Ackermann, I Albu, F W Böcker, R Virchow, T L W Bischoff, K von Voit, and other western European pioneers of nutritional science reached Poland in the mid-nineteenth century. Polish translations of some of these works soon began to be published. For example, in 1870 and 1879 Libieg's *O wartosci pozywney pokarmow* [Nutritional value of foods] and *Notatki dotyczace hygieny pokarmowej* [Notes concerning food hygiene], and in 1880 Karl Reclam's *Nauka zachowania zdrowia i zdolnosci do pracy* [The science of retaining health and fitness for work] appeared in Polish. Most probably, the professional curiosity of some Polish physicians was responsible for the turning of their attention towards the newly emerging knowledge. Soon, original works written by Poles also appeared, for example, *Notatki tyczace sie hygieny pokarmowej* [Notes concerning food hygiene] by W Kleczkowski was published in 1879 and *O zywieniu sie i pokarmach* [On feeding and food] by H Nusbaum and L Necki in 1887.

The first step towards a large-scale propagation of the new knowledge concerning food hygiene and nutrition was the establishment of the magazine *Zdrowie* [Health] in 1878. The magazine did not have a popular character, but was rather aimed at institutions and individuals in some way involved in the matter of public health: physicians, sanitary inspectors, and official social surveyors who specialised in dietary matters.

On the initiative of the chief editor of *Zdrowie*, a doctor of medicine J Polak, and under the patronage of Countess Augustowa Potocka, the first Hygienic Exhibition took place in Warsaw in 1887.[1] The exhibition was divided into Biological, Architectural, Educational, Clinical, Industrial, and Statistical sections. The Physio-chemical part of the Biological section was almost entirely devoted to nutrition and food hygiene. Next to educational tables, lectures and brochures, new products such as Graham bread, meat extracts, canned and instant soups, and enamel cooking utensils were displayed and sold.[2] A similar, second, Hygienic Exhibition in Warsaw was organised in 1896.[3]

During both exhibitions efforts were made to establish an association which would act for improvement of public health, like those already active in Western Europe. The Warsaw Hygienic Association (Warszawskie Towarzystwo Higjeniczne) was finally founded in March 1898. A year later the total membership of the Association exceeded 500, and from July 1900 *Zdrowie* became the organ of the association.[4] The magazine not only gave an account of the activities of the Association, but also reported on the activities of related organisations.[5]

Nutritional conditions for the Polish population in the late nineteenth and early twentieth centuries were generally worse than in Western Europe. For example, according to a study from the turn of the century, the average Polish male servant was then 60.7 kg in weight and 166 cm in height, while a German servant weighed 70 kg and was 167.7 cm tall.[6] The nutritional standard of the Polish peasantry and industrial workers was low. Dembinska's calculations imply that an English industrial worker around 1863 consumed twice as much meat as Polish worker, and almost four times as much around 1890. Around the turn of the century, only 44.6 per cent of workers in a wool factory in Czestochowa were regarded as well fed, and in the jute sacks factory in Bleszyn the figure was even smaller – ten per cent.[7] This poor nourishment of the Polish lower classes was reflected in the poor physical condition of conscripts. In the period between 1865 and 1870, 18.2 per cent of men drafted from the territory of the Polish Kingdom were considered unfit for service. In 1910, this dropped to 6.7 per cent, but only 51.8 per cent were drafted and the rest were classified as reserve.[8] Sobczak points out that although the energy food supply within the Polish population improved greatly throughout the nineteenth century,[9] this improvement should be seen as a reflection of economic growth rather than as the spread of nutritional advice.

The growing interest among physicians and bureaucrats in dietary matters, and in particular in the poor nourishment of the lowest social orders observed in the late nineteenth century,[10] was reflected in the columns of *Zdrowie*. The magazine included articles treating specific dietary problems, such as nourishment in hospitals and sanatoria,[11] and published reports examining the diet of the lowest social orders. In fact, the diet of the Polish people had already become a matter of inquiry for the physicians and sanitary inspectors from the 1870s.[12] Open inquiry and on-the-spot personal observations, the new methods practised in England, France, Germany, Switzerland and Russia, attracted Polish investigators.[13] *Zdrowie* published many such dietary surveys. For example, *Przyczynek do wiadomosci o zywieniu sie ludu wiejskiego* [Information about the diet of peasantry] by K Chelchowski, published in 1890, *Plan badania warunkow zywienia sie ludnosci miejskiej* [The plan of research into the dietary conditions of the urban population] by S Sterling, and *Z badan nad zywieniem sie Zydow malomiasteczkowych* [Study on the diet of provincial Jews] by Koskowski, both published in 1897.[14] In 1902 the magazine included a report on the dietary conditions of manorial servants in Plonsk region,[15] and in 1908 published the result of a similar survey conducted among Jewish communities in small settlements.[16] At the same time, Dr Peltyn investigated the diet of peasants.[17] Based on the collected data, he pointed out that there was almost no difference in the consumption habits of the more and less affluent peasantry. An average daily intake calculated by Peltyn was: 139 g protein, 60 g fat, 855 g carbohydrates.

Zdrowie also included advice on the improvement of the diet of the poorest strata of the Polish population. For example, in 1880 a series of articles concerning the feeding of the poor by philanthropic institutions was published.[18] The author advised institutions on how to provide proper nourishment at the lowest cost, and gave recipes for nourishing soups along with examples of cheap and healthy menus.

We may presume that activity in relation to improving hygienic and nutritional conditions in the Polish Kingdom in the late nineteenth century resulted merely in the spread of knowledge in medical circles and amongst the mainly male individuals involved professionally in the matter of public health. It seems unlikely that neither the two Hygienic Exhibitions from 1887 and 1896, nor the Household Exhibition, organised by the Warsaw Hygienic Association in 1905,[19] influenced the dietary patterns of the population. Rather, these events should be viewed as the important starting point for the awakening of nutritional consciousness amongst middle-class women.

MIDDLE-CLASS WOMEN c 1900

In the mid-nineteenth century, Polish cuisine entered a period of radical change. Foreign influences, in particular Italian and French, had entered the kitchen of the élite from the sixteenth century onwards. However, from the second half of the nineteenth century we can talk about westernisation of the Polish middle-class cookery. This extensive westernisation was to a certain extent conditioned by fashion. However, social changes initiated by the Industrial Revolution, in particular the growing urban middle-class, were also responsible for the adoption of foreign dishes in Polish middle-class kitchens. Poland's Industrial Revolution was not spectacular by European standards.[20] Nonetheless, industrialisation and urbanisation had similar consequences for dietary matters as in other western European states, such as growing household literature.

A serious change in the availability of printed household literature, which took place in the early nineteenth century, had a great impact on the modernisation of the Polish diet.[21] A trend for imitating foreign cookery began with the use of French, German, and Austrian cookery books in Polish households. Soon, many translations of French and Italian books appeared on the Polish market.[22] Culinary reformers who influenced the diet of the urban upper- and middle-classes from the late nineteenth century onwards, such as M Disslowa, J Izdebska, M Norkowska and M Gruszecka, popularised European and American dishes through publications, lectures, and cooking demonstrations organised by women's clubs and newly emerging schools of cookery. Along with foreign recipes the new 'scientific' attitude towards cookery was adopted from abroad.

Magazines were the most important means for the diffusion of nutritional knowledge outside medical circles, and the relation between food, drink and health began to be featured in their columns long before the arrival of hygienic exhibitions. Semi-scientific advice on diet was included in various magazines between the 1830s and the 1880s, for example, *Pamietnik Rolniczo-Technologiczny* [Farming and Technology Diary], *Pamietnik Domowy* [Home Diary], *Opiekun Domowy* [Home Guardian], *Gospodyni Wiejska* [Rural Housekeeper], and *Gospodyni Wiejska i Miejska* [Rural and Urban Housekeeper].[23] The first editions of the magazine *Bluszcz* [Ivy] from 1865 included a series of articles by Dr Plaskowski dealing with mineral waters.[24] The same author published a series of articles about food and digestion in the 1870 editions of the magazine.[25] In 1867, *Bluszcz* published an article about Liebig's artificial food, and in 1896 a series of articles on nutrition by Dr Kaminski.[26] The second Warsaw Hygienic Exhibition was also covered extensively by the magazine.[27] Support from the scientists was important for the reformers of Polish middle-class cookery in providing scientific justification for their actions towards the improvement of the Polish diet.

The number of articles dealing with nutrition increased considerably after the turn of the twentieth century. The women's magazine *Dobra Gospodyni* [Good Housekeeper] – one of the cheapest on the market and aimed at rural as well as urban middle-class women – often popularised the knowledge disseminated by the Warsaw Hygienic Association. For example, a series of articles under the joint title *O zywieniu niemowlat* [About feeding infants], based on two public lectures given by Dr Baczkiewicz under the auspices of the Warsaw Hygienic Association in November 1900, was published in the magazine in 1902.[28] The article *Jak nalezy urzdzic zycie codzienne, aby dlugo pozostac zdrowym i zdolnym do pracy?* [How does one arrange one's daily life in order to stay healthy and fit for work for a long time?], was a summary of the article by Dr Chodecki published in *Zdrowie* in 1911 and included in a 1912 edition of *Dobra Gospodyni*.[29] A public lecture of the Warsaw Hygienic Association dealing with household education, delivered in October 1902, was published in the columns of *Dobra Gospodyni* in January 1903.[30] The magazine featured a relatively high number of articles dealing with nutrition until 1915, when its publication was interrupted by World War I.[31]

Of course, we can never be sure what affect these articles had on the diet of the middle classes. However, the fact that the life-span of women's magazines was very sensitive to readers' approval of their contents, suggests that articles dealing with nutrition enjoyed popularity.

Dietary advice was usually featured in the health and hygiene columns of women's magazines rather than in cookery columns. Generally speaking, nutritional knowledge was only marginally included in popular household advice,[32] and was seen as being related to medicine rather than to cooking.[33] Although the importance of nutritional knowledge for household work was increasingly emphasised in the publications aimed at middle-class housewives,[34] until the 1920s such knowledge was not perceived as an integral part of cookery.

The Warsaw food exhibitions played an important role in the spread of knowledge concerning proper nourishment. Their main purpose was to introduce technological novelties from Western Europe, and to stimulate domestic food production based on Western models. Nevertheless, nutritional matters received attention as well. The first Warsaw Food Exhibition was organised in 1885 by the author of many best-selling cookery books, L Cwierczakiewiczowa, and the restaurant owner, Reyner. It was supported financially by the Warsaw Philanthropic Association (Warszawskie Towarzystwo Dobroczynnosci), and attracted more than ten thousand visitors. Several more exhibitions were organised in the first decade of the twentieth century, the most successful being that of 1902, visited by seventy thousand people.[35]

WIDER SECTIONS OF SOCIETY c 1920

New trends in the popularisation of nutritional knowledge were set in the 1920s. Efforts to reach lower social classes with nutritional advice were observed. Various activities of local character gave way to more nationally co-ordinated actions, and the matter of proper nourishment began to be clearly linked with the idea of modern cookery and propagated as part of household education. The issue of the improvement of dietary conditions in rural Poland also began to receive more attention.[36]

Existing magazines began to change their profiles. *Bluszcz* and *Dobra Gospodyni* continued to feature articles dealing with nutrition,[37] including the recent discovery of vitamins.[38] However, *Bluszcz* changed its entertaining character and became involved in women's social activities. It reported, for example, the actions of the Housewives' Association (Zwiazek Pan Domu). This emerged from various middle-class women's organisations, and aimed at popularising the modern methods of housekeeping, including its health aspect. Lectures, demonstrations, courses and exhibitions were organised by the branches of the association in many Polish cities.[39] *Zdrowie*, in turn, began to be involved in national-scale issues, for example the debate concerning hygiene and nutrition education in schools.[40] New magazines dealing with health issues emerged as well, for example *Higjena ciala i sport* [Body Hygiene and Sport] published in the city of Lwow. It was first published in 1925, and included many articles aiming at popularising nutritional knowledge.[41] The magazine also dealt with the dietary conditions of the citizens of the town.[42]

The number of books dealing with nutritional issues increased in the 1920s and the 1930s,[43] and popular cookery manuals began to contain more information concerning digestion and the nutritional value of foods than those published a few decades earlier.[44] Nutritional advice was also spread via radio transmissions.[45]

Probably the most remarkable changes occurred in the field of household education. The underdevelopment of household education in the Polish Kingdom, and the necessity of establishing non-professional domestic science courses for young women, were often pointed out by physicians and culinary reformers.[46] Although women of means could afford cookery courses, which began to be organised at the end of the nineteenth century by L Cwierczakiewiczowa, M Norkowska, and other famous instructors,[47] cookery advice did not reach the working classes, in cities or in the country. Some actions towards improving the dietary habits of the lower social orders were made, usually in the form of housekeeping brochures and courses.[48] However, they had a limited effect on the general picture of the badly nourished Polish working class. Elementary domestic science education in France, Germany, Belgium and Scandinavia was seen as the model to be learned from.

From the 1920s onwards, slowly but persistently the subject of household management was included in the curriculum of the last years of elementary schooling. One- or two-year domestic science schools for elementary school graduates were also emerging.[49] Domestic science education in the Polish Republic, which included an extensive amount of knowledge concerning healthy food preparation, began to flourish under the scientific and organisational leadership of the Household Institute (Instytut Gospodarstwa Domowego). This institute emerged in 1930 as the result of the joint efforts of the Household Management Section of the Scientific Management Institute (Sekcja Gospodarstwa Domowego Instytutu Naukowej Organizacji), the Council General of the Women's Household Education (Rada Naczelna Gospodarczego Ksztalcenia Kobiet) and other organisations.[50] The Institute organised cookery presentations and lectures on proper nourishment, conducted research in the field of cookery, hygiene and nutrition, developed new teaching methods for the instructors of modern housekeeping, and was involved in the reform of mass catering. All these activities were propagated throughout the country via the network of the Housewives Association, co-operating with the Institute. Its revolutionary educational methods received attention even outside the country.[51]

From 1932, the Household Institute and the Housewives Association jointly published a monthly journal, *Pani Domu* (The Lady of the House). The magazine was originally published by the Household Management Section of the Scientific Management Institute as *Organizacja Gospodarstwa Domowego* [Household Management]. Its columns included information about the latest discoveries in the field of nutritional science, cookery, and household management. Articles that appeared in the magazine were often later compiled into textbooks and guides for housekeeping reformers.

In the 1930s, particular attention was given to the education of rural women from the lower social orders in household skills, hygiene, and nutrition. Although the dietary conditions of peasant households were extensively studied from the 1870s onwards, not much was done in order to improve them. There are indications that this was partly due to the arrogance of the male bureaucrats towards women's household work.[52] The first female section of the Central Farming Association (Centralne Towarzystwo Rolnicze) emerged in 1920, but for financial reasons started its educational activities four years later. In the 1930s various projects aimed at bolstering the peasants' diet began. The General Council for Women's Household Education (Rada Naczelna Gospodarczego Ksztalcenia Kobiet) organised correspondence household courses,[53] and courses and presentations were organised on the spot by regional Rural Housekeepers' Circles of the Central Association of Farming Organisations and Circles (Kola Gospodyn Wiejskich Centralnego Towarzystwa Organizacyj i Kolek Rolniczych).[54]

The Housekeepers' Circles emerged in 1933 as the result of the fusion of seven regional rural women's organisations.[55] Various regional activities of the Circles were reported in its organ, the magazine *Przodownica* [Headwoman]. The magazine appeared every two weeks from 1930 to 1939, for the first three years as a free supplement for women to the rural magazine *Przewodnik Gospodarski* [Farming Guide]. The magazine included articles dealing with important issues of rural life, and had an 'advice column' where questions from the readers were answered. In 1935, the Housekeepers' Circles also published an elementary household book with the title *Ksiazka Gospodyni Wiejskiej* [The Book of the Rural Housekeeper]. It included, besides recipes and advice on hygiene, a twelve-page article about nourishment and digestion.[56]

The government was directly and indirectly involved in the efforts to disseminate nutritional knowledge among the population. The Household Institute worked on the modernisation of household equipment in co-operation with the Ministry of Industry and Commerce. The members of the government regularly attended lectures and other public activities of the Institute, and its educational improvements were supported by the Ministry of Education. Rationalisation and modernisation of Polish households were regarded as important elements of the state's welfare.[57]

The government was involved in the propagation of educational publications. For example, a note about the Polish translation of the book, *How to Live*, by Fisher and Fisk, first published in New York in 1915, was sent to all provincial administration offices in December 1927 by the Medical Service Department of the Ministry of the Interior. The book treated the matters of health preservation, hygiene and nourishment in a popular and practical way.

Exhibitions dealing with hygiene and nutrition were supported financially by the state. For example, the Hygiene-and-Consumption Exhibition in Warsaw in 1926 was organised under the protectorate of the Ministry of Industry and Commerce.[58] The International Sanitary-Hygienic Exhibition, one of the biggest and most important exhibitions in Poland, was organised in 1927 under the patronage of the President of the Polish Republic, and ran simultaneously with the International Congress of Military Medicine and Pharmacology, taking place in Warsaw at that time.[59]

The government also established several national institutions dealing with nourishment, such as the National School of Hygiene (Panstwowa Szkola Hygieny) and the National School of Household Work (Panstwowa Szkola Pracy Domowej).

CONCLUSIONS

In the time span covered by this paper I distinguished three somewhat overlapping stages in the dissemination of nutritional knowledge in pre-World War II Poland. The nineteenth century was when the organisational ground for the application and propagation of nutritional knowledge was laid, and the pioneering period for the study of dietary conditions of the population. The last decade of the nineteenth century marked the beginning of the propagation of nutritional knowledge on a wider scale, mainly among middle-class women, and this activity continued to flourish during the following decades. After the period of instability caused by World War I and the establishment of the Polish Republic, efforts to create a national network for dietary education, including the lower social strata, were observed and became characteristic for the late 1920s and the 1930s. The study of the reception of these activities by the general public lay outside the scope of my investigation.

Did the political situation play a role in the dissemination of nutritional knowledge among the Polish population? Generally speaking, the first two stages discussed here, were the results of private initiative, or eventually of the initiative of voluntary organisations. No governmental agencies were involved in the propagation of nutritional knowledge in Poland before the 1920s. On the contrary, the deliberate policy of the annexing powers to destroy Polish culture and learning forced many Polish scientists to study and work abroad.[60] However, as Leslie argues, the fact of partition gave Poles a deeper appreciation of the culture of other countries in continental Europe,[61] and this might have been one of the factors responsible for the vigorous adoption of foreign knowledge by Polish physicians.

Western Europe served as the model of advancement for the Polish intelligentsia, and dietary matters were no exception. Polish obscurity in the field of nutritional and hygienic conditions was to be changed through the application of western European science. The Polish intellectual élite were involved in the propagation of the new knowledge with the aim of improving the health of the population through proper nourishment. The reason behind their enthusiasm was not strictly scientific. The tragic failure of the insurrection in the Polish Kingdom in 1863 gave birth to the so-called 'organic movement', the new idea of fighting for independence through the improvement of the nation both spiritually and physically. Hygiene and proper nourishment were the means of pulling Polish society from its backward state and making it compatible with the 'civilised' nations of the West.[62]

> It was not until the latter part of the century that the idea of organic progress through mass self-improvement achieved the status of theory. The works of Auguste Comte, John Stuart Mill and Charles Darwin appeared to hold special relevance to the Polish problem. [sic] The Romantic concept of the nation as spirit or divine body had given way to the concept of the nation as an organism.[63]

It remains a matter of speculation whether various activities described in this paper, which emerged out of private initiative, would have been more effective in the political situation of the independent nation state. It can also be plausibly argued that, on the contrary, the interest in dietary reform would have been weaker in independent Poland, considering the fact that the 'organic movement' often formed the ideological backbone of the actions aiming at the diffusion of nutritional knowledge.

It is also difficult to judge whether the creation of the Polish Republic in 1918, which meant the beginning of the government's involvement in matters of public nutrition, was an important factor in the increased effort to reach the lower social strata with nutritional advice. The new tendencies in the 1920s were certainly the continuation of the pioneering work done before, and private initiative still continued to play an important role in putting reforms forward. The impetus given by World War I to food and nutritional studies,[64] as well as the development of the 'newer knowledge of nutrition', should not be overlooked either. Moreover, the changing social role of women, with their increased involvement in social and educational issues, certainly influenced the character of Polish household education.

Considering the involvement of various governments in dietary reforms during World War I,[65] it seems that the government of the Polish Republic from its outset lagged behind in relation to these matters. A separate study, however, is needed to compare the level of state participation in the dissemination of nutritional knowledge in the 1930s between Poland and other countries. At any rate, the Polish case indicates that the diffusion of nutritional knowledge is not a strictly scientific, economic, and social matter, but involves political and ideological factors as well.

ACKNOWLEDGEMENTS

This research was supported financially by the Ajinomoto Foundation for Dietary Culture in Tokyo. During the collection of material, I received much help from Beata Meller, former Director of the Historical Museum of Warsaw. I am also very grateful to Peter Scholliers for his valuable comments on the earlier version of this paper.

BIBLIOGRAPHY

Anon. *Katalog Wystawy Hygjenicznej* [The Catalogue of the Hygienic Exhibition], Warszawa, 1887.

Antoszka. *Upominek dla matek i gospodyn* [A Gift for Mothers and Housekeepers], Warszawa, 1896.

Biehler, M. *Hygiena Dziecka* [Child hygiene], Warszawa, 1916.

Bielicka, Z. Kursy gospodarstwa domowego przy Schronisku Dzieci Marji [Household courses at Mary's children's shelter], *Dobra Gospodyni*, 14 (1914), 89–90.

Bleszynski, J. Instytuty gospodarstwa kobiecego [Household institutes], *Dobra Gospodyni*, 7 (1907), 361–362.

Chodecki, W. Czy jesc chleb bialy, czy razowy? [Which bread should we eat, white or wholemeal], *Dobra Gospodyni*, 16 (1925), 43.

Cwierczakiewiczowa, L. *365 Obiadow* [365 Dinners], Krakow, 1985, facsimile of the 23rd edn from 1911.

Czerny-Biernatowa, Z and Strasburger, M. *Organizacja i metody pracy w szkolnictwie gospodarczym zenskim* [Organisation and Methods of Work in Household Education for Females], Lwow-Warszawak, 1930.

Czerny, Z and Strasburger, M. *Teorja Przyrzadzania Potraw* [The Theory of Food Preparation], Lwow-Warszawa, 1936.

Czerny, Z and Strasburger, M. *Zywienie Rodziny* [Feeding the Family], Warszawa, 1948.

Dembinska, M. Z badan nad dziennymi racjami zywnosciowymi robotnikow przemyslowych w Krolestwie Polskim w drugiej pol. XIX w. [Daily food consumption patterns of Polish workers in the second half of the 19th century], *Kwartalnik Historii Kultury Materialnej*, 27 (1979), 145-156.

Editorial. O Warszawskim Towarzystwie Higjenicznem [About the Warsaw Hygienic Association], *Zdrowie*, (1900), 168–172.

Editorial. Kilka slow o biblioteczce podrecznej [A few words about the reference library], *Dobra Gospodyni*, 1 (1901), no 23.

Editorial. Nadzwyczajne posiedzenie w sprawach hygienicznych w Towarzystwie Lekarskim Czestochowskiem [Extraordinary meeting for hygienic matters of the Medical Association of Czestochowa], *Zdrowie*, (1902), 576–577.

Editorial. Wystawa Hygieniczno-Spozywcza w Lodzi [Hygiene-and-food exhibition in Lodz], *Dobra Gospodyni*, 3 (1903), 34.

Editorial. Wystawa gospodarstwa domowego [Household exhibition], *Dobra Gospodyni*, 5 (1905), 11.

Gillespie, C C. *Dictionary of Scientific Biography*, New York, 1972–76.

Gruszecka, M. *366 obiadow: Praktyczna Ksiazka Kucharska* [366 Dinners: Practical Cookery Book], Krakow, 1895.

Harvey, M. *Tajemnice powodzenia w zyciu* [Secrets of Life's Success], Krakow, 1908.

Huberowa, J. Dzialalnosc instytucji gospodarczych i oswiatowych w Polsce na polu naukowej organizacjii w zakresie gospodarstwa domowego w latach 1928–1934 [Activities of economic and educational institutions in Poland in the field of scientific organisation of the household 1928–1934], *Przeglad Organizacji*, 9 (1935).

Ihnatowicz, E. Koniec wieku w kuchni [The end of the century in the kitchen], *Wiedza I Czlowiek*, 22 (1995), 1–4.

Instytut Gospodarstwa Domowego. *Wytyczne pracy w Kolach Gospodyn Wiejskich* [Directions of Work in Rural Housekeepers' Circles], Warszawa, 1938.

Izdebska, J. *Mloda Gosposia* [Young Housekeeper], Warszawa, 1894.

Jakimiak, B. Posiedzenie z dnia 4 maja 1901 r. [Meeting of May 4, 1901], *Zdrowie*, (1901), 638–639.

Jaworski, J. Szkoly gospodarstwa domowego [Household schools], *Dobra Gospodyni*, 3 (1903), 2–3.

Kacprzak, M. Pokarmy spozywcze [Articles of food], *Ksiazka Gospodyni Wiejskiej*, (1935), 173–185.

Karaffa-Korbutt, K. O metodyce nauczania higjeny w szkolach srednich [Methodology of teaching hygiene in secondary schools], *Zdrowie* (1926) 483–499.

Koryzna, H. Wskazowki dietetyczne sprzed stu lat [Nutritional advice from a hundred years ago], *Pani Domu*, (1937), 348.

Koskowski, B. Warunki hygieniczne w malych osadach i sposob zywienia sie ich mieszkancow, glownie Zydow [Hygienic conditions in small settlements and food habits of their inhabitants, mainly Jews], *Zdrowie*, (1908), 676–682.

Kowecka, E. Pozywienie [Food]. In *Historia Kultury Materialnej w zarysie 5* [Outline of the History of Material Culture, vol 5], Warszawa, 1978, 343–385.

Kozlowski, St. Zaklad dyetetyczny w Ojcowie [Dietary sanatorium in Ojcow], *Zdrowie*, (1910), 689–703.

Ks, L. *Szczescie domowe* [Home Happiness], Gladbach-Leipzig, 1882.

Landaw, H. O zywieniu chorych w szpitalach Warszawskich [Feeding the sick in Warsaw hospitals], *Zdrowie*, (1901), 75–102.

Leskiewiczowa, J. Kwestionariusz w sprawie zywienia sie ludzi w Galicji [Questionnaire concerning the folk diet in Galicia], *Kwartalnik Historii Kultury Materialnej*, 26 (1978), 179–191.

Leslie, R F, ed. *The History of Poland since 1863*, Cambridge, 1980.

Lutostanski, B. Slowo w sprawie zywienia ubogich w czasach panujacego glodu: Najtansze obiady [About feeding the poor in the time of hunger: the cheapest meals], *Zdrowie*, (1880), 25–28, 41–43, 53–54, 61–64.

Malewski, B. O zywieniu dyetetycznym chorych w zakladzie leczniczym w Grodzisku [About the diet of the sick at the infirmary in Grodzisk], *Zdrowie*, (1910), 382.

Meller, B. Warszawskie wystawy spozywcze w koncu XIX i poczatkach XX wieku [Warsaw Culinary Exhibitions at the end of the 19th and beginning of the 20th century], *Kwartalnik Historii Kultury Materialnej*, 30 (1982), 225–232.

Meller, B. Ksiazki kucharskie w XIX wieku [Cookery books in the nineteenth century], In *Wokol stolu i kuchni*, Warszawa, 1994, 81–89.

Naake Naleski, W. Odzywianie sie mieszkancow Lwowa w latach 1910–1922 [Diet of the citizens of Lwow between 1910 and 1922], *Higjena Ciala i Sport*, 2, (1926) no 14; 16; 18; 19.

Norkowska, M. *Najnowsza kuchnia wytworna i gospodarska* [The Newest Refined and Plain Cookery], Warszawa, 1903.

Ochorowicz-Monatowa, M. *Uniwersalna Ksiazka Kucharska* [Universal cookery book], Warszawa, 1995, facsimile c 1930 edn.

Oldziejewski, K. *Wystawy Powszechne, ich historja, organizacja, polozenie prawne I wartosc spoleczno-gospodarcza* [Public Exhibitions, their History, Organisation, Legislation and Socio-economical Value], Poznan, 1928.

Rothfeld, J. Brak apetytu u dzieci szkolnych [Lack of appetite among school children], *Higjena Ciala i Sport*, 3, 22 (1927), 17–18.

Rutkowski, L, Odzywianie sluzby dworskiej w powiecie Plonskim w roku 1898 [Diet of manorial servants in Plonsk district in the year 1898], *Zdrowie* (1902), 217–226

Sarysz-Stokowska, M. Kola Gospodyn Wiejskich [Rural Housekeepers' Circles], *Bluszcz*, 69 (1933) no 33, 16–17.

Sobczak, T. *Przelom w konsumpcji spozywczej w Krolestwie Polskim w XIX wieku* [The Turning Point in Consumption of Food in the Polish Kingdom in the 19th century], Wroclaw, 1968.

Sobczak, T. Pozywienie [Food]. In *Historia Kultury Materialnej w zarysie*, 6 [Outline of the History of Material Culture, vol 6], Warszawa, 1978, 405–426.

Szeliga, E. *Nowy kucharz doskonaly* [New Perfect Cook], Krakow, 1929.

Szkola E F. Gospodarstwa domowego dla panien p Marty Norkowskiej w Warszawie [Marta Norkowska's household school for ladies in Warsaw], *Dobra Gospodyni*, 6 (1906), 2.

Teich, M. Science and food during the Great War: Britain and Germany. In *The Science and Culture of Nutrition, 1840-1940*, Amsterdam-Atlanta, 1995, 213–234.

Todhunter, E N. Chronology of some events in the development and application of the science of nutrition, *Nutrition Reviews*, 34 (1976), 353–365.

Wl Tr. Szkoly gospodarstwa domowego [Household schools], *Dobra Gospodyni*, 8 (1908), 345–346.

Wyrobek, E. *Nowoczesna Kuchnia Domowa* [Modern Home Cookery], Katowice, 1931.

Zamoyski, A. *The Polish Way: A thousand-year history of the Poles and their culture*, London, 1987.

NOTES

1 Anon, 1887, 1–3.
2 ibid, 21–24.
3 Oldziejewski, 1928, 47.
4 Editorial, 1900, 169.
5 Editorial, 1902.
6 Rutkowski, 1902, 226.
7 Sobczak, 1978, 426; Dembinska, 1979, 150.
8 Sobczak, 1978, 425.
9 Sobczak, 1968, 254.
10 Dembinska, 1979, 146.
11 Landaw, 1901, Malewski, 1910, Kozlowski, 1910.
12 Leskiewiczowa, 1978, 179.
13 Dembinska, 146.
14 ibid, 146.
15 Rutkowski, 1902.
16 Koskowski, 1908.
17 Jakimiak, 1901.
18 Lutostanski, 1880.
19 Editorial, 1905.
20 Zamoyski, 1987, 310.
21 Meller, 1994, 81.
22 ibid, 85.
23 Koryzna, 1937.
24 *Bluszcz*, 1 (1865), 159; 164; 172.
25 *Bluszcz*, 6 (1870), 120; 128; 144.
26 *Bluszcz*, 3 (1867), 228; *Bluszcz*, 32 (1896), 237; 245; 255.
27 *Bluszcz*, 32 (1896), 163; 178; 187; 194; 203; 215.
28 *Dobra Gospodyni*, 2 (1902), no 29; 30; 31; 32; 34; 38; 40; 41; 43; 44; 46; 48; 50.
29 see *Dobra Gospodyn*, 12 (1912), 147 and *Zdrowie* (1911), 865-881.
30 Jaworski 1903.
31 The nature of the dietary advice can be judged from the titles of the articles: *Slow pare o pokarmach* [A few words about food], 1 (1901) no 13; *Rady dla osob otylych* [Advice for obese persons], 1 (1901) no 19; *Kuchnia djetyczno-hygieniczna, jej sposoby i znaczenie* [Hygienic and nourishing cookery, its

methods and its significance], 2 (1902) no 8, 10, 11, 12, 15, 21; *Wplyw roznorodney zywnosci na ludzi i zwierzeta* [The impact of various foods on human beings and animals], 2 (1902) no 9; *Jak karmic niemowleta* [How to feed infants], 3 (1903) no 22, 23; *Jak odzywiac dzieci nasze* [How to feed our children], 4 (1904) no 14, 18, 19; *Wartosc odzywcza piwa* [Nutritional value of beer], 7 (1907) no 4; *Wartosc odzywcza owocu* [Nutritional value of fruit], 7 (1907) no 7; *Kuracja glodowa* [Hunger treatment], 7 (1907) no 10; *Kuracja owocowa* [Fruit treatment], 7 (1907) no 11; *Mleko Bulgarskie (jogurt)* [Bulgarian milk (joghurt)], 7 (1907) no 13; *Poziomki* [Wild strawberries], 7 (1907) no 26; *Lecznicze znaczenie owocow* [Medicinal significance of fruit], 7 (1907) no 37; *Lecznicze znaczenie czarnych jagod* [Medicinal significance of black currants], 7 (1907) no 38 ; *Mleko dla dzieci* [Milk for children], 8 (1908) no 12, 13; *Chleb* [Bread], 8 (1908) no 16; *Jak odzywiac mlodziez* [How to feed the young], 8 (1908) no 46; *Trawienie i zdrowie* [Digestion and health], 9 (1909) no 6; *Wartosc owocow* [The value of fruit], 11 (1911) no 12; *Wplyw kawy na organizm* [The impact of coffee on the body], 11 (1911) no 16; *Ja dlugo pozostac mlodym* [How to stay young longer], 12 (1912) no 4; *Karmienie niemowlat* [Feeding infants], 12 (1912) no 13; *O czestosci przyjmowania pokarmow w ciagu dnia* [About the frequency of eating during the day], 12 (1912) no 46; *Pozywienie plynne i picie podczas jedzenia* [Liquid food and drinking during meals], 12 (1912) no 51; *Sok cytrynowy jako srodek leczniczy* [Lemon juice as medicine], 14 (1914) no 6; *O glodzie i apetycie* [About hunger and appetite], 14 (1914) no 7; *Kuchnia djetetyczna dla osob pracujacych fizycznie i umyslowo* [Dietetic cookery for white-collar and blue-collar workers], 14 (1914) no 8; *Mleko dla niemowlat* [Milk for infants], 14 (1914) no 15; *Pozywienie ludzkie dawniej i dzis* [Human food now and then], 14 (1914) no 16; *Wartosc odzywcza chleba* [Nutritional value of bread], 14 (1914) no 19; *Ile i jak sie u nas jada* [How much and how we eat], 14 (1914) no 21; *Czy owoce sa zdrowe?* [Is fruit healthy?], 14 (1914) no 22, 23; *Kawa i herbata* [Coffee and tea], 14 (1914) no 24; *Ogolne uwagi o pozywieniu* [General remarks about food], 14 (1914) no 32-33; *Poznajemy wartosc pokarmow* [We learn about value of food], 14 (1914) no 48-49; *Wartosc pozywna sera i jaj* [Nutritional value of cheese and eggs], 14 (1914) no 50-51.

32 see Cwierczakiewiczowa, 1985; Norkowska, 1903; Gruszecka, 1895; Izdebska, 1894.

33 see Harvey, 1908, 46–53 and Biehler, 1916, 67–118.

34 For example, a bride-to-be was advised to equip her new household with a reference library which, among other items, included *Dyetetyka Dziecka* [Child Dietetics] by Dr Mejewski, and *Jak sie mamy zywic* [How Should We Feed Ourselves?] by Weigheldt (Editorial), 1901.

35 Meller, 1982, 226, 230.

36 Nutritional advice spread via lectures, exhibitions, and publications reached mainly the upper and the middle-classes, particularly in the urban areas, although in 1900 almost 70 per cent of the population still lived in the country. Zamoyski, 316–317.

37 For example, *Harmonia i ekonomia odzywiania* [Harmony and economy of diet], *Bluszcz*, 69 (1933) no 2; *Kartofle jako pokarm i srodek leczniczy* [Potatoes as food and medicine], *Bluszcz*, 69 (1933) no 3; *Higjena pokarmow*

[Food hygiene], *Bluszcz*, 69 (1933) no 9, 10, 20; *Krajowe jablka jako zrodlo witamin* [Polish apples as a source of vitamins], *Bluszcz*, 69 (1933) no 23; *Na letni brak apetytu* [Remedies for the lack of appetite in summer], *Bluszcz*, 69 (1933) no 27.

38 Chodecki, 1925.

39 Huberowa, 1935, 3–4.

40 Karaffa-Korbutt, 1926.

41 For example, *O witaminach czyli czynnikach deplniajacych pozywienie* [About vitamins, or supplementing elements in feeding], 1 (1925) no 2; *O walce z otyloscia* [Fighting with obesity], 1 (1925) no 6; *Kilka uwag o racjinalnym odzywianiu* [A few remarks about sensible eating], 1 (1925) no 7, 2 (1926) no 9; *O dlugowiecznosci: Odzywianie* [About longevity: Food], 3 (1925) no 7.

42 For example, Naake-Naleski, 1926; Rothfeld, 1927.

43 For example: Kader, *Teorja kaloryczna* [Calorific Theory],Wilno, 1922; Opienski *Zywienie i pozywienie* [Nourishment and Food], Lwow-Warszawa, 1929; Kramsztyk, *Nowe kierunki w nauce of zywieniu* [New Directions in Nutritional Science], Warszawa 1929; Kaplan, *O wspolczesnej wiedzy djetetycznej* [Modern Nutritional Knowledge], Wilno 1931; Strasburger and Czerny-Biernatowa, *Higjena odzywiania wraz a wskazowkami gospodarczemi* [Food Hygiene with Economical Indications], Warszawa, 1932; A. Szczygiel, *Zywienie jako zagadnienie ekonomiczne i socjalne* [Feeding as an Economical and Social Issue], Warszawa, 1936.

44 For example, Szeliga, 1929; Ochorowicz Monatowa, c 1930; Wyrobek, 1931.

45 *Pani Domu* (1932), 37; (1935), 253; (1938), 438.

46 Jaworski, 1903; Bleszynski, 1907; Bielicka, 1914.

47 E F, 1906.

48 See Ks L, 1882; Antoszka, 1896.

49 Czerny-Biernatowa and Strasburger, 1930, 24–26.

50 Huberowa, 1935, 1.

51 ibid, 2.

52 Sarysz-Stokowska, 1933.

53 Huberowa, 1935, 4.

54 *Instytut Gospodarstwa Domowego* (1938).

55 *Bluszcz*, 69 (1933), no 41.

56 Kacprzak, 1935.

57 *Pani Domu* (1935), no 4.

58 Oldziejewski, 1928, 95.

59 ibid, 95–96.

60. For example, Casimir Funk, born in Warsaw in 1884, studied in Bern and worked at the Pasteur Institute, the Wiesbaden Municipal Hospital, the University of Berlin, and the Lister Institute in London before he emigrated to the United States in 1915. Gillespie, 1972–76.

61 Leslie, 1980, 62.

62 Ihnatowicz, 1995, 1–2; Meller, 1982, 225.

63 Zamoyski, 1987, 316–17.

64 Todhunter, 1976, 361.

65 See for example, Teich, 1995.

'What the body needs': developments in medical advice, nutritional science and industrial production in the twentieth century

Annemarie de Knecht-van Eekelen and
Anneke H. van Otterloo

Just one hundred years ago a standard German work on dietary therapies – written by the German physician Ernst von Leyden (1832-1910) – was published under the title *Handbuch der Ernährungstherapie und Diätetik*. Von Leyden, professor in internal medicine and director of the 'Erste Medizinische Klinik' in Berlin, was one of the leading clinicians from the Berlin school of medicine which set the tone in Europe during the second half of the nineteenth century. Berlin had taken over this role from Vienna, so Von Leyden propagated – according to the Berlin ideas – his positivistic therapy-related approach against the therapeutic nihilism of the Second Viennese Clinic. Because of the almost complete lack of specific medication for internal diseases, Von Leyden directed his research to a hygienic-dietetic treatment of patients, especially of those with some internal disease.[1] He wrote on this choice:

> In a lot of cases the patient's diet will be a support of other therapy only; in other cases, however, the diet gives the lead and the diet alone can support life and restore health; in these cases the medication only supports the dietary therapy.[2]

The chapters in Von Leyden's *Handbuch* were written by 27 prominent professors from the German-speaking medical world and it can be regarded as the first complete overview of nutrition and dietetics, containing the results of physiological and chemical research during the nineteenth century. Indeed, during the preceding years some other books on nutrition had been published in the German language, but in none of these was the science of nutrition integrated in a clinical approach in the way Von Leyden and his collaborators had done.

However, this *Handbuch* can be seen as an interval between two periods: on the one hand the old Hippocratic approach of nutrition and diet was set aside, on the other hand the new science of nutrition still showed many gaps in its structure. Important elements of knowledge – such as the existence of vitamins and the structure of proteins – were totally lacking, while data on other dietary topics was rather scanty. In many cases no clear-cut relations between diet and disease could be established.

The *Handbuch*, especially the phrase quoted above, and the comments given from a contemporary point of view, may serve as a vivid image of the type of problems that are studied in this article. These concern the changing relations between the state of medical knowledge, nutritional insights, pharmaceutical development and dietary advice.

THE PROBLEM

For centuries the opinion was held that a moderate and diversified diet offers the optimal guarantee for maintaining health. Since the medieval period the *Regimen* of Salerno had been the leading document, containing generally accepted health prescriptions. If, in spite of these preventive measures, illnesses did occur, they could possibly be cured with the aid of dietary advice. This option was wholly dependent on the prevailing opinions about the origin, the nature and the course of a particular illness. The less clear the aetiology of an illness was, the more one's hope was put on the positive effects of certain dietary prescriptions. Thus many diets and food prescriptions had been circulating for a great many disorders. Among those, dietary advice for illnesses of the intestines (stomach, bowels, kidneys, bladder) had always taken an important place. Other illnesses, which had been counteracted for a long time by dietary rules, were those leading to a general wasting away, such as tuberculosis and hormonal disorders, for instance diabetes. Dietary prescriptions had also been formulated for blood complaints, fevers and neuroses.

The modernization of the medical sciences, which took place in The Netherlands from about the 1850s onwards, led to new initiatives. One of the indications of this important renewal consisted in the foundation of the professional 'Dutch Society for the Advancement of Medicine' in 1849. Several modern academic types of laboratory research came into being, among which the chemical and bacteriological investigations were of greatest importance. At the end of the nineteenth century ideas about the causes of some illnesses had undergone far-reaching changes; theories could be founded on research results. This situation of rapid growth of scientific medical knowledge continued in the twentieth century, with varying speed for different diseases.

An important aspect of this development in the medical – and adjoining biological and chemical – sciences, consisted in the increasing differentiation and specialization of knowledge concerning the special parts, organs and functions of the body, for instance the function of the metabolism. This was one of the incentives for the growth and further development of a separate science of nutrition after World War II. Another incentive was the increasing insight into the structure and composition of foodstuffs by chemical and microbiological investigation.[3]

In this article we will focus on the remarkable changes in medical and nutritional dietary advice concerning the cure and prevention of illnesses during the twentieth century. How can this interesting development be described and interpreted from a historical and sociological point of view? Our approach is as follows. First we will specify briefly the social context and some long-term social trends, to which changes in dietary advice may be connected. Next, these trends will be illustrated by means of two cases, tuberculosis and coronary heart disease. These cases jointly cover the whole century, occurring respectively roughly before and after World War II. Finally, some concluding remarks will be made.

THE SOCIAL CONTEXT

Since the 1890s, about the time the *Handbuch* was published, several developments which had already started much earlier in the century accelerated substantially under the impetus of new economic growth in The Netherlands. Industrialization of food production was on its way, and the establishment of many modern industries goes back to this decennium. Modernization also took place in the (medical) sciences, especially in the form of an increasing differentiation and specialization of knowledge.

Research in the field of food and nutrition was obviously of particular importance for advice in dietary treatment of illnesses. The relationship between food and health was seen as complicated; biological and chemical research nevertheless slowly succeeded in offering some understanding of the quality and quantity of food needed. Problems as to the composition and the amount of food deemed necessary for the maintenance of health could be solved in this way. These insights were based on opinions about the average quantity of nutrients and the energy-value of food-intake per day in relation to age, sex, etc. Nutritional research, which was done in an increasingly sophisticated manner, provided data on 'necessary' nutrients. Details on the chemical structures of the main groups of carbohydrates, fats and proteins became available, and a new group – the vitamins – was discovered.

The fundamental knowledge about human nutritional needs, undernourishment and (later on) over-nourishment, opened the possibility for a second type of research. Investigations were made into the detrimental effects of certain foods and nutrients on health. Examples are the research into carcinogenic substances and into the undesirable presence of certain nutrients in food, in relation to cardio-vascular diseases. All these types of research have led to advice about the choice of foods and nutrients. Such advice concerns the equation of food with energy, as well as the omission of certain elements.

The increase of knowledge about food and nutrition and other relevant medical fields, such as pharmacology, had a far-reaching influence on changes in the role of diet in the treatment of illnesses in the period studied.

Although this statement may be obvious, it is useful to realize that this process got entangled with at least two other important long-term trends. Firstly, we aim at the use of medicines as a treatment of illnesses; this method increasingly began to take the place of diet. Secondly, the curing of illnesses with the help of dietary advice was replaced in the long run by (partly diet-supported) measures of prevention. In this last case one may think of industrially produced 'healthy' foods and of food supplements like nutriceuticals.

Moreover, the two changes in treatment from diet to medicine and from cure to prevention have not been dependent only on the growth of scientific knowledge. They rely on, additionally, the presence of another societal development, that is to say the expansion of the food and pharmaceutical industries. In the decennia after World War II in particular, these industries began to apply the new medical and chemical knowledge with ever-increasing speed. Companies started to equip their own laboratories, while employing their own researchers in order to be able to sell their products, preferably using health claims. Doctors, therefore, lost their exclusive authority to give dietary advice in the case of health problems. In the course of the century other social groups, in addition to doctors and other health functionaries, presented themselves as influential parties in the field of diet and health. Private organizations, the government and, last but not least, the patients and consumers themselves, all obtained a more or less influential opinion in questions of diet and health. The developments mentioned belong to the complicated and changing social context which must be taken into account when trying to answer the question we have posed on the remarkable twentieth century evolution of dietary advice.

Finally, we cannot remain silent on a more general and well-known change in the conditions of Dutch society. The expansion of the food trade and food industry was a part of the general economic revival in The Netherlands. The improvement in the standard of living since the 1890s – with ups and downs in the first half of the century – was intimately related to this development. Both have been prominent factors in a social change that is crucial for the discussion on diet and health: the evolution from scarcity of food into plenty.[4] In connection with this fundamental historical change, the prevalence of deficiency-related illnesses decreased very rapidly. However, the frequency of other affluence-related disorders increased.

TWO CASE-STUDIES AND THEIR SOURCES

To illustrate the broad trends mentioned above, we will present two case-studies: one refers to diet for patients with tuberculosis or pulmonary consumption as this disease was called, the other is about the diet of patients with coronary complaints. They are examples of the change from dietetical to medicinal treatment and of the development of dietetic cure to dietetic prevention. The study on tuberculosis starts around the beginning of the twentieth century and concentrates on the 'Dutch Health-resort for Poor Patients with Pulmonary Consumption' in Davos (Switzerland).[5] After a short introduction on different strategies in the treatment of this disease, we will focus on the importance of diet in the cure of these patients. The study closes after World War II; at a time when the possibility of medical treatment with specific medication of the antibiotic *streptomycin* was introduced. In 1946 the tuberculostatic properties of *para-amino-salycil-acid* (PAS) were discovered and in 1952 *isoniazide* was introduced. *Isoniazide* together with *rifampicin*, first synthesized in 1956, are today's most important medicines in the treatment of tuberculosis.[6]

The possibility of effective medical treatment does not mean that the disease has been eradicated in The Netherlands. On the contrary, during the last ten years there has been a significant increase in the number of patients with tuberculosis in our country. Largely, this is caused by the immigration of people from third world countries. However, ambulant treatment with the above mentioned medicines during a period of nine months cures the patient definitively. Hospital treatment is needed in some special cases only; for instance if there is a social indication or a complex disease pattern.[7]

The case-study on coronary heart diseases may be considered in certain respects to be the opposite of the former one. While tuberculosis was a wasting disease – often related to poor conditions of life – coronary heart diseases are associated with an affluent life style. Of course, diseases of heart and blood vessels are not new, but as they gradually came to be regarded as the main cause of mortality in the second half of the twentieth century, the interest in the cure and prevention of these diseases increased. Because no real cure is as yet available – surgery takes away symptoms only and medication has to be taken permanently – the main topic is prevention. Change of diet plays the most important role in all prevention campaigns.

To get some idea of how dietary advice was linked to scientific insights and how nutritionists, physicians, industries and the government have tried to influence the consumer's behaviour on this matter, relevant medical and nutritionists' journals are a good source. In addition, scientific and popular books on diet may be 'goldmines' of information.

In the discussion of tuberculosis we will use Von Leyden's *Handbuch* as the starting-point of the scientific approach to dietetics. Even though there is no Dutch translation of this volume, it can be argued that – because of the strong relationship between Dutch and German physicians – the *Handbuch* had the same position in The Netherlands as it had in the German-speaking world. Medical books and journals from the German speaking countries were widely used in The Netherlands and many German professors were teaching medicine in our universities at the end of the nineteenth century. Moreover, we have also used the archives of the 'Dutch Health-resort for Poor Patients with Pulmonary Consumption' in Davos (Switzerland).

For our case-study on coronary diseases and the changing opinions on diet and nutrition we studied both scientific and popular books. The principal sources used were: the *Nederlands Tijdschrift voor Geneeskunde* (Dutch Medical Journal), the leading journal for physicians which was first published in 1857, and the journal *Voeding* (Nutrition) which started publication in 1939. Both journals are still on the market.

The first case: pulmonary consumption

TAKING THE CURE FOR PULMONARY CONSUMPTION

After Robert Koch's (1843–1910) announcement (1882) of his finding the tuberculosis bacteria, little changed in the therapy of 'the number 1 people's disease', as consumption was called in The Netherlands. The tuberculosis bacteria could be found in the patients, but destroying these pathogens was not yet possible. Until 1945 the treatment of tuberculosis was characterized by a symptomatic treatment as no medication against the bacteria itself existed. Two directions can be discerned in this treatment: one propagated the isolation of patients in health-resorts in some unpolluted environment – woods, seashore or mountains – far from the unhealthy cities; the other promoted home treatment supervised by consultation bureaux.[8] Both directions developed in The Netherlands, first as private enterprises and charities, later with some government support, but still organised by a 'Central Society', an association of private initiatives. Preferences for home treatment of patients with consumption or for treatment in a health-resort depended on the different opinions about the aetiology of the disease.

Around the turn of the century consumption was seen not only as a disease of the proletariat, caused by poor social-economic circumstances and genetic weakening of the lower classes, but also of adolescents, young intellectuals with a delicate frame and a certain disposition for this illness. Mass treatment in a – mostly expensive – health-resort was not a realistic possibility, because of the large numbers of patients with low incomes. In The Netherlands some societies were established to exploit what were called 'people's health-resorts', but the number of patients who could be treated in these institutions was only a drop in the ocean. A special task of these institutions was – in the eyes of the members of these societies and the leading physicians – the education of the lower-class patients in how to live a clean and healthy life. It is obvious that this goal could not be reached as long as treatment in this type of establishment was limited to the middle and higher social classes.

From 1900 onwards the first health-resorts were established in The Netherlands, but some years before there had already been a Dutch initiative in Davos (Switzerland). This initiative dates from 1890 when J A Wijnhoff (1854–1921), physician in the Town Hospital in Utrecht, spoke in a meeting of the Dutch medical society. He was in favour of 'climate therapy' in people's health-resorts. By 'climate therapy' he meant the use of hydro-therapy, open air treatment, gymnastics and 'strengthening food' in 'bracing air'. This could be found in the mountains, and in The Netherlands too. In his opinion labourers did not belong in hospitals but in these health-resorts, which could be founded by charities.[9]

During the second half of the nineteenth century Davos was well known as a place to take a cure for pulmonary consumption, but a stay there was quite expensive. Nevertheless, there was a considerable number of wealthy Dutch tuberculosis patients who wanted to do more for their poorer fellow patients in an exclusively Dutch health-resort. In 1896 a society was founded to exploit such a home. In 1897 – over a century ago – the 'Nederlandsch Sanatorium voor minvermogende longlijders te Davos-Platz' (Dutch Health-resort for Poor Patients with Pulmonary Consumption) opened its doors. Today there still exists a Dutch clinic in Davos, no longer for patients with pulmonary consumption, but for the treatment of asthma. Davos always had a hard time to prove its superior value above the health-resorts in The Netherlands. In fact, only by its high altitude did it differ from health-resorts in the Low Countries. Nevertheless, favourable reports on the cure in Davos were published, especially because of its bond regime.

IDEAS ON THE NUTRITION OF PATIENTS WITH PULMONARY CONSUMPTION

An idea of the cure for patients with consumption is given in the 1898 lecture of Henri Johan Adriaan van Voornveld (1869–1943), who for some years already had a private practice in Davos. He can be seen as an authority in the field of cures for consumption. For many years he worked as medical supervisor of the Dutch health-resort.[10] In his opinion pulmonary consumption is not exclusively a disease of the lungs, but of the body as a whole. So the patient can only recover when he adapts his way of life. A healthy life includes a lot of fresh air and of course a healthy diet. In fact, this is the old Hippocratic approach to illness in which the balance between the 'six non-naturals' – among which the diet is the most important – is disturbed.

A healthy diet in Van Voornveld's view is an 'ample' diet containing a combination of meat, vegetables, fruit and farinaceous foods. All of these foods should be offered in large amounts, as the patient should eat in fact more than he feels able to. Moreover, he should eat slowly and drink little by little. Milk (only cooked milk should be used) – one of the essentials in the diet – 'has to be sipped; a glass of milk may not be emptied in less than ten minutes'.

For more details on this diet we can study the chapter on 'Ernährungstherapie bei Lungenkrankheiten' (Dietary therapy in pulmonary consumption) in Von Leyden's *Handbuch*. It was written by an expert in this field, the physician Peter Dettweiler (1837–1904), director of the 'erste Volks-heilstätte für unbemiddelte Lungenkranke' (first people's health-resort for poor patients with pulmonary consumption) in Falkenstein i.T., established by him in 1876. Dettweiler was a pupil of the German physician Hermann Brehmer who is said to have introduced the 'Sanatoriums Frischluft Liegekur'.[11] In his chapter in the *Handbuch* Dettweiler published lengthy tables with foods (arranged according to quantities: of the total, of protein, fat, carbohydrates and calories) used in his health-resort. He also gave examples of a week's menu and of individual ratios. According to his regime there was a meal at 08.00 and 10.00 in the morning and at 13.00 and 19.00. At 16.00 and 21.00 some glasses of milk had to be taken. Eight glasses of milk a day was normal. The use of large quantities of butter strikes us in these menus, as well as the recommendation for strong liquors, a combination that – according to Dettweiler – had several advantages:

> For patients with pulmonary consumption a diet with a lot of fat is advised, especially plenty of butter of a good quality and cream should be used, and bacon can be advised as well [. . .] Some strong liquor along with fat food is good for the digestion.[12]

For Dettweiler alcohol was not only a stimulant, but also a source of extra calories, and he even asserted the effect of alcohol as a febrifuge.

MILK

However, milk and milk products were the real 'pièce-de-résistance' in these diets; milk was used as such and in all kinds of combinations: as hot cocoa, in tea or coffee, in porridge etc. Dettweiler also gave the instruction to sip the milk or even to use a spoon to eat it. There is no explanation given for this, but in my opinion [AdK] one thought was to promote the digestion of the milk, as the slow ingestion would stimulate the production and secretion of digestive juices.

The use of milk for patients with pulmonary consumption was not an invention of Dettweiler. In some older literature – for instance in popular health handbooks – one can read: 'Animal food, with some fat and salt, seems to be most advisable; of course milk is the first choice.'[13] Or in another book by the same author

> The patient should take care to have good blood and to do this he needs nourishing foods, easy to digest and with a considerable amount of fat and salt; the best food is milk.[14]

Returning to Davos, we see the use of Dettweiler's directions, not only in the Dutch health-resort, but in the cure in general. Dettweiler's directions fitted nicely into the ideas of one of the leading Swiss physicians, Alexander Spengler (1827–1901), who was the initiator of the development of Davos as **the** place to take the cure.[15] Spengler – who together with the Dutch business man Willem Jan Holsboer (1834–1898) – developed Davos from a sleepy village to a leading 'Kurort', wrote about his patient's diet:

> The diet should be hearty and easy to digest: meat, milk, eggs, fat, fat produc-
> ers and wine are the basic ingredients. A diet with meat is the best when it is
> prepared in the right way; game is the first choice. Ample use of milk has to be
> planned and adapted according to individual needs.[16]

Moreover, Karl Turban (1856–1935), the 'auctor intellectualis' of the cure in Davos, studied in Dettweiler's clinic in Falkenstein. Turban introduced a regimen of six meals a day, with one to two litres of milk (which was said to be of especially good quality in Davos) and little salt and spices.[17] Indeed, in the Dutch health-resort notes were taken on the amount of milk and the number of eggs a patient should consume. In the Davos archive I [AdK] found a paper from 1906 showing that each of the 35 patients who were treated there at that time, had his/her own prescription of the number of eggs and mugs of milk: these varied from two to seven mugs of milk (mostly five) and one to two eggs a day.

On the whole very few data on the diet were found in the Davos' archive. Letters from 1900 show that some products were ordered in The Netherlands, for instance from the 'Hollandsche Conservenfabriek' (Alblasserdam) (Dutch Canning Factory) and the 'Cacao- en Chocolaad-fabrikanten De Erve H de Jong' (Wormerveer) (Cocoa and Chocolate Factory) to supply 'De Jong's cocoa', while 70 kilos of stockfish, six Gouda and six Leiden cheeses were ordered from 'J de Graeff export and import' (Amsterdam).

A 'Dutch meal' was prepared, which meant that large quantities of cooked vegetables and fruit were served, and that the evening meal consisted of bread and butter next to some hot dish. A large amount of fat was used and a litre of milk a day was necessary to reach the prescribed daily amount of 3500 cal. No main changes occurred in this diet until World War II. Only during World War I did some problems arise with the distribution of foods, while prices rose considerably. Nevertheless, one could report that the situation was under control.[18] It was possible to import more butter, cheese, sugar, beans and peas from The Netherlands. A rationing of bread was organised as late as October 1917 and lasted until 1919, so the period of want was relatively short.[19] In World War II the food supply came under pressure again. During that period the health-resort took to gardening and produced cabbages, carrots, turnips and leeks for its own kitchen.[20]

During the early years after the War patients could be sent to Davos thanks to financing from the 'Don Suisse pour des victimes de la guerre', a Swiss initiative. In July 1948 this funding came to an end and from that moment the Dutch health-resort got into increasing financial problems, because of a lack of patients. Around 1950, many health-resorts in Davos had to close down as their cure for pulmonary consumption had become obsolete. Tuberculosis had become an ordinary infectious disease to be

treated with antibiotics. The Dutch clinic survived, but had to change to
other patients and another type of care.

SOME CONCLUSIONS ON THE CASE OF
PULMONARY CONSUMPTION

There is an important body of literature on the treatment of tuberculosis
in the inter-war period. However, most articles were written on the surgical treatment of the disease, the X-ray diagnosis, the organisation of the
consultation bureaux and health-resorts, and the selection of patients for
treatment or cure. In one of the few Dutch books for physicians written
on patients' diets the physician Pieter Johannes de Bruïne Ploos van Amstel
(1864–1939) discussed the 'Gerson's, Hermannsdorfer and Sauerbruch diet'
for patients with pulmonary consumption, a diet without any salt. This
type of diet was based on the assumption that tuberculosis caused an excess
of sodium and a shortage of calcium in the patient's body. Gerson's diet
was slightly modified by Adolf Herrmannsdorfer and supported by the well
known German professor of surgery Ferdinand Sauerbruch (1875–1951).[21]
However, these ideas did not get any foothold in the diet of the Davos'
patients. Their diet remained unchanged for over 50 years. In the health-
resort one even sees no influence of the introduction of the vitamin concept
in the science of nutrition. This could be explained by the fact that patients
taking the cure had no deficient diet; indeed, just the contrary. Sunshine,
milk, vegetables, fruit – all these sources of vitamins were an essential part
of their daily cure. So no change was needed there.

Another striking fact is that – at least in the study described – industrially
prepared foods played hardly any role in the diet. All ingredients were those
of an ordinary Dutch meal as it was prepared before World War II. Bread
and butter, soup, a main course with meat, potatoes and vegetables, and
a dessert – this was not special. The addition of extra milk, cream, butter,
wines and spirits was thought necessary to increase the patient's calorie
intake, but these products were not specially prepared for these patients.
Cocoa was an extra addition to the patient's diet, as cocoa was thought to
give strength. Moreover, cocoa – as cocoa drink – made the consumption of
more milk possible. No special industrially prepared food for tuberculosis
patients is mentioned; I did not come across any 'anti-tuberculosis chocolate', 'pulmonary consumption preventing margarine' or anything of that
kind.

As antibiotic treatment appeared quite suddenly, from one moment to
another pulmonary consumption was looked on as an infection for which a
dietary regimen was no longer needed. In the prevention of tuberculosis the
diet played no part either; the X-ray programme, scanning the population
at risk, was the new method to trace infected individuals. Not only did the
health-resorts close their doors or change to another type of patient, but the
system of consultation bureaux for tuberculosis – monitoring home treat-

ment – lost their function too. But, luckily for them, other diseases took over the role of tuberculosis, so new programmes were developed. One of these was the prevention of the coronary heart diseases.

The second case: coronary heart diseases

THE RELATION BETWEEN OBESITY AND DISEASE

For some past centuries a relation between obesity and disease – especially chronic diseases – was known to exist. The first systematic study on this relation, however, dates from the years before World War II. In the period 1938–1943 an inquiry was held among 2,400 inhabitants of a Baltimore district (USA) about the prevalence of chronic illnesses. Height and weight of these people were measured and statistics were used to correlate these data with their complaints. The conclusion was that

> obesity could be a predisposing factor to explain the significant relation to the occurrence of these diseases (namely coronary heart diseases, hypertension, arthritis and diabetes.[22]

This rather carefully formulated proposition set the scene for subsequent research all over the world. On the one hand campaigns were started to persuade people to reduce calorie intake, and on the other more research was needed to specify those factors in the diet which could cause this relation with coronary heart diseases. In research priority was given to the relation between cholesterol and lipids in the diet and coronary heart diseases. This research was stimulated by the finding that coronary heart diseases had taken over the role from tuberculosis: they had become the number one cause of death. In 1910 only nine per cent of deaths were attributed to heart and vascular diseases. This number increased to sixteen per cent in 1930, 37 per cent in 1950 and 45 per cent in 1970. From the 1970s onwards a slow decrease can be noted to 40 per cent in 1992. In absolute figures: 12,068 men and 9,026 women died in 1992 of coronary diseases.[23]

CHOLESTEROL AND LIPIDS: RESEARCH, INDUSTRY AND PUBLIC OPINION

Pathological anatomical research – as was carried out at the beginning of the twentieth century – showed, by colouring of the preparations, that arteriosclerotic changes of the vascular wall contained lipid substances. Analyses of these lipids demonstrated the presence of cholesterol. So from 1910 on cholesterol was judged the most suspect factor for the development of arteriosclerosis. The idea was that the digested cholesterol (especially present in animal foodstuffs) would enter the vascular wall and accumulate there. In the 1940s, however, Ancel Keys and his collaborators in the USA showed that the cholesterol level of the blood is not permanently influenced by cholesterol in the diet. Together with increasing knowledge on the mechanism of production of cholesterol by the human liver and the feedback mechanism to keep standard levels of blood cholesterol, the views on cholesterol intake changed. Already in the 1950s cholesterol intake could no longer be seen as the main cause of arteriosclerosis.

Researchers started looking for other ingredients in the diet that could be responsible for the fatty degeneration of the vascular wall. In 1956 H M Sinclair suggested an unbalanced ratio between saturated and unsaturated fatty acids as the cause of arteriosclerosis. Chemical research of blood vessels indeed showed increased levels of linoleic acid. However, these were only some of the findings from the 1950s, and others showed contradictory results. This resulted in an unclear discussion on the pros and cons of dietary products that claimed to lower the risk of vascular diseases. There was no 'communis opinio' among chemists, nutritionists and physicians. One party stated that the intake of poly-unsaturated fatty acids decreases the levels of cholesterol and lipids in the blood, while saturated fatty acids increase these levels. In their opinion a diet with more poly-unsaturated fatty acids would have a beneficial effect on health. Their opponents did not believe in a relation between blood cholesterol levels and the development of arteriosclerosis.

For the food industry the findings on fatty acids were sufficient to start research on oils with cholesterol-lowering properties. In 1960 several products were marketed: the Calvé factory in Delft started with vegetable oils – maize-oil with 34–62 per cent and sunflower oil with 51–68 per cent linoleic acid – but even more important was the spreadable fat Becel, a Unilever product.[24] The technological possibilities of using these fats in margarine had just been developed. For a long time unsaturated fatty acids had been unsuitable because of their weak structure and their changing into saturated fatty acids during the production process. Unilever had tested Becel on 70 of its employees and indeed had found a 20 per cent decrease of blood cholesterol levels, with which result they started their advertising campaign (Fig 1).[25] With the margarine industry in the camp of the adherents of the poly-unsaturated fatty acids, the dairy industry found itself in the opposite camp.[26]

In The Netherlands the first real debate on dietary lipids and arteriosclerosis dates from the 1960s. In this debate the views of the different experts were heavily influenced by their position in the world of nutrition. Indeed, two opponents can be discerned: the dairy industry on the one side and the margarine industry on the other. When we read the text of a lecture held by the chemist C J F Böttcher, professor at Leiden University, on the occasion of 'Dairy Day 1961', entitled 'Do food lipids play a role in the occurrence of arteriosclerosis and coronary thrombosis?', we have to ask ourselves: to which camp does Böttcher belong?[27] One can not presume that a **Dairy Day**

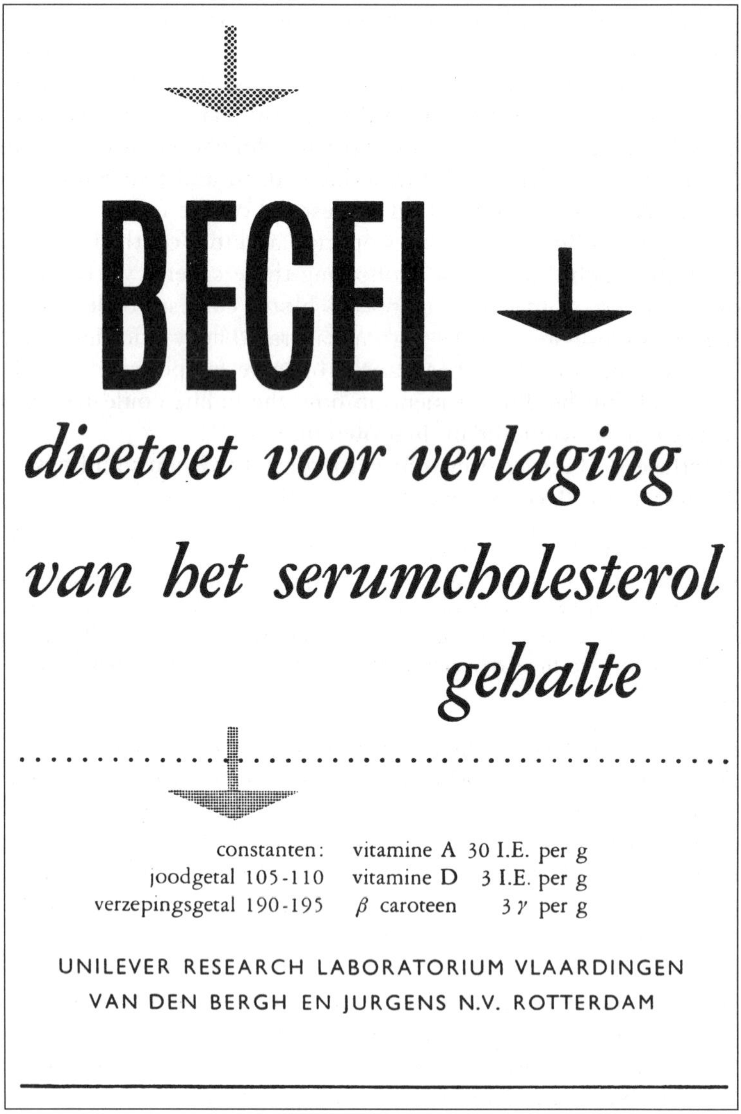

BECEL

dieetvet voor verlaging

van het serumcholesterol

gehalte

constanten:	vitamine A 30 I.E. per g
joodgetal 105-110	vitamine D 3 I.E. per g
verzepingsgetal 190-195	β caroteen 3 γ per g

UNILEVER RESEARCH LABORATORIUM VLAARDINGEN

VAN DEN BERGH EN JURGENS N.V. ROTTERDAM

Fig. 1. *First advertisement for Becel 'dietary fat for lowering the blood cholesterol level' in the* Dutch Medical Journal *17 December 1960.*

is the place to hear all the pros of margarine. Certainly, we do not. Böttcher even stated that 'animal food was put in an unfavourable light'. In his opinion the relation between blood cholesterol and arteriosclerosis was rendered out of date by new research, and he stressed the finding of the differences in fatty acid composition of the vascular wall. He did not see enough arguments to choose for a prevalence of either vegetable or animal foodstuffs. His advice to the public was to reduce the dietary intake of fats and carbohydrate as a whole, an advice as old as the Hippocratic doctrine on temperance.

The same Hippocratic view was held by the physician S A ten Bokkel Huinink, also one of the speakers at this meeting. He drew attention to the results of his colleague, physician J J Groen, who had studied the daily diet of monks from Trappist and Benedictine orders, and had found a significant influence of the level of blood cholesterol on the incidence of arteriosclerosis.[28] In Ten Bokkel Huinink's opinion and that of 'the large majority of physicians'- as he stated – the following three criteria were relevant for the origin of arteriosclerosis: increased blood cholesterol levels, obesity and high blood pressure. A diet with unsaturated fatty acids he found dubious and even unsafe. 'We physicians propagate temperance', Ten Bokkel Huinink said; but he did not mention how the public could be convinced that a frugal meal would be in their own interest.[29]

Nevertheless, Unilever drew more attention to Groen's findings in their advertisements for Becel, stating:

> Becel lowers the blood cholesterol level without a distressing diet. Prof dr J J Groen says this: 'Especially it has to be expected that introducing food habits lowering the blood cholesterol level, shall eliminate one of the main causes of myocardial infarction'. [...] Becel is a very important ingredient of a therapeutic diet [...] Becel also fits extremely well in a preventive diet for potential patients. (Fig 2)

The view of one of his colleagues, the Amsterdam specialist in internal medicine M Koster, who had worked with Groen on this topic, was somewhat different, but led to the same advice. Koster did believe in a causal relation between a high caloric intake and coronary problems, but – as did Böttcher – not in blood cholesterol as a specific factor. Therefore he discarded the use of any special cholesterol-lowering diet or of medication that supposedly would lower the blood cholesterol level.[30]

In the 1960s, nevertheless, an important part of the scientific research in The Netherlands concentrated on the role of cholesterol in the diet. A study by the 'Nederlands Instituut voor Volksvoeding' (Dutch Institute for People's Nutrition) showed in 1962 no significant correlation between dietary fat and blood cholesterol in the elderly, not even a relation between body weight and blood cholesterol.[31] One may wonder if these were the results required by the provider of the research grant, the 'Royal Industries T Duyvis Jz', manufacturers of all types of mayonnaise and other products with a significant fat content. The fact that this industry subsidized research in this field, however, shows how important the matter already was. In this case the food industry acted ahead of other groups concerned, namely the nutritionists and physicians, and the consumers.

In the marketing of margarine, health claims for certain constituents had always been a strong weapon against butter. As soon as the possibility existed to produce margarines with a low fat content and especially with

Becel verlaagt het serum-cholesterol gehalte zonder deprimerend dieet

Prof. Dr. J. J. Groen zegt dit: „In het bijzonder is te verwachten dat invoering van voedingsgewoonten, die het serum-cholesterol (en triglyceride) tot daling zullen brengen, althans één der belangrijkste causale wortels aan de pathogenese van het myocard infarkt zouden ontnemen."

In Becel dieetmargarine is de verhouding poly-onverzadigde: verzadigde vetzuren optimaal, namelijk 2,5 :1. De rest van de vetzuursamenstelling is enkelvoudig onverzadigd en dus neutraal. Daarom vormt Becel een zeer belangrijk onderdeel van een **therapeutisch dieet** voor hart- en vaatpatiënten. Bovendien heeft Becel een prettige psychologische werking, omdat Uw patiënt zijn tafelvrijheid behoudt. Want Becel smeert, smaakt, bakt en braadt als gewone margarine.
Ook in een **preventief dieet** voor potentiële hart- en vaatpatiënten past Becel uitstekend.

BECEL SIGNALEMENT: Becel bestaat voor ca 90% uit zuivere zonnebloemolie en bevat dus 50-55% cis-cis-linolzuur; ongezouten; zuiver plantaardig. Voor Uw patiënt in blikjes van 250 gram verkrijgbaar bij apotheken, drogisten en vele levensmiddelenzaken.

Dieetvoorschriften en wetenschappelijke informatie worden U gaarne op aanvraag toegezonden door Van den Bergh & Jurgens N.V., Postbus 590, Rotterdam.

becel
DIEETMARGARINE DIE UW PATIËNT ZIJN TAFELVRIJHEID LAAT

Fig. 2. *Advertisement for Becel using a quotation from Professor Groen in the* Dutch Medical Journal *6 May 1967.*

a low content of saturated fatty acids, the margarine industry wanted to profit from the ideas on the relation between certain lipids and arteriosclerosis. With claims such as 'the highest percentage of poly-unsaturated fatty acids', 'the lowest percentage of saturated fatty acids' and 'produced from 100 per cent golden maize oil', special dietary margarine was marketed.[32] Even though the producers themselves were not so sure about the health effects of poly-unsaturated fatty acids, they stated that the consumption of margarine with more cis-cis-linoleic acid would not do any harm. But more research was needed.[33]

The public got more and more interested in this problem too, and addressed themselves to the supposed experts, namely the physicians. The fact that quite a number of questions were asked on this topic and published in the *Nederlands Tijdschrift voor Geneeskunde* (Dutch Medical Journal), shows that the medical world was uncertain about what advice they should give. Most questions concerned the influence of some foodstuff on the blood cholesterol level: for instance a diet with fish[34] or the use of a special oil. The answers were not always very clear. Indeed, eating fish was advised because of the presence of fish oil, consisting of poly-unsaturated fatty acids, and these were supposed to cause 'an important decrease of blood cholesterol'. About another oil (ground nut oil) the experts were not sure: it had long saturated chains, which were supposed to be harmful, but 'until now [...] there is no indication of a special influence of these on the process of arteriosclerosis'.[35]

Consumers, organised in the 'Consumentenbond' (Consumers' Association), already took part in this discussion at an early stage. We find the Consumers' Association on the side of those physicians who propagate temperance, recommending the reduction of dietary fat as a whole. The Consumers' Association had made analyses of the levels of poly-unsaturated fatty acids in different dietetic margarines – such as Becel, Vegana and Diät-san – and was not convinced that the constituents would really contribute to a decreased chance of developing arteriosclerosis.[36]

To conclude this part we can state that in the 1960s most physicians stressed the use of a low-calorie diet to prevent obesity. In this diet a choice of foods with a high content of poly-unsaturated fatty acid was advisable, but they were not in favour of the use of special products to lower cholesterol. The consumers were uncertain about this matter. The Consumers' Association took the side of the physicians and was sceptical about the claims of some new types of dietetic margarine. 'Eat less' was the soundest advice.

FAT ON THE POLITICAL AGENDA

During the 1960s the Dutch government became concerned about the changing food pattern in The Netherlands. The 1968 report of a 'Commissie van de Voedingsraad ter oriëntering omtrent de Voeding en Voedingstoestand in Nederland (Oriënteringscommissie)' (Orientating Committee) – published both in the journal for nutrition *Voeding* and in the medical journal *Nederlands Tijdschrift voor Geneeskunde* – showed an overall increase of the use of fats and a decrease of protein and carbohydrate consumption in that decade.[37] These fats mainly consisted of saturated fatty acids. According to nutritionist De Wijn (later professor of nutrition in Leiden University) one could not be absolutely sure about the role of the different dietary elements on the development of arteriosclerosis, but in his view there was an 'accumulation of signs' that a diet with less fat and more (poly)-unsaturated fatty acids would have a 'positive influence' on the prevention of arteriosclerosis by lowering the blood cholesterol.

Based on the opinion of the Orientating Committee the 'Voedingsraad' (Nutrition Board), an advisory board of the ministries of health and of agriculture, devised the following guidelines for the public:

- fat intake should be diminished,
- butter, margarine and animal fat should be replaced by products containing poly-unsaturated fatty acids such as vegetable oil,
- skimmed milk should be used instead of full-cream milk.

The next step was to get more political support for this advice. In 1973 the 'Voedingsraad' published again on this matter in an answer to the question of the ministry of health: 'Are advice and/or measures needed regarding the amount and/or the constituents of fat in the diet of the Dutch population?'[38] To answer this a special committee had been formed with expert nutritionists and physicians. Among the physicians were Groen and Koster, whose ideas have been mentioned before, but also the emeritus professor in internal medicine F S P van Buchem (1897–1979), who had started a large, long-term epidemiological study on nutrition and arteriosclerosis in Zutphen (The Netherlands) in 1960. This study is still running and is part of the 'Seven Countries Study'; in 1978 the direction of the Zutphen Study was taken over by the epidemiologist D Kromhout, now working in the RIVM (State Institute for Health and Environment).[39]

The interesting thing in the advice of the 'Voedingsraad' is the fact that the eighteen members of the committee did not reach an agreement. After elaborate discussions two recommendations were published: a majority and a minority recommendation. The majority recommendation consisted of two parts: 1) Proposals for the composition of people's nutrition; and 2) Guidelines to change the diet of the Dutch population. The proposals were especially on the reduction of calorie intake to prevent obesity, the reduction of the total fat intake and of saturated fats in particular, and an increase of linoleic acid to reduce the risk of arteriosclerosis. This part of the majority recommendation was the crucial point which was not supported by the one person who had formulated his minority recommendation. From the text published in *Voeding* one can not see whose recommendation it was. However, from a publication in the *Nederlands Tijdschrift voor Geneeskunde* one gets the strong feeling that it was Van Buchem.[40] The criticism in the minority recommendation was namely focused on fat and fatty acids. In his view the present knowledge on this matter was not decisive enough to give a dietary advice to the population as a whole. Groups at risk – those with an elevated blood cholesterol – could already be determined and for them the physician could advise the use of special dietary products with poly-unsaturated fatty acids. As one can read in his article, Van Buchem used the results of his Zutphen study to argue that arteriosclerosis has a multi-factorial cause. He had not found enough arguments to pinpoint the level of blood cholesterol as the main cause of coronary problems. His colleague Koster, also a member of the committee, disagreed with Van Buchem, as his reaction in the same journal showed.[41] In Koster's view the indications were strong enough to direct the recommendation towards the population as a whole.

In retrospect Van Buchem's position was a sound one – indeed there was no unanimous result of research – and one may wonder about the fact that in The Netherlands – with a tradition of governmental non-intervention – seventeen committee members agreed on directives so manifestly attempting to influence the nutrition of the population.

INDUSTRIAL PRODUCTS: POLY-UNSATURATED FATTY ACIDS AND LINOLEIC ACID

To achieve their goals the committee had drawn up the following proposals (remember this was in the beginning of the 1970s): people were to decrease their food intake, to choose fats with a high percentage of poly-unsaturated fatty acids and linoleic acid, to use skimmed milk and dairy products, to eat whole wheat products, to use no more than two to three eggs/week and few animal organs (liver, kidney).

According to the views of the 'Voedingsraad' the guidelines could be introduced to the public only when:

- industrial products with a low fat content, enriched with linoleic acid, are available at a reasonable price and can be discerned easily from other products (by labelling);
- legal objectives against these products are withdrawn;
- press, television and all other media support the campaign;
- healthy products are available in the army, in hospitals, in canteens, restaurants etc;
- the new science of nutrition is taught in all schools and universities.

The industries producing the products mentioned had the best laughs. Unilever, producer of Becel, advertised this fat in the journal *Voeding* (1974) using these views, but – wisely – taking them not from the Committee's advice but from American sources (Fig 3). Their position became even stronger as it took till 1986 before any governmental action was taken. In *Voeding* (1980) we can find a two page Unilever advertisement discussing the pros of linoleic acid (Fig 4). They stated that the effect of linoleic acid in lowering the blood cholesterol level 'had been accepted for quite some time' and that there was the 'general advice to increase the intake of linoleic acid to *c* one third of the total fat consumption'.

THE NUTRITIONISTS

It was a hard time for the nutritionists. The government took no action, so some of the leading nutritionists, such as the Wageningen professor in nutrition, J G A J Hautvast, and R J J Hermus, working at CIVO (Central Institute for Nutrition Research), tried to generate some action.[42] They made an analysis of the health paragraphs in the programmes of the Dutch political parties and came to the conclusion that none of the parties in power had

Verklaring

door de
Food and Nutrition Board en de
American Medical Association
in juli 1972 in de
Verenigde Staten afgelegd:

,, Er is overvloedig bewijsmateriaal waarin aangetoond wordt, dat de kans op het ontstaan van hart- en vaatziekten verband houdt met een hoog gehalte aan cholesterol in het bloed.

Deze kans is - wanneer men de andere genoemde risicofactoren buiten beschouwing laat - betrekkelijk gering bij een plasmacholesterolspiegel beneden de 220 mg%, maar stijgt met iedere verhoging van de plasmacholesterolwaarde.

Ongeveer een derde van de Amerikaanse mannen, en een minder exact bekend gedeelte der vrouwen, heeft een plasmacholesterolwaarde van 220 mg% of lager bij gebruik van normale voeding. Ander materiaal bewijst dat het cholesterolgehalte van het bloed van de meeste mensen verlaagd kan worden door geëigende voedings maatregelen.

In het algemeen kan deze verlaging het gemakkelijkst bereikt worden door gedeeltelijke vervanging van verzadigde vetzuren, door meervoudig onverzadigde vetzuren - en door een vermindering van het gebruik van voedingsmiddelen, die veel cholesterol bevatten.

Voorlopige gegevens wijzen erop, dat een consequent en gedurende een aantal jaren volgehouden cholesterol-verlagend dieet, het aantal hartaanvallen bij mannen van middelbare leeftijd kan verminderen.

Zoals te verwachten is bij een dergelijke chronische ziekte, lijkt vroegtijdig ingrijpen effektiever dan ingrijpen wanneer de afwijking reeds manifest is."

• Bron: Nutrition Reviews October 1972 vol. 30 No. 10

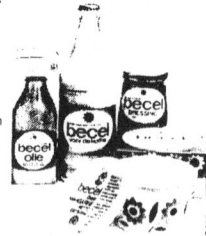

Becel - voor een serumcholesterolverlagend dieet

Fig. 3. *Advertisement for Becel in the journal* Voeding *(1974) using a statement from the* Food and Nutrition Board and the American Medical Association.

any ideas on this topic. In their opinion the government showed little vision on the nutrition issue. They pointed to the physicians too, who were not prepared to act according to a nutrition strategy and hardly had any feeling for the importance of nutrition for people's health.

This seems not the best way to convince physicians of their responsibilities. And certainly not the heading of a subsequent article in this medical journal in 1980: 'Nutrition and coronary heart diseases, a ramshackle pie in the sky?'[43] This was written by the most influential cardiologist of the day, the Utrecht professor in cardiology F L Meijler. He asked for more dis-

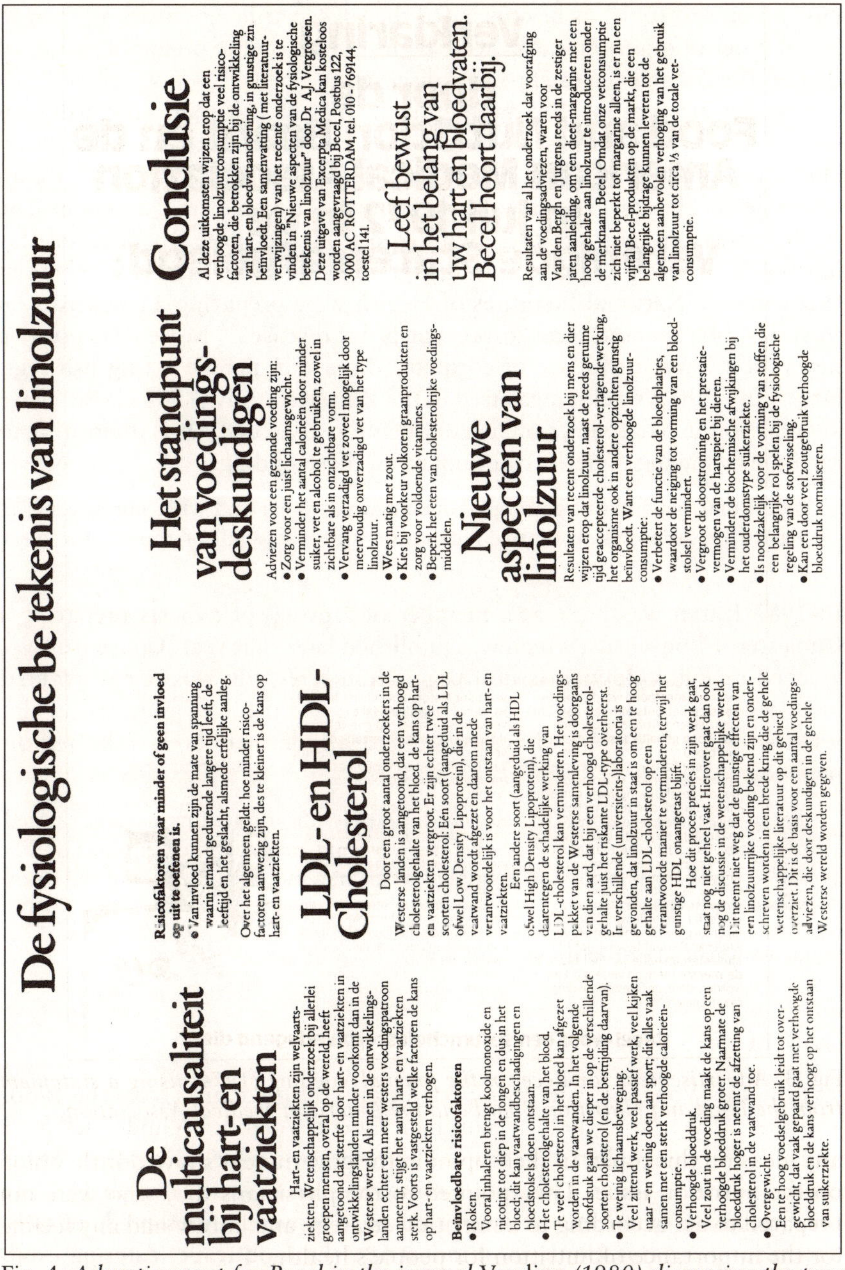

Fig. 4. *Advertisement for Becel in the journal* Voeding *(1980) discussing the pros of linoleic acid.*

cussion on this topic, as he concluded that in scientific literature an increasing number of question marks were being placed on the predictory value of diet on the occurrence of coronary diseases.

Another attempt in 1985 by the biochemist M B Katan, now professor in nutrition in Wageningen University, to show the need for a consensus on cholesterol, had more effect and the topic returned to the agendas. Katan was able to give an overview of data on blood cholesterol levels in The Netherlands and compare these with data from the USA. Dutch blood cholesterol levels were considerably higher than those in the USA, where at that time the National Institutes of Health were preparing a consensus on 'lowering blood cholesterol to prevent heart disease'.[44] Moreover, positive news on a lower incidence of coronary disease in people eating fish regularly (200–300 g/week), measured in the Zutphen study (1960–1980), gave support to the older views on fish oil mentioned earlier.[45] It is interesting to read the following American comment on these findings:

> We all may get tired of getting advice on what to eat and what not to eat. [...] put it [the supposed preventive factor] in a one-a-day pill or capsule for everybody.[46]

In 1987 Katan was back as a member of a group of experts preparing a Cholesterol Consensus, which was published later that year. Consensus was reached on the following issues: population screening was not warranted, but classification of individuals with an increased risk was indicated. A cholesterol level < 5 mmol/l was considered ideal. Elevated levels indicated the need for:

> dietary intervention (fat 30 per cent, ratio poly-unsaturated:mono-unsaturated: saturated 1:1:1, cholesterol < 300 mg/day) and medical intervention [...] The whole population is advised to adhere to the nutritional guidelines of the Dutch Nutrition Board.[47]

What were these guidelines?

GUIDELINES FOR A GOOD DIET

In 1986 the 'Voedingsraad' formulated again the guidelines from the 1960s and the 1970s. Now these 'Richtlijnen Goede Voeding' (Guidelines for a Good Diet) were taken over by the government, which created a 'Stuurgroep Goede Voeding' (Steering Committee for a Good Diet) in 1987. In the Steering Committee all interested parties were represented, namely: agricultural organisations, food industries, the food trade, catering establishments, the Consumers' Organisation, physicians (by means of the Dutch Heart Foundation), nutritionists and the different ministries involved. This Steering Committee organised a four-year public campaign on the theme 'Let op vet' (Watch out for fat) starting in 1991.[48] The campaign concentrated on the following recommendations:

- use a variety of food products;
- use less fat, especially saturated fat, and enough poly-unsaturated fat;
- use less cholesterol;
- use more complex carbohydrates, especially starch and fibres, and less sugars;
- use less alcohol;
- use less salt.

The goal of this campaign was to reduce people's fat intake from 40 per cent to 30–35 per cent while the ratio of saturated to unsaturated fat should be changed to 1:1 instead of the 2:1 found in the 'Voedsel Consumptie Peiling' (Food Consumption Measurement) 1987/1988. Close reading shows some interesting differences from the guidelines from 1973: the word 'replacement' is not used, so butter, margarine and animal fat keep their place (even though it is a smaller one), enrichment with linoleic acid is not mentioned, and there is no specification of food products.

The campaign started, notwithstanding that some doubts – based on nutrition research – were expressed on the influence of a high fat intake, of cholesterol and of poly-unsaturated fats on coronary heart diseases. The government even asked the 'Voedingsraad' if the goals should be revised, but this board stuck to the views once taken. Their argument was the following:

> The Guidelines for a Good Diet will again and again be confronted with new views in the science of nutrition. As soon as the guidelines have been rendered out of date by the results of scientific research they will be adjusted. [...] The Guidelines for a Good Diet are meant for the Dutch population as a whole and are not directed towards a relation between diet and disease only. They want to prevent disease. Therefore the Council on Nutrition sees little reason to change the advice concerning the consumption of fat.[49]

The key point in this statement is the difference made between the functions of dietary advice: is it directed to prevention or to therapy? The conclusion was that the government may take action to prevent diseases, but that therapy is a more individual based problem to be solved by the patient and his physician.

THE PHYSICIANS

At last the physicians took more action. Also in 1991 the 'Nederlands Huisartsen Genootschap' (Society of GPs) introduced the so called 'NHG-Standard for Cholesterol'. At the end of the same year the consensus on cholesterol was revised.[50] The consensus and the NHG-standard had the same objectives and the NHG was represented in the consensus group. The 'NHG-Standard for Cholesterol' consisted of guidelines for the GP on how to trace and treat hypercholesterolemia. Blood cholesterol level should be measured in all patients aged 18–65 years with one of the following characteristics of a patient at risk:

- signs of familial hypercholesterolemia;
- experience of a coronary disease;
- a coronary disease of the nearest kin;
- hypertension;
- diabetes mellitus;
- familial hyperlipidaemia.

The blood cholesterol should be measured at least twice with a 1–2 weeks' interval. If the level is > 5 mmol/l, a diet according to the Guidelines for a Good Diet should be prescribed for six months. Levels of 5.1 to 6.4 mmol/l are not to be treated any further. When higher levels do not decrease with a diet only, medication should be added. The 'NHG-Standard Cholesterol' did not advocate the prescription of cholesterol decreasing medicines by the GP.

After four years the use of the 'NHG-Standard Cholesterol' was evaluated. The conclusion was that GPs did know about the Standard, but that they used it only partly. They often (72 per cent) did not measure blood cholesterol levels in patients with the above named characteristics, yet on the other hand they did measure these levels in others for whom it was not needed (56 per cent). They often measured only once and they rarely used the Guidelines for a Good Diet.[51] The conclusion of the editor of the *Heart Bulletin* was that the Standard needed revision.[52] For the future not a diet, which 'often is not enough', but treatment with medicines was emphasized, as there was already a choice of medicines available. He mentioned *pravastatin, simvastatin, cholestyramin, colestipol, gemfibrozil* and *acipimox.*[53]

In 1995 the physicians of the 'Nederlandse Hartstichting' (Dutch Heart Foundation) made preparations for a new cholesterol consensus. The medical director of the Foundation, G Jambroes, wanted to make people more responsible for their own health. In his view people should measure their own cholesterol so they would learn that an increased blood cholesterol level may be their own problem and not only their neighbour's. He stated:

> For too long a pedantic profession has withheld from the public the methods to judge for themselves on this matter and then to take appropriate measures.[54]

He had in mind the development of a cholesterol-testing method, which could be used by everyone, just like a thermometer. He admitted that it would not be an easy task to give instructions to the public, but in his view this was the only strategy suitable for a modern society.

THE PUBLIC

Does the public want to know anything about a blood cholesterol level? The answer seems to be: 'yes and no': yes – as long as it is a general medical topic; no – when it comes too close, concerning one's own health with consequences such as using a diet or taking pills for the rest of one's life. People have become more and more informed on medical issues. During the last two decades journals, magazines and especially television-programmes have presented an increasing number of issues on diseases and their cures. This type of information, together with the health claims of industrial food products, often causes a feeling of uncertainty. In that case some people turn to the 'Voorlichtingsbureau voor de Voeding' (Information Bureau on Nutrition) for advice. In 1988 this Bureau published a series of questions asked – pointing at the large number of questions on diet and health.[55] On coronary diseases the public asked (among several questions on the use of salt) the questions (Q); but the answers (A) are also interesting, as they show a strong propaganda for the use of linoleic acid:

- Q: *What should I use for frying: fat or oil?*
  A: Oil rich in linoleic acid such as soybean oil, sunflower oil, maize oil and safflower oil.
- Q: *Is it better to use vegetable margarine?*
  A: No, vegetable does not mean a high content of linoleic acid. Margarines rich in linoleic acid are those packed in tubs and the dietary margarines.
- Q: *Do dietary products prevent one from having a heart attack?*
  A: This cannot be said. Having a heart attack depends not only on nutrition. If the diet is a healthy one no special products are needed. A healthy life style adds to the prevention of coronary diseases.
- Q: *I am using a diet low in cholesterol. Eggs are not allowed. Can I eat egg-white?*
  A: Views have changed. Most important is the reduction of the total fat intake; secondly poly-unsaturated fat should be used (linoleic acid); thirdly products rich in cholesterol can be used, but not too often: a whole egg (yolk and white) a week is no problem.

Simple messages have a big impact on the public, but research does not come up with simple answers. Researchers often complain that their results are presented to the public at too early a stage; on the other hand they themselves want to be the first to make their findings known. In this situation no clear-cut information reached the people, as was stated by the editor of the leading journal on nutrition *Voeding* in 1994. Under the title 'Fat: a signal with a lot of background noise' he discussed the presentation of some results of medical research on heart diseases.[56] The role of cholesterol in particular was shown to be in doubt, as he cited from headings such as 'Cholesterol not determining for the chance of a heart attack'. He saw the undermining of the position of cholesterol as a trend, also to be noticed in Germany and in England, pushed by the agriculture lobby and dairy industry. In his view nutritionists had to prevent that the press 'gets rattled', because this was not favourable for the general public. He asked for more unbiased information.

Of course people's uncertainty does not diminish with more information when the results keep on being as contradictory as they have been during the last few decades. New research solves some questions but raises other new ones. Changing scientific opinions diminishes people's faith in so-called scientific 'truths'. In that situation the message of the industry in advertisements has more influence than the subtle approach of non-profit organisations. This effect is shown in the results of the 'Watch out for fat' campaign.

The campaign results were closely followed and a series of studies evaluating people's fat intake were published. In 1995, in the last year of the campaign, the outcome was not so favourable. Even though the campaign was fairly well known (by 47 per cent of the population) only a small minority of people had changed their diet. Most people had the idea that the campaign was not directed to themselves, as they did not consider their own fat intake as high.[57] As a cause of the disappointing effect of the campaign, the researchers pinpointed the rivalry between non-profit public information and advertising by the food industries. In their opinion – as is the general view – advertisements have a much larger impact on the public than information. In this case however, one wonders why the researchers mention this topic, as during the same period the food industry marketed more and more 'light' products that could have supported the 'Watch out for Fat' campaign.

THE CASE OF CORONARY HEART DISEASES: A NEVER ENDING STORY?

Comparing the case-study of coronary heart diseases with the one on tuberculosis we do not have such a happy ending. Coronary heart diseases seem to have no simple cause – at least no one has found one yet – which can be treated with some medicine. Prevention, changing life style, a life-long thinking about your health and diet, are the same issues as are used in the fight against tuberculosis. How easy it would be if a 'coronary heart disease bacteria' were found and also some antibiotic to cure all the problems. As we recently saw with the example of the discovery of a bacterium *Helicobacter pylori*, causing gastric ulcers, it may even be a possibility. Gastric ulcers have long been thought to be related to life style and personality-characteristics and were cured with milk diets, so why not a bacterium (or a virus) causing degeneration of the blood vessel walls?

At the moment, however, we still find ourselves in the middle of an increasing number of often contradictory data. Even the 'Seven Countries Study', the epidemiological study on coronary heart diseases which started in 1958, does not come up with a simple, single piece of advice. An evaluation of the 40 years the study has been running shows that it provides 'an insight into the relation between life-style and health', but not one cause of disease. The poly-unsaturated fatty acids have kept their place as protectors against coronary heart diseases, but now they have got company from 'flavonoids', complex chemical structures present in tea, apples, onions and red wine.[58] These findings seem to be more in favour of the Dutch producers of vegetables and fruits and the French wine merchants than of the general public. The same can be said on the health claims for olive oil which have just been accepted by European nutritionists.[59] The comment of the editor of *Voeding* on this case is somewhat cynical: the campaign for olive oil is in the first place a commercial enterprise. Olive oil has a marginal place in the Dutch diet because of its price and its taste, so what is the idea?[60] And is it the use of olive oil which reduces mortality from coronary heart diseases in Mediterranean countries, or is it the diet as a whole or even the life style as such?

For the general public it is difficult to know what to do when messages on the use of special products and diets are contradictory. A recent discussion between physicians in the *Nederlands Tijdschrift voor Geneeskunde*, with one article by C P M Boot entitled 'A cholesterol-decreasing diet is not sensible' and another by A F H Stalenhoef 'Cholesterol-decreasing nutrition surely is sensible' shows clearly the difference between 'diet' and 'nutrition'. Boot stresses the ineffectiveness of an individual 'medicalized' diet to lower cholesterol and supports the view that only changing the lifestyle of the population as a whole would have an effect on the incidence of coronary diseases.[61] Stalenhoef only partly agrees as he thinks it also inevitable to treat patients with a cholesterol-decreasing diet and he is less sceptical about patients sticking to their diet. It is not unimportant in this discussion that Boot is a GP and Stalenhoef a professor of internal medicine. One can state that people coming to a GP's practice are less likely to act as a 'patient' than the people treated by a specialist; or in other words the specialist sees a selection of severe cases, people who are more likely to follow medical advice. Anyway, even Stalenhoef agrees that 'in individual cases the results of dietary advice are often disappointing'.[62] Concluding, we can say that the Hippocratic advice still seems the sound one: keep the balance in all you do and you will live a healthy life.

CONCLUDING REMARKS

In the above description of the twentieth century history of medical dietary advice on the cure and prevention of diseases in The Netherlands, we have shown several interrelated changes, the most remarkable of which are the following. Within the period of 100 years we have seen diseases come and go with changing socio-economic and cultural conditions. In the first of our two case-studies medical advice changed from a cure using diet to a cure using medicines; in the second case-study advice changed from a dietary cure to prevention using a diet as medicines remain lacking. The fight against pulmonary consumption has been a success story, which cannot be said of the battle against cardiovascular diseases. The conclusion forces itself upon us that, if no clear-cut empirically based causal relationships are demonstrated between disease and lifestyle or other types of exposure to health-risks, the classic dietary rules of moderation still hold. The interesting thing is, however, that dietary health claims as such have attained a dynamic of their own in which several influential parties in society are involved.

To get an idea of the scope of this dynamic it is important to realize that the developments described above have taken place in the larger framework of the modernization and industrialization of Dutch (and other western) societies. A most fundamental condition and incentive to these general trends was the process of economic growth which in The Netherlands got a new impulse from the 1890s onwards. Through industrialization and the improvement of means of transport, both the food supply and the purchasing power of the population increased considerably. An implication of this development – which contains a complex change which only can be touched upon here – was the overcoming of scarcity and the availability of plenty of food. With this historical watershed, the problems of the relation of disease to diet and life styles have fundamentally changed in character.

One of the important economic sectors which has contributed to economic and social welfare has been the food industry at national and international level. The expansion and intensification of agriculture, livestock production and of the mechanization and 'chemicalisation' of food in factories has been an important source of economic wealth.[63] At the same time this development has now resulted in an ever-increasing response of food producers to the continuing rise in quantitative and qualitative demands and expectations of food consumers. Enough food to eat and food of a good quality certainly has contributed to the health of the population and the near victory over infectious diseases, were it not for the so-called welfare and chronic diseases. The relatively high level of contemporary life-expectancy of the population envisages a life longer than ever before. This long life is expected to be spent being as healthy as possible and it is in this cultural climate that dietary health claims of products, maintained by the food producers concerned, may be a successful selling argument. The sound scientific base of the health claim of a product is therefore of enormous interest to the food companies.

Another conclusion from our study is that the type of dietary advice, given by physicians and nutritionists, seems to reflect precisely the state of knowledge and technology at that given moment. This may be a self-evident judgement, but to our mind it focuses attention on one of the most important groups in society, relevant to the question of medical dietary advice we have brought up in this article. We refer to the group of medical and other scientists and technologists doing research on nutrition and pharmacy in different areas of society: universities, industrial companies and state- or consumer-financed laboratories. The rapid evolution of medical science and its different offshoots into many specialisms – among which are nutritional and pharmaceutical science – are most akin to our topic.

Scientific communities, however, do have many differences of opinion and, what is more, they have different interests as well, obviously connected to various social positions and customers. The social pressures to achieve substantial findings, contributing to the treatment of illnesses, may be one of the causes of the all too rapid public proclamation of health claims and dietary advice that have to be withdrawn later. Despite the fact that much insight into the connection between illness, health and nutrition has been gained, the two cases we have dealt with illustrate the limits of scientific nutritional science as a sound foundation of medical dietary advice in different ways. Diet finally appears to be of more general than specific importance to health. As soon as medical and pharmaceutical knowledge about the causes and remedies of illnesses is available, the need for dietary discipline seems to disappear to the background.

Pulmonary consumption appeared to be an infectious disease, easily cured by medical treatment. It turned out finally that this illness had more to do with the lack of medicinal therapy than with a deficient diet or a poor lifestyle. No wonder, though, that in a society in which scarcity in many respects was no exception, the relation between these social factors and tuberculosis was seen. In particular, since the 1960s this socio-economic situation has changed completely and even turned into affluence. Now coronary heart diseases are believed to be related to an affluent life style and an over-indulgent diet. Decisive results of scientific medical and nutritional research to give clear dietary advice, however, are as yet lacking.

Ironically the demand for health and health-care in western societies has increased instead of decreased with the rise in the welfare and life-expectancies of their populations. This is one of the reasons why many social groups and parties other than doctors and scientific researchers have entered the arena of health, diet and nutrition. We have already mentioned the producers; the role of the government as a controlling authority on food safety and other rules of food law has also substantially increased in the period studied. The recent emancipation of consumers and patients and their position opposite producers and doctors has resulted in new and sometimes strong voices in the field of nutrition. All the social groups mentioned have gained power over the previously nearly exclusive authority of doctors. Dietary advice is given by many experts outside the medical branch, not particularly aiming at health, but for instance for slimming or performance in sports. The slimming trend now may be a source of new illnesses like anorexia.

Thus the striving for physical and psychological health has taken first place in Dutch public opinion on important personal topics. Since the 1960s health is a much more attractive life-goal than a 'strong belief' or a 'happy marriage', which used to throw most weight on the scale of life-goals only a few decennia ago.[64] One may perceive this cultural change as a process of 'sacralization' of health. In our post-modern and individualized contemporary society the hypothesis might be made that we ourselves are the only responsible authorities left to maintain our health, with or without dietary rules.

BIBLIOGRAPHY

Advies inzake de vraag: 'Zijn er adviezen en/of maatregelen gewenst ten aanzien van de hoeveelheid en/of aard der vetten in de Voeding van de Nederlandse bevolking?' (Advice as to the question: 'Are advice or measures asked for concerning the quantity and/or type of fat in the nutrition of Dutch people?'), *Voeding*, 34 (1973), 552–62.

Bericht [News], *Voeding*, 22 (1961), 357–8; from *Consumentengids*, 9 (1961), 122–3.

Bleiker, M A, et al. *Leerboek der tuberculosebestrijding* (Handbook for the Fight against Tuberculosis), 's-Gravenhage, 1984.

Bock, C E. *Het boek van den gezonden en van den zieken mensch* (The Book for the Healthy and the Ill Man), Amsterdam, 1872; *De huisdokter voor stad en land. Gezondheidsleer voor het volk* (The Physician for Town and Country. Hygiene for the people), Groningen, 1884.

Bokkel Huinink, S A ten. Klinische aspecten bij ziekte der bloedvaten (Clinical aspects of diseases of the blood vessels), *Voeding*, 22 (1961), 372–7.

Boldingh, J. Wetenschappelijk onderzoek (Scientific research). In Stuijvenberg, J H. *Honderd Jaar Margarine 1869-1969* (One Hundred Years of Margarine 1869–1969), 's-Gravenhage, 1969, 120–82.

Boot, C P M. Een cholesterolverlagend dieet is niet zinvol (A cholesterol-decreasing diet is not sensible), *Nederlands Tijdschrift voor Geneeskunde*, 141 (1997), 2539–42.

Böttcher, C J F. Spelen voedingsvetten een rol bij het optreden van atherosclerose en coronair-trombose? (Do dietary fats have an influence on arteriosclerosis and coronary thrombosis), *Voeding*, 22 (1961), 409–15.

Brevarium. Cholesterol en voedingsvetten (Cholesterol and dietary fats), *Voeding*, 21 (1960), 173–4.

Bruijn, R de. *Een Hollands huis in Zwitserland. 90 jaar Nederlands astmacentrum DAVOS 1897–1987* (A Dutch House in Switzerland. 90 years of the Dutch Centre for Asthma Davos 1897–1987), Leiden, 1987.

Bruïne Ploos van Amstel, P J de and Neuberg J. *Dieet-behandeling* (Dietetic Therapy), Amsterdam, 1937.

Buchem, F S P van. Pathogenese en preventie van atherosclerose en atherosclerotisch complicaties (Pathogenesis and prevention of arteriosclerosis and arteriosclerotic complications), *Nederlands Tijdschrift voor Geneeskunde*, 115 (1971), 1311–18.

De campagne 'Let op Vet' (The campaign 'Watch out for Fat'), *Voeding*, 52 (1991), 37–44.

Chotkowski, L A. *What's new in medicine. More than 250 of the biggest health stories of the decade*, Santa Fe, 1991.

Daal, M van. *De tuberculosebestrijding in Nederland tussen 1900 en 1910 aan de hand van het Nederlandsch Tijdschrift voor Geneeskunde* (The Fight against Tuberculosis in the Netherlands between 1900 and 1910 Seen from the Dutch Medical Journal), Typescript, Amsterdam, 1992.

Daal, M van and Knecht-van Eekelen, A de. Over aetiologie en therapie van tuberculose: het debat in Nederland (1900–1910) (On the aetiology and therapy of tuberculosis: the debate in the Netherlands (1900–1910)), *Gewina*, 15 (1992), 211–33.

Daal, M J W G van and Knecht-van Eekelen, A de. *Johannes Juda Groen (1903–1990). Een arts op zoek naar het ware welzijn* (Johannes Juda Groen (1903–1990). A physician looking for the true well-being), Rotterdam, 1994.

Dalderup, L M and Appeldoorn, W C A. Vetgebruik, gewicht en cholesterolgehalte van het serum van een groep bejaarden (Use of fat, body weight and cholesterol level of the blood serum of a group of elderly people), *Voeding*, 23 (1962), 513–8.

Dettweiler, P. Ernährungstherapie bei Lungenkrankheiten. In Leyden E von, ed. *Handbuch der Ernährungstherapie und Diätetik*. Part 2, Leipzig, 1897, 1–42.

Dieetvet Becel (Dietary fat Becel), *Voeding*, 21 (1960), 521.

Drenth, B B van and Weijden, T van der. Cholesterol in de huisartspraktijk, van eigen aard naar standaard (Cholesterol in the GP practice, from own idea to standard), *Hart Bulletin*, 26 (1995), 85–8.

Erkelens, D W. Cholesterol-consensus in Nederland (Cholesterol consensus in The Netherlands), *Nederlands Tijdschrift voor Geneeskunde*, 131 (1987), 1564–9; Herziening consensus cholesterol (Revision of cholesterol consensus), *Nederlands Tijdschrift voor Geneeskunde*, 135 (1991), 2337–40.

Frazer, A C. Aspecten van Voeding en voedingswaarden (Aspects of nutrition and nutritional values). In Stuijvenberg, J H. *Honderd jaar margarine 1869–1969* (One Hundred Years of Margarine 1869–1969), 's-Gravenhage, 1969, 183–230.

Gerritsen, W J. Vetten: signaal met veel ruis (Fat: signal with a lot of background noise), *Voeding*, 55 7/8 (1994), 4; Geoliede gezondheid (Oiled health), *Voeding*, 58/6 (1997/1), 4; Voor gezondheidsclaims olijfolie voldoende onderbouwing (For health claims of olive oil enough evidence), *Voeding*, 58/6 (1997/2), 18-19.

GHI Bulletin. Longtuberculose (Lung tuberculosis), Rijswijk, 1987.

Hart- en vaatziekten in Nederland. Cijfers over ziekte en sterfte (Heart and Coronary Diseases in The Netherlands. Figures on disease and mortality), Den Haag, 1994.

Hautvast, J G A J and Hermus, R J J. Een voedsel- en voedingsbeleid in Nederland; bestrijding van de gevolgen van de welvaart. I (A food and nutrition policy in The Netherlands: fighting the effects of affluence), *Nederlands Tijdschrift voor Geneeskunde*, 123 (1979), 939–44; De overheid geeft nog weinig blijk van visie op dit specifieke terrein. II (The government still shows little vision on this special topic), 975-85.

Hemel, A e a. Evaluatie Let op Vet-campagne 1994 (Evaluation 'Watch out for Fat' Campaign 1994), *Voeding*, 56/9 (1995), 12–15.

Herrmannsdorfer, Mimicia and Adolf. *Praktische Anleitung zur Kochsalzfreien Ernährung Tuberkulöser. Mit einem Geleitwort von F. Sauerbruch*, Leipzig, 1930.

Hoogerbrugge, N. De NHG-Standaard Cholesterol 1991. Vier jaar later gezien door een internist (The NHG-Standard Cholesterol. Four years later seen by a specialist for internal diseases), *Hart Bulletin*, 26 (1995), 82–4.

Jaarverslagen (Annual reports) from the Nederlandsch Sanatorium voor minvermogende longlijders te Davos-Platz (Dutch health-resort for poor patients with pulmonary consumption, (1897–1950).

Jambroes, G. Cholesterol, *Hart Bulletin*, 26 (1995), 116–17.

Katan, M B. Een consensus over cholesterol? (A consensus on cholesterol?) *Nederlands Tijdschrift voor Geneeskunde*, 129 (1985), 2490-2.

Knecht-van Eekelen, A de. *Naar een rationele zuigelingen voeding. Voedingsleer en kindergeneeskunde in Nederland 1840–1914* (Towards a Rational Infant Feeding. The science of nutrition and pediatrics in The Netherlands 1840–1914), Nijmegen, 1984.

Knecht-van Eekelen, A de. Men kan van tuberculose genezen: Opvattingen over oorzaak en therapie rond de eeuwwisseling (One may be cured from tuberculosis: Ideas on cause and therapy around the turn of the century), *Tijdschrift voor Geschiedenis der Verpleegkunde*, 2/1 (1995), 3–10; Geschiedenis van het genezen; de behandeling van tuberculose in Nederland rond 1900 (History of therapy; the treatment of tuberculosis in The Netherlands around 1900), *Nederlands Tijdschrift voor Geneeskunde*, 140 (1996), 2195–9.

Knuiman, J T and Katan, M B. Cholesterolniveaus in serum in Nederland in vergelijking met die in de Verenigde Staten (Cholesterol levels in blood serum in The Netherlands compared to those in the US), *Nederlands Tijdschrift voor Geneeskunde*, 129 (1985), 2500–5.

Koster, M. Dieet-therapie bij hypercholesterolemie en hyperlipemie (Dietary therapy in cases of hyper-cholesterolemia and hyper-lipemia), *Nederlands Tijdschrift voor Geneeskunde*, 111 (1967), 954–5; review of *Controversy in internal medicine*, Philadelphia/London, 1966; Ingezonden. Pathogenese en preventie van atherosclerose en atherosclerotisch complicaties (Letters to the editor. Pathogenesis and prevention of arteriosclerosis and arteriosclerotic complications), *Nederlands Tijdschrift voor Geneeskunde*, 115 (1971), 1664–5.

Kromhout, D. Zestig jaar NIVV en negentig jaar cholesterol (60 years NIVV and 90 years cholesterol), *Voeding*, 40 (1979), 230–3; Het belang van vis in de voeding (The significance of fish in the diet), *Nederlands Tijdschrift voor Geneeskunde*, 129 (1985), 2493–5; De Zeven-landenstudie: 40 jaar onderzoek naar coronaire hartziekten (The seven-countries study: 40 years of coronary diseases), *Nederlands Tijdschrift voor Geneeskunde*, 141 (1997), 7–9.

Leyden, E von, ed. *Handbuch der Ernährungstherapie und Diätetik*. 2 Parts, Leipzig, 1897.

Meijler, F L. Voeding en coronaire hartziekten, een bouwvallig luchtkasteel? (Nutrition and coronary heart diseases, a ramshackle castle in the air?), *Nederlands Tijdschrift voor Geneeskunde*, 124 (1980), 1694–5.

Otterloo, A H van. *Eten en eetlust in Nederland (1840–1990). Een historisch-sociologische studie* (Diet and Appetite in The Netherlands (1840–1990). A historical-sociological study), Amsterdam, 1990.

Rebsamen, H and Stutz, W. *Davos. INSA Inventar der neueren Schweizer Architektur 1850–1920*, Davos, 1983.

Redactie, eds. Wederom cholesterol (Cholesterol again), *Hart Bulletin*, 26 (1995), 81.

Sociaal en Cultureel Rapport 1996 (Social and Cultural Report 1996), Rijswijk, 1996.

Spengler, A. *Die Landschaft Davos als Kurort gegen Lungenschwindsucht. Klimatologisch-medizinische Skizze*, Davos: Hugo Richter, 1899[2], reprint from the first edition of 1869.

Stalenhoef, A F H. Cholesterolverlagende voeding is wel zinvol (Cholesterol-decreasing nutrition surely is sensible], *Nederlands Tijdschrift voor Geneeskunde*, 141 (1997), 2543–5.

Stuijvenberg, J H. *Honderd jaar margarine 1869–1969* (One Hundred Years of Margarine 1869–1969), 's-Gravenhage, 1969.

Tousley, R D. Marketing. In Stuijvenberg, J H. *Honderd jaar margarine 1869–1969* (One Hundred Years of Margarine 1869-1969), 's-Gravenhage, 1969, 231–284.

Turban, K. Lebenskampf. Die Selbstbiographie eines Arztes, Sonderheft der *Acta Davosiana*, 3 nr 10 (1935).

Voorlichtingsbureau voor de Voeding (Nutrition information service). *De meest voorkomende vragen aan de Voedingstelefoon* (Questions Asked Most at the Nutrition Telephone), Utrecht/Antwerpen, 1988, 108–9.

Voornveld, H J A van. *Tuberculose* (Tuberculosis), Amsterdam, 1898.

Vraag en antwoord (Questions and answers), Vissoorten en cholesterol-arm dieet (Fish species and diet low in cholesterol), *Nederlands Tijdschrift voor Geneeskunde*, 113 (1969), 2152.

Vraag en antwoord (Questions and answers), Arachide-olie in plaats van andere onverzadigde vetzuren als middel om het serumcholesterol te verlagen (Arachid oil replacing other unsaturatd fatty acids in order to decrease serum cholesterol), *Nederlands Tijdschrift voor Geneeskunde*, 114 (1970), 1376.

Wijn, J F de. Het verband tussen het samengaan van verschillende chronische ziektetoestanden bij eenzelfde persoon en de samenhang daarvan met zwaarlijvigheid (The relation between different chronic diseases and overweight in the same person), *Voeding*, 15 (1954), 264–6; A discussion of: Downes J. Association of the chronic diseases in the same person and their associations with overweight, *The Milbank Memorial Fund Quarterly*, 31 (1953), 125–40; De veranderingen in het Nederlandse Voedingspatroon (Changes in the Dutch food pattern), *Voeding*, 29 (1968), 490–504; De veranderingen in het Nederlandse Voedingspatroon (Changes in the Dutch food pattern), *Nederlands Tijdschrift voor Geneeskunde*, 113 (1969), 899–906.

Wijnhoff, J A. Phthisis-behandeling in ons klimaat (Treatment of pulmonary tuberculosis in our climate), *Nederlandsch Tijdschrift voor Geneeskunde*, Second Series 26 II (1890), 65–7.

Winau, R. *Medizin in Berlin*, Berlin/New York, 1987.

NOTES

1 Winau, 1987, 198–200.
2 Von Leyden, 1897, V.
3 De Knecht-van Eekelen, 1984, 17–22; Van Otterloo, 1990, 38–40, 54–59.
4 Van Otterloo, 1990.
5 De Bruijn, 1987.
6 Bleiker et al, 1984, V. 71 etc.
7 *GHI Bulletin*, 1987, 13.
8 Van Daal, 1992; Van Daal & De Knecht-van Eekelen, 1992, 211–33; De Knecht-van Eekelen, 1995, 3–10; De Knecht-van Eekelen, 1996, 2195–99.
9 Wijnhoff, 1890, 66.
10 Van Voornveld, 1898.
11 De Bruijn, 1987, 10.
12 Dettweiler, 1898, 27, 29.
13 Bock, 1872, 439.
14 Bock, 1884, 166.
15 Rebsamen & Stutz, 1983, 346.
16 Spengler, 1899, 67.
17 Turban, 1935.
18 *Jaarverslag*, (1916), 10.

19 *Jaarverslag*, (1917), 15.
20 *Jaarverslag*, (1942), 12.
21 De Bruïne Ploos van Amstel & J Neuberg, 1937, 175–182; Herrmannsdorfer, 1930.
22 De Wijn, 1954, 264–6.
23 *Hart- en vaatziekten*, 1994.
24 Boldingh, 1969, 173.
25 Brevarium, 1960, 173–4.
26 Diectvet, 1960, 521.
27 Böttcher, 1961, 409–15.
28 Van Daal & De Knecht-van Eekelen, 1994, 91–2, 116–20, 158–61.
29 Ten Bokkel Huinink, 1961, 372–7.
30 Koster, 1967, 954–5.
31 Dalderup & Appeldoorn, 1962, 513–18.
32 Tousley, 1969, 267.
33 Frazer, 1969, 223.
34 Vraag en antwoord, 1969, 2152.
35 *ibid*, 1970, 1376.
36 Bericht, 1961, 357–8.
37 De Wijn, 1968, 490–504; 1969, 905.
38 Advies, 1973, 552–62.
39 Kromhout, 1970, 232.
40 Van Buchem, 1971, 1316.
41 Koster, 1971, 1665.
42 Hautvast & Hermus, 1979, 981.
43 Meijler, 1980, 1695.
44 Katan, 1985, 2492; Knuiman & Katan, 1985, 2500–5.
45 Kromhout, 1985, 2493–5.
46 Chotkowski, 1991, 21–2.
47 Erkelens, 1987, 1564–9.
48 Campagne Let op Vet, 1991, 37–44.
49 *ibid*, 38.
50 Erkelens, 1991, 2337–40.
51 Drenth, 1995, 85–8.
52 Redactie, 1995, 81.
53 Hoogerbrugge, 1995, 82–4.
54 Jambroes, 1995, 117.
55 Voorlichtingsbureau, 1988, 108–9.
56 Gerritsen, 1994, 4.
57 Hemel, 1995, 12–15.
58 Kromhout, 1997, 7–9.
59 Gerritsen, 1997b, 18–19.
60 *ibid*, 1997a, 4.
61 Boot, 1997, 2542.
62 Stalenhoef, 1997, 2544.
63 Van Otterloo, 1990, 52–89.
64 *Sociaal en Cultureel Rapport*, 1996, 466.

9 Food culture of the less affluent Slovene urban population and efforts for its improvement: the case of the Maribor Municipality (1900–1940)

Maja Godina-Golija

The nineteenth century was a period of rapid population growth in Slovenia, especially in its cities. The century was marked by swift urbanization and by the completion of the railway between Vienna and Trieste. The latter thus connected all major Slovene towns and brought about a period of intense economic development. World War I slowed the growth of Slovene towns to a certain extent, but the quickly developing industry after the end of the War caused them to expand again in the 1930s and 1940s. In the first half of the nineteenth century the population of Slovene towns consisted mainly of small tradesmen, manufacturers, trade shop workers and domestics. Less important and less numerous was a group of noblemen and wealthy townsmen, those who worked in liberal professions, manufacturing, higher-ranking soldiers, and politicians. This was the time when Slovene towns were still provincial, lagging behind the rapid industrial development of Western and Central European towns. Emil Korytko, a refugee from Poland, sent in 1837 the following letter from Ljubljana to his parents in Poland:

> Yet we find it difficult to live here not only because of high prices. Wasting our time is perhaps even harder to bear. I had expected to find a factory or a company of some kind here. But there is nothing here. There is an English refinery nobody is allowed to visit because of the secrecy of its products, another one burned down, and there is nothing more . . . Even though I occasionally read books in the library which is not very large and study languages at home, most of the time I am just wasting my time. I am very sorry that there are no factories or factory owners here. I should like to get to learn a trade.[1]

In the last third of the nineteenth century larger industrial companies with several thousand employees were opened in Slovene towns. Ljubljana acquired in 1871 a tobacco factory with over 1,000 employees, and Maribor a railway machine company in 1863 which gave work to more than 1,000 domestic and foreign workers.[2]

The period after World War I, especially the 1930s, brought about a marked industrial development, and industrial workers started to represent

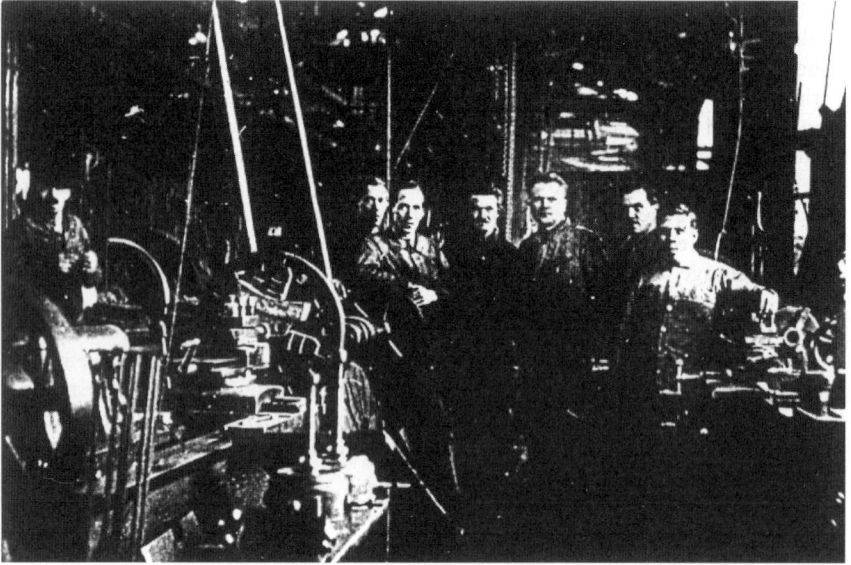

Fig. 1. *Workers of the State Railway Workshops in Maribor (1930)*

a significant social group in Slovene towns. Based on the past research into the food culture of the population of the urban Slovene centres,[3] it is possible to conclude that food culture depended largely upon the social and financial position of an individual. Unlike the situation in villages, regional origin was of lesser importance.[4] Most urban families had enough food before World War II but there were many ways of saving money where food was concerned. Often they wanted to save for other, more obvious, expenses such as new clothes or house furnishings at the expense of food.[5] They bought only the most essential food for their everyday meals: flour, salt, groats, semolina, chicory coffee, sugar, and certain spices. Only occasionally they bought a delicacy such as coffee, salami, cheese, fresh meat of good quality, candy, more expensive fruit, citrus fruits, and sweets.

Because of this, meals were most often modest and rather monotonous, largely depending upon the seasonal foods grown in gardens and in hired fields, or upon those which were bought in outdoor markets at low prices.[6]

Before World War II urban Slovene families that suffered an actual shortage of food were rare, and the reasons for it were most often unemployment, alcoholism, or an illness in the family. Food in particular is a cultural element which reflects even the smallest economic oscillations very quickly.[7] On such occasions more expensive food was replaced with the less expensive, for instance bread was replaced with corn mush, or chicory coffee with cheaper soups such as brown flour soup.

Malnutrition and monotonous food was reflected in the poor health of the less affluent urban population, especially workers. The Slovenec newspaper wrote in 1941 the following:

The Maribor Workers' Insurance Company physicians have been noticing an alarming phenomenon. Formerly, they hardly encountered a worker who had been working in the Maribor Textile Factory for several years. Now, however, these workers come seeking help in increasing frequency. It is obvious that the majority of them have digestive organ problems, are anaemic, suffer from consumption or similar diseases of a social nature. The cause for all of this is malnutrition. Most workers who come here to be cured live in the vicinity of Maribor. Each morning they pedal their bicycles from great distances to Maribor to work, returning in the evening. With them they bring only a piece of bread, they buy some sausage and – if there is any money left – a small bottle of apple cider. This is their only food for the whole day. Female workers are even worse off. Day after day they bring with them to the factory a bottle of weak coffee sweetened with saccharin, drinking it with their piece of bread. No wonder their body grows weak and starts decaying after years of such life, its immune system no longer working. What is needed is social help in the form of the factory kitchen, but this initiative unfortunately went to sleep again.[8]

Before World War II the food culture of most of the Slovene population relied heavily on vegetables. Aside from bread, mush (corn, buckwheat, or wheat) was made from cereals, while polenta was consumed in the coastal region. Supper consisted of grits with milk, or rice. Pap and porridge had been almost abandoned by this time. Dishes made from legumes and root vegetables formed the basis of Maribor inhabitants' meals. Beans were consumed throughout the year. Most often they were eaten shelled and prepared in soups, gravies, salads, or boiled and with an addition of cracklings. In the summer string beans were very popular, while peas and lentils were less widespread. Among the most popular were numerous potato dishes. Cabbage, turnips, and kale were very important vegetables in poorer families and were eaten fresh in salads, or cooked in soups and gravies. In winter sauerkraut and turnips were frequently prepared as well.[9]

Meat and dairy dishes were of lesser importance, but were an important element of meals on festive days when even poorer households prepared one or several meat dishes. Their number and, above all, the quality, price and the manner of its preparation reflected the financial status of individual families. Wealthier families ate the choicest cuts such as sirloin steak or roast veal, roast pork, roast beef, veal cutlets, capons, etc. Less affluent households prepared less expensive meat, for instance beef or smoked pork, most often cooked in the cheapest way possible, that is boiled.[10] The water was later used for soup as well.

Even though meals were uniform and simply prepared, the greater part of the income in most poorer town households was used for buying food. About one half was spent on food, one third on rent, and the rest went for new clothes, shoes, and other expenses.[11] The lack of money was behind the infrequent consumption of meat, delicatessen items, sugar, coffee, citrus fruits, and sweets. Compared with wages of that period, the price of these items was extremely high. In the mid-1930s a factory worker with an average wage of 3 dinars had to work between 0.66 to 1 hour for 1 litre of milk,

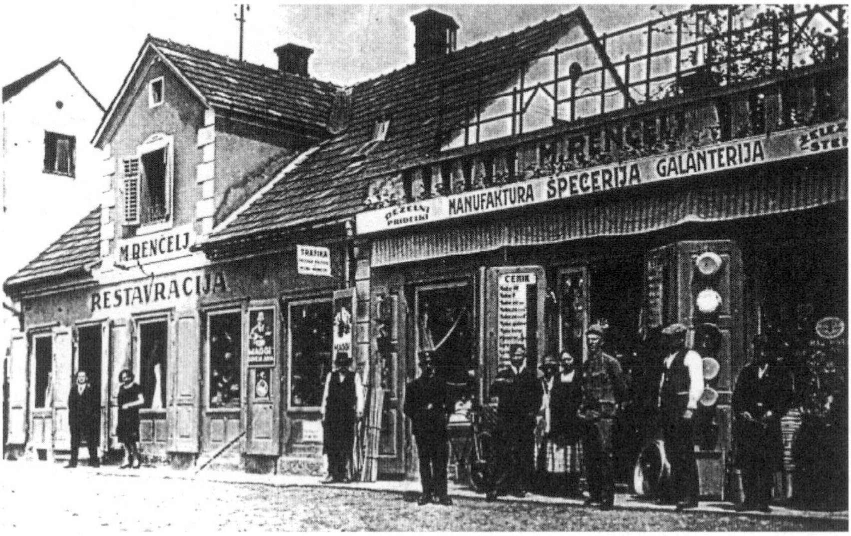

Fig. 2. *Former grocery store in the suburbs of Maribor (1932)*

from 4.6 to 5 hours for a kilo of sugar, between 3.3 to 4.6 hours for 1 kilo of pork, and as many as 23.3 hours for 1 kilo of coffee.[12]

A former grocery store salesperson reminisces thus about his work before World War II:

> Citrus fruits were sold only before holidays, but lemons were always available. They were sold apiece, cost between 1 and 1.5 dinars, and were bought only by the more affluent. For Christmas they bought oranges, one for each person, and oranges were sold apiece as well . . . People did not buy sweets, for instance waffles or cookies, in larger quantities. These were sold apiece too. One waffle cost half a dinar, for instance. We sold candy by 2 or by 5 dekagrams. People were very poor so other things had to be weighed as well and were not bought in larger quantities. Thus we were selling $1/8$ of a kilo of sugar, or $1/12$ of a litre of oil. A five-kilogram packet of coffee was sold to different buyers by dekagrams and lasted us two months.'[13]

The food culture of the urban Slovene population before World War II thus depended upon the financial and social position of each individual. These were not reflected only in the quantity of food consumed which had been characteristic of earlier periods of human society, but above all in the composition and quality of meals. Wealthier families consumed better and more expensive cuts of meat, fish and vegetables, while more substantial, greasy, and cheaper foods (mush with cracklings, beans and cabbage, less expensive smoked pork and beef) were served in poorer families on an everyday basis.[14] Regional as well as temporal dimensions of food culture were of lesser importance. These were mainly preserved in the manner of preparation of dishes and in the composition of festive meals which reflected a strong attachment to the home and dishes of one's childhood, and which were prepared almost identically in the new surroundings as well.[15]

THE TOWN OF MARIBOR – AN INDUSTRIAL CENTRE WITH NUMEROUS SOCIAL AND HEALTH PROBLEMS

Prior to 1918 Maribor was mainly a natural trade and commercial centre. Among the trades the production of goods for the needs of the local inhabitants prevailed. The largest share of the commercial trade comprised agricultural products including wine and timber from the surrounding area. At this time the brewer's industry, leather trade and the milling industry were important in the industrial line, which after 1918 began to decline.[16] Intensive industrialization of the town began with the construction of the Fala water power plant at the end of World War I. In the 1920s and 1930s the machine factory of the Southern Railway was joined by some other industries, particularly the textile industry. The importance of trade and commerce in the town's economy continued to decline, and Maribor became one of the most important industrial centres of old Yugoslavia.[17] Due to the growth of the textile industry it was named the 'Yugoslav Manchester'. Of the 33,921 inhabitants living in Maribor in 1931, 30.9 per cent were employed in industry and trade. An important share of the inhabitants was still employed in shops, banks and traffic (29.9 per cent); other activities were of little importance.

The financial situation of the majority of Maribor's inhabitants was poor, for their employers often abused the laws on both the length of a working day and the lowest wage. The worst situations were found in some of the textile factories and we can find numerous reports in the newspapers of that time:

> It happened in Ehrlich Braun's factory that a female employee who earned 120 dinars a fortnight asked for a pay increase because she had to look after herself and her two children – the foreman snapped her head off saying that 1 dinar for bread and 1 dinar for onions was sufficient for one day for her.[18]

Consequently nourishment in most homes was poor and monotonous. The combination of food did not differ from the already ascertained nourishment of the other poor urban dwellers throughout Slovenia. Under exceptional conditions, for example during World War I, during the economic crisis at the beginning of the 1930s, and during bad winters, the nourishment of this group was much worse. It was during these times that the most important form of public kitchens and workers' canteens began. With the help of the municipality of Maribor and donations from some organisations they were able to prepare meals for the poorest group of Maribor's inhabitants, mainly children.

In 1916, during World War I, the town army kitchen began to function and was then stopped in August 1919.[19] In 1925 the town public kitchen

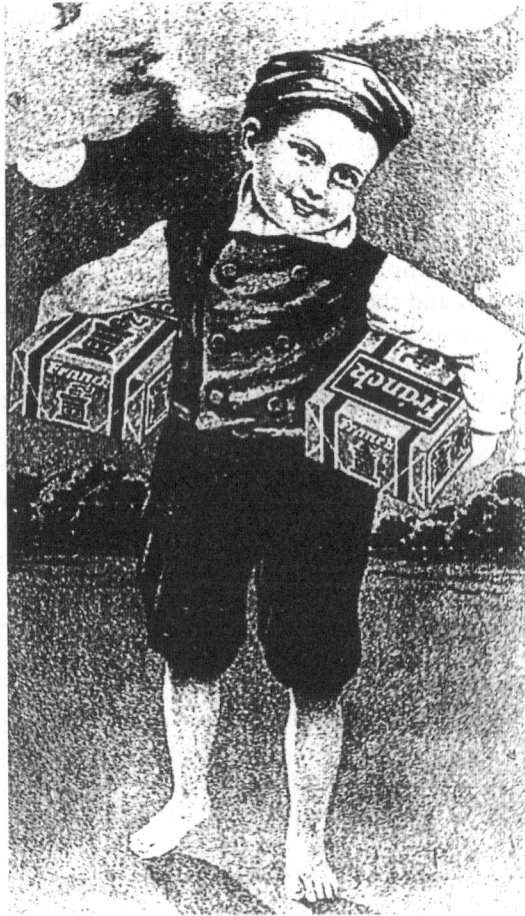

Fig. 3. *Advertisement for chicory coffee (1922)*

was founded where food was prepared for the town's poor. They were given food free of charge, and when there was a large number to feed they were given food-cards.[20] By the end of the 1920s the public kitchen was preparing 200 good mid-day meals, which were mainly distributed free of charge. Only a few people paid the sum of 4 dinars for their meal. The food prepared in the town public kitchen was similar to the food eaten at that time by the majority of the less wealthy inhabitants of Maribor. During the week there were barley groats with pork, pickled cabbage and hard maize mush, pickled cabbage and beans, potatoes, rice and beans; and on Sundays there was the popular beef soup with meat. As was reported in the newspapers of that time the kitchen was successfully managed by Mr Sterlet, who was greatly helped by the then caretaker, Karel Dermelj. The people of Maribor could see them everyday at the market place buying food for the public kitchen. The caretaker was the one to barter over prices, which was a custom of that time.[21] The work of the public kitchen did not change until the beginning of World War II. During all those years warm meals and bread were distributed free of charge to the poor of Maribor. In 1925 it prepared 25,703 meals, and by 1937 the number had grown to 125,183. Expenses were covered by money from the town municipality's budget.[22]

Besides the public kitchen, warm mid-day meals for the poor were also prepared by the Karitas association. Here sixty people were given food free of charge or for the price of 2 dinars. The food they prepared was bought only with money given by individuals supporting the cause. Also the cloister of teaching nuns and the Franciscan monastery in Maribor distributed warm food to about sixty people every day.[23]

Occasionally warm meals were prepared by other organizations and associations. During the winter warm rooms were organized, where the poor visitors were served with warm drinks and bread in the morning and evening. In the terrible winter of 1929 three tea kitchens were organized in town. Here the unemployed and poor children were given tea and bread three times a day. A journalist in the Marburger Zeitung newspaper wrote in February 1929 that two tea kitchens distributed 1,400 and 1,700 portions on Sunday and Monday; and, on Wednesday, when the third tea kitchen was opened, 3,050 portions were given out. He also wrote that the warm rooms, where mainly the unemployed gathered, were also well visited.[24]

In the winter of 1932, during the economic crisis, in the warm room on Razlagova Street, more than 1,000 people were given a warm cup of milk and some bread in the mornings,[25] but in the evenings the number was much lower. In the 1920s and 1930s warm meals were organized in schools for children from poor families. In this way the pupils of Maribor in 1920 were given warm meals from the American aid action for European children. The Red Cross also had kitchens in schools where they provided warm lunches for the most needy children.[26] In the 1930s, within the frame of the health centre, school milk kitchens were also functioning. There, poor children in Maribor's secondary, grammar, primary schools and kindergarten were given a quarter of a litre of first class, pasteurised milk every day. This activity was supported by the town municipality.[27] Despite these forms of organized help for adults and children, it is necessary to emphasize that help was received by only a small number of those in need.

The rapid growth of industry in the town, mainly textiles, brought an increase in the number of women being employed, who did not have enough time to prepare warm food. In 1930 the Worker's Chamber, the public employment agency and the municipality founded a public kitchen in rooms on Slomšek square. It was a non-profit making, charitable institution which prepared meals mainly for families where both parents were employed. Those interested were offered a choice of A, B and C meals, which differed in the quantity of food and therefore the price. The most expensive was the C ticket which included breakfast, lunch (soup, two vegetables, meat and hasty-pudding) and supper which cost 16.30 dinars. The cheapest was A and included only a lunch of soup, meat and vegetables.[28] Due to the interest in this kind of feeding the public kitchens expanded in 1935.[29]

There were no other public kitchens or canteens at this time in Maribor. After finishing work employees did not have a warm meal, and the situation was likewise in kindergartens and schools. Only the owner of the textile factory, Josip Hutter, at the end of the 1930s set up a dining room for his employees. Here they could warm up food they brought with them and eat it in peace and quiet away from the textile machines. Besides this, as I already mentioned, the well established distribution of milk or warm meals among the needy and sick children was organized by the health centre and Red Cross. Children and youths brought their mid-morning snack to school with them; usually it was only a piece of bread and an apple. During the school break the school attendants also sold bread rolls for snacks. Only the better off pupils were able to afford them as most of the rolls were too expensive. Bakers, bringing their bread and rolls in baskets, sold them in front of schools and factories. However, for the majority of people bread rolls, pretzels, salted and other biscuits were too expensive and so they purchased them only occasionally.

The efforts made by the town municipality in Maribor and some other charitable organizations for improving the nutrition of the needy prior to World War II were limited especially to some forms of preparation and distribution of food for the poorest group of citizens (eg the unemployed) and needy children (public kitchen, Karitas association kitchen, Red Cross kitchen). The help given by these organisations was received by only a small segment of the inhabitants. A large number of industrial workers and their families, according to the doctors of that time, were sick with illness of a social character and also because of poor and monotonous food, and did not receive any help from the municipality. Efforts to get factories to organize factory canteens did not materialize. As there was no set time for a work break in most factories prior to World War II, employees had to eat their snack standing up while working. This was extremely unhealthy in the textile factories where the workers' clothes and hands were covered in fibre particles, as well as being in the air they breathed, and were eaten together with their food.

Only the establishment of the public kitchens under the patronage of the Workers' Chamber, the public employment agency and the town municipality show that the period prior to World War II with its growing industrialization also introduced new ideas of the eating of food and drink away from home. With the lack of time to prepare hot food at home, this era also shaped some new relations between the social economics and social cultures phenomena.[30]

BIBLIOGRAPHY

Borba (The struggle newspaper), 1934.

Burnett, John. *Plenty & want. A social history of food in England from 1850 to the present day*, London, 1989.

Godina, Maja. *Iz mariborskih predmestij* (From Maribor's Suburbs), Maribor, 1992; *Prehrana v Mariboru v dvajsetih in tridesetih letih 20. stoletja*. (Food culture in Maribor during the Twenties and Thirties of the 20th Century), Maribor, 1996.

Židov, Nena, Ljubljanski živilski trg in prehrana meščanov v dvajsetih in tridesetih letih 20 stoletja (Ljubljana's market place and citizen's food in the 1920s and 1930s). *Traditiones*, 25 (1996), 229–239.

Korytko, Emil. *Korespondenca z družino (1836–1838)* (Correspondence with a Family (1836–1838)), Ljubljana, 1983.

Kremenšek, Slavko. *Etnološko proučevanje Ljubljane novejše dobe* (Ethnological Study of Ljubljana's New Era), Ljubljana, 1980.

Krug-Richter, Barbara. Kaiserliche Tafelfreunden – bürgerliche Esskultur? *Rheinisch- westfälische Zeitschrift für Volkskunde*, 38 (1993).

Kržičnik, Ermin. *Gospodarski razvoj Maribora* (Maribor's Economic Development), Maribor, 1956.

Leskovec, Antoša. Razvoj gospodarstva v Mariboru 1752–1941. V *Maribor skozi stoletja* (Economic Growth in Maribor 1752–1941. In Maribor through the century), Maribor, 1991, 313–514.

Makarovič, Gorazd. Prehrana v 19. stoletju na Slovenskem. (The food culture during the 19th century in Slovenia), *Slovenski etnograf*, 33–34 (1988–1990), 127–205.

Marburger Zeitung (The Marburg newspaper) 1919, 1929, 1939.

Mariborski Veernik Jutra (Maribor's evening-paper) 1929, 1930, 1932, 1936.

Novak, Anka. Hrana v Šenčurju (Food in Šenčurj), *Traditiones*, 15 (1986), 121–163.

Slovenec (Slovene newspaper), 1941.

Sterle, Meta. Prehrana na Loškem (The food culture in Loška), *Loški razgledi*, 34 (1987), 105–161.

Teuteberg Hans J, Wiegelmann G. *Der Wandel der Nahrungsgewohnheiten unter dem Einfluss der Industrialisierung*, Göttingen, 1972.

Tolksdorf, Ullrich. Der Schnellimbiss und the World of Ronald McDonald's. *Kieler Blätter zur Volkskunde*, 12 (1981).

Wiegelmann, Günter. *Alltags-und Festspeisen. Wandel und gegenwartige Stellung*, Marburg, 1967.

Žagar, Janja. *Oblačilna kultura delavcev v Ljubljani med prvo in drugo svetovno vojno* (The Dress Culture of Workers in Ljubljana between the First and Second World Wars), Ljubljana, 1994.

NOTES

1 Korytko, 1983, 35.
2 Godina, 1992, 17; Kremenšek, 1980, 24.
3 Godina, 1996; Makarovič, 1991; Novak, 1986; Sterle, 1987; Židov, 1996.

4 Godina, 1996, 150.
5 Žagar, 1994, 135.
6 Godina, 1992, 75.
7 Wiegelmann, 1967, 14.
8 *Slovenec*, 69 (1941), 11.1, 7.
9 Godina, 1996, 66.
10 ibid, 82.
11 Godina, 1992, 99.
12 ibid, 76.
13 Richter, 1993, 132.
14 Richter, 1993, 132.
15 Godina, 1991, 79.
16 Leskovec, 1991, 369.
17 Kržičnik, 1956, 35.
18 *Borba*, 2 (1934), 28.7, 4.
19 *Marburger Zeitung*, 79 (1939), 20.10, 4.
20 *Marburger Zeitung*, 59 (1919), 20.7, 2.
21 Maribor's *Večernik Jutra*, 3 (1929), 9.3, 3.
22 Regional archives Maribor, Town Hall Maribor, document 2495.
23 In those places.
24 *Marburger Zeitung*, 69 (1929), 9.3, 3.
25 Maribor's *Večernik Jutra*, 6 (1932), 27.1, 2.
26 Regional archives, Chronicle on girls' schools 1, during 1919–1941.
27 Regional archives Maribor, Town Council Maribor, document 22135.
28 Maribor's *Večernik Jutra*, 4 (1930), 16.7, 2.
29 Maribor's *Večernik Jutra*, 10 (1936), 27.2, 3.
30 Tolksdorf, 1981, 121.

10 Symbols in the rhetoric on diet and health – Norway 1930: the relation between science and the performance of daily chores

Inger Johanne Lyngø

'A housewife should not have to be a scientist to ensure that her family has a healthy diet', wrote the renowned doyenne of Norwegian cookery, Henriette Schønberg Erken, in a book published in 1939.[1] In this paper, where I will focus on symbols as mediated through scientific knowledge, this quotation touches on some of the themes I will examine: the relationship between theory and practice or, rather, the relationship between abstract natural science and the performance of daily chores. The overarching issue is how things are given new meaning. I intend to examine concrete expressions in order to analyse them, for the literal meaning of terms and things is inadequate. This does not mean that I will focus on what things mean, their significance: rather, my task is to focus on the interplay between things and meanings.

THE 'NORWEGIAN' DIET

A housewife should thus not have to be a scientist. Her duties are bound to practical matters, first and foremost to preparing food for her family. However, especially in the twentieth century, it is science, or more precisely, the science of nutrition which determines the premises for how this chore is performed. In the middle of the nineteenth century the science of nutrition had its breakthrough, the 'discovery of the different nutrients being an essential underpinning for this.'[2] This was also the breakthrough for modern chemistry. The roots of the great *'grautstrid'* [porridge war] in Norway in the 1860s between Peder Christen Asbjørnsen (the first collector of folktales in Norway) and Eilert Sundt (a pioneer in Norwegian sociology) are grounded in the knowledge that emerged from this discovery. The 'porridge war' was a power struggle to determine who was in the right, common people or the experts.[3] Nevertheless, the science of nutrition did not gain larger influence until this century. This became most apparent in the 1930s, when nutrition became an official project. During this period the Norwegian people became 'more wholesome, healthier and stronger',[4] and this was attributed to dietary changes. Tall and healthy children became signs and symbols, showing that diets were moving in the right direction. The origins of semiotics come to mind in this context, more precisely the interpretation of illness symptoms. But we can say that this has been turned upside down, as it were, becoming rather the interpretation of the symbols of good health. Diets constituted perhaps the most important element of the public hygiene project which was so important during this period. Preparing food is thus not merely a matter of feeding hungry mouths or exhibiting status. A housewife, meaning 'the Norwegian housewife irrespective of class',[5] was obliged to ensure that her family had a healthy and correct diet, without this meaning that greater expenses had to be incurred. It was possible for people from *any* class, rural and urban, to have a correct diet. A healthy diet need not necessarily be an expensive diet. The important message was that knowhow was more important than money.

Thus a housewife would have to acquire know-how, she had to *know*, and she had to establish conscious attitudes concerning the food she would prepare and serve her family. The rhetoric about diets and nutrition naturally saw housewives as the target group, as manifested in numerous articles on diet and nutrition issues in magazines for women and housewives. Even in health magazines and manuals on proper living, articles on food and food preparation abound, and here as well the authors address women: 'Not only the older, more experienced housewife but also the young, inexperienced housewives-to-be carry a heavy responsibility on their shoulders'.[6] It was no longer sufficient to simply follow tradition in the sense that 'what my mother did, I will do'; housewives in the 1930s were expected to prepare and serve food based on other premises: 'It is quite common to hear the objection that people through the ages have coped without knowing much about correct and healthy diets, but the truth is really that in the "good old days" our forebears were much worse of with respect to sickness and mortality than we are today'.[7]

Social science research had established facts about the Norwegian diet, the insights of nutritional science had determined how to improve this diet, and social economists endeavoured to find ways to implement this diet within a realistic financial framework. National diet plans were drawn up, some even building exclusively on domestic produce.[8] Diets also became a business issue, so agriculture enjoyed a strong position. The general diet also became a political issue when a Norwegian nutrition policy was established.[9] As the magazine *Liv og Sundhet* [Life and Health] puts it, 'a campaign was mobilised' for new and improved diets.

> To turn around the eating habits of an entire population is the most difficult task imaginable. There is no field where people are more conservative . . . The head of the Department of Hygiene at the University has sounded the alarm and is spearheading the work to reform our national nutritional habits. This work must be supported by all those who are working for better health conditions in our country . . . There must be a general mobilisation for a field campaign to change the eating habits of the Norwegian people.[10]

Many people took part in this campaign and, in addition to the official bodies mentioned above, Ms Schønberg Erken was an important figurehead. In 1939 she said that thanks to 'the propaganda of recent decades for a better way of living' diets had improved,[11] but she added that matters were still not good enough, and the rural areas of the country especially were lagging behind. In the middle of the 1930s it was determined that tooth cavities were caused by improper diets, and thereafter having tall, sound and healthy children was no longer sufficient, and now teeth also had to be perfect. 'Let it be stated that if anyone should claim that diets in Norway are sound, this is patently untrue as long as teeth are in the state they are, and if a housewife or father of a family claims that the diet is good, let every member of the family display their teeth'.[12] Time was now ripe for a *proper* and *enduring* change of diets in *all* Norwegian homes',[13] and housewives were important collaborators in this work. 'It is of the utmost national importance that housewives know their profession, and they must understand and know that the health and vitality of the nation greatly depends on them', she said as she travelled around the country making speeches and giving demonstrations, producing cookery books both small and large, writing articles and recipes in weekly and housewives' magazines, and also managing her own cookery classes at Hamar, a small city in southern Norway. Posterity probably knows her best for her 'complete Norwegian cookery book', first published in 1914 with frequent reprints, which taught several generations of Norwegian women to cook.

SCIENCE, THINGS AND MEANINGS

How the knowledge of nutritional science found its way out of the laboratories and was given concrete design leading to the transformation of our daily lives is really a story about mediation. I want to focus on this aspect. By studying the rhetoric, or rather the various rhetorics that emerged after the first health magazine was established in 1881 and through the years up to World War II, when *one* rhetoric gained sway, I hope to give general impressions about cultural matters and processes in our time, especially concerning how natural science influences day-to-day life. My project basically deals with how science becomes a cultural matter, and in this context mediation takes on significance. How did the mediation act? What kind of symbols were created? My intention is to examine how things may take on new meanings and the relationships between things, symbols and meaning. There is much literature on this topic, and it is thus easy to wander off track. In ethnology it is not primarily theoretical aspects of such issues that are interesting, rather how these manifest themselves in the material sense. I shall elaborate on this by examining some advertisements for milk and dairy products. The advertisements I refer to are taken from the periodical *Liv og Sundhet* which was published in the period 1935 to 1939 up to twelve issues each year. This magazine may be taken as an example of the period's official attitude on diets and nutrition. It has a clear informative perspective, and even its advertising was approved by the editors who were all central figures in the health and school systems. The editor-in-chief was Carl Schiøtz, a prime mover in the social hygiene project. As head of the school health service in Oslo he instigated a series of important reforms, of which it will suffice in this context to mention the famous 'Oslo breakfast'. From 1932 until his death in 1938, he was also professor of hygiene at the University of Oslo. The magazine printed a number of articles about milk and dairy products, hence I chose this as the context for my interpretation of the advertisements.

FIVE ADVERTISEMENTS

Liv og Sundhet is not primarily a women's magazine, but it nevertheless addresses itself more or less directly to the Norwegian housewife, or perhaps it might be more appropriate to say the Norwegian mistress of the house. Many magazine articles about food and cookery emphasise that the housewife does not have to be a 'scientist'. Preparing food is a concrete act, admittedly during this period to be built on scientific insight, but it was not really necessary to know something about these insights themselves. The housewife's know-how was to be applied in practice, to the selection of food, preparation methods and eating habits, which she would have to perform *correctly*. She had to be taught to *see* the same things, but not in the same way. When teaching the nutritional science message on diet and health, great emphasis was placed on the visual aspect.

On the last few pages of each issue of the magazine we find advertisements for a plethora of products, but the advertisements for milk and dairy products stand out from the rest. This advertising does not consist of simple line-art like the other advertisements, but uses big, beautiful photographs which, with interspersed text, fill a whole page. Roland Barthes says that the significance of a picture in advertising is wholly intentional. The meaning of symbols is displayed as clearly as possible. 'If the picture contains symbols, we may take it for granted that in advertising these symbols will be complete, intentionally designed for optimal readability'.[14] These advertisements, of which there are in total 34, may be divided into three main categories: people of varying ages and varying situations who drink milk or say they drink milk; 'still life' compositions; and pictures of animals, nature and the environment. Some consist of text only, and the amount of text in the others varies, from a few words to big blocks of text representing different genres. They run the gamut from tales of the 'Once upon a time' variety to texts with scientific information displaying tables and graphs. This last type is represented only a few times. Recurrent words in the headlines are national, scientific or rational.

It is not always so clear whether the advertisement is for butter, cheese or milk. In one sense it is for all of them. '1 litre milk, half of it to drink,

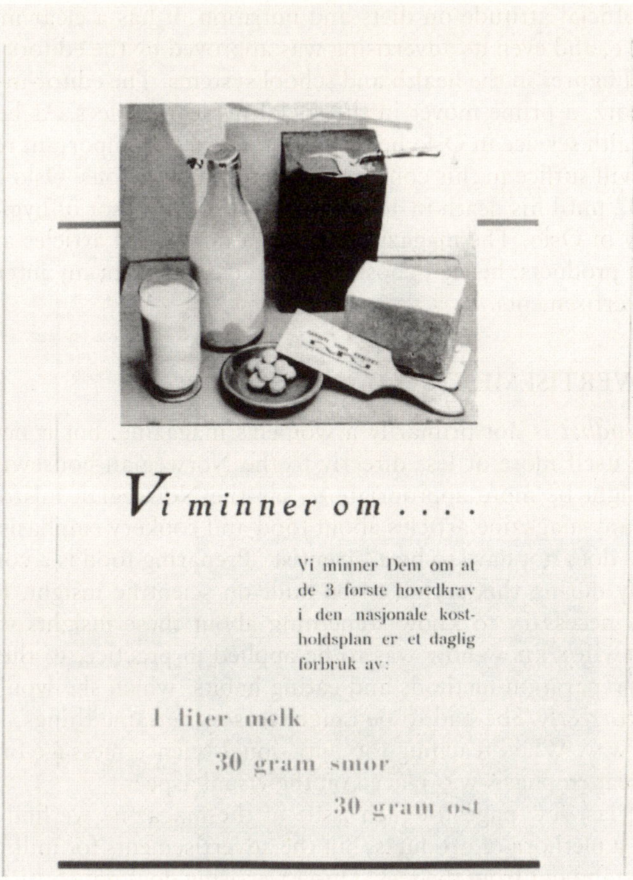

Fig. 1. *Liv og Sundhet* [Life and Health] *(1936), 7.*

30 grams of butter, and 30 grams of cheese' was the recommended quantity which should be part of everybody's daily diet, and this is what we see in the pictures. Fresh milk in clean sparkling glasses, or in bottles, catches the eye. This is what is focused on, dominating both the pictures and the text.

I shall now examine more closely five of these advertisements which have been selected because they deal with and support largely the same theme. The pictures do not show only milk and dairy products, but also a particular meal.[15]

One advertisement carries a picture of milk, cheese and butter (Fig 1). The milk is poured into a glass, on top of one of the two blocks of cheese sits a cheese slicer holding half a slice of cheese, the butter is displayed as small pats on a little saucer. 'We remind you . . .' the headline below the picture says, and it is eminently clear that the message of this advertisement is that milk, cheese and butter should be included as important elements in the daily diet, which is also emphasised in the text. The glass of milk sug-

Kostholdet.

et

nasjonalt

problem.

Det er så lett å glemme, — når man diskuterer kostholdsspørsmål, — at dette i bund og grunn er et nasjonalt problem.

Vi vet nok at eskimoene kan skape et sundt kosthold ut fra de næringsmidler de har, at innbyggerne på Tristan da Cunha kan sette sammen et sundt kosthold ut fra de næringsmidler de har, at italienerne kan gjøre det samme, ut fra sitt grunnlag o. s. v., o. s. v.

Vi kan dog ikke blindt overføre enkelte løsrevne sannheter fra andre folks ernæring. Vi må sette dem i relasjon til de næringsmidler som står til tjeneste i den daglige norske folke-ernæring. Spørsmålet er igrunnen heller ikke i sin innerste kjerne de for-

skjellige næringsmidler, mer hvilket utvalg blandt næringsmidlene vi skal gjøre for å skaffe best mulig og sikrest mulig de riktige næringsstoffer.

I et norsk tidsmessig kosthold, hvor de moderne, almengyldige ernæringsprinsipper er innpasset og omsatt i praksis, er et av de første grunnkrav: Tilstrekkelig melk. Melk er vårt mest allsidig sammensatte næringsmiddel og av den grunn står den på første ns i våre forskjellige næringsplaner. En økning i forbruk av melk og melkprodukter betyr at man gjør hele folkets kosthold bedre og vi vet alle at dette er en høist aktuell opgave for de fleste hjem.

Hovedkravene til det daglige kosthold er blandt annet et forbruk pr. individ av:

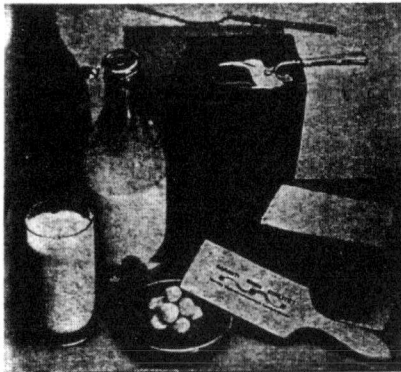

1 liter melk,
(til mat og drikke)

30 gr. smør,

30 gr. ost.

Fig 2. *Liv og Sundhet* [Life and Health] *(1937), 2.*

gests that some of the daily milk should be drunk. Even if there is no bread in the picture, we 'see' it anyway. Bread, cheese and butter belong together, the half slice of cheese in the slicer further underlining this. When we see the picture we know that the slice of bread is not far away. It is there even though we do not see it. Bread has an 'invisible presence' in the picture.

The same picture is used in a later issue, but in another context (Fig 2). The picture has been moved to the bottom of the page, and above it there is a fair amount of text. 'Our diet, a national problem' is stated in big letters in a separate column, and the text tells us that in the world at large people have always composed their diets based on the given surroundings. However, what is most important is not the kind of food that exists, but the kind of food we select. Milk, especially fresh milk as a drink, is emphasised as our most important food stuff. The text underlines that at least half a litre should be drunk.

Kostholdet er grunnlaget for vår helse.

Når man tidligere snakket om forbindelse mellem ernæring og helse så mente man med dette — bare for noen årtier tilbake — hovedsakelig det at enkelte fordøielsessykdommer skulde behandles med «diet». Vi vet nu at det er kostholdet — maten vi spiser — som er *grunnlaget* for en sterk, god helse.

Det er ikke lenger bare kjennskapet til matlagning i den forstand å lage «god» mat som er avgjørende. Det er kjennskapet til ernæringslæren som er det viktigste. Men vi vet også at får vi tilstrekkelig av de næringsmidler som verner helsen vår — vernekosten — da er det i grunnen det samme hvad vi spiser utenom dette.

I vernekosten — «protective foods» er det viktigste melk og melkeprodukter. Betydningen av hver dag hele året gjennem å få tilført tilstrekkelige mengder av disse ting kan derfor vanskelig overvurderes.

Alle moderne ernæringsplaner har som det første krav: tilstrekkelig melk. Og grunnen til dette er enkel nok. Melken er nemlig det mest allsidig sammensatte næringsmiddel vi kjenner. En økning i forbruket av melk og melkeprodukter betyr at man gjør hele folkets kosthold bedre og vi vet alle at dette er en høist aktuell opgave for de fleste hjem.

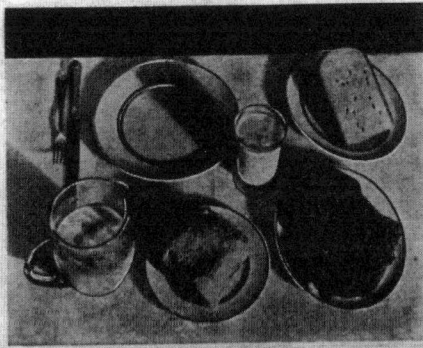

La MELKEN, SMØRET og OSTEN *innta en bred plass på Deres frokostbord.*

Fig 3. *Liv og Sundhet* [Life and Health] *(1937), 3-4.*

These two advertisements do not merely say something about milk being our most important article of food. They also state something about a particular situation, which is not visible in the picture itself, not even as a shadow, but is nevertheless present. The uncovered cheese, the half-opened milk bottle, the half-finished slice of cheese, the small pats of butter and the 'invisible' bread state something about a particular meal. Though neither the text not the picture say anything 'directly' about this meal, it is nevertheless entirely obvious that the picture presents associations of the 'Oslo breakfast'. If we look at the next issue, we find a picture of this meal.

A little picture at the bottom of this advertisement depicts a nicely laid breakfast table for one person (Fig 3). This bird's-eye-view picture shows us milk in a glass and a jug, butter, cheese and bread, everything laid ready for the first meal of the day. 'Let milk, butter and cheese enjoy favoured positions on your breakfast table' says the text alongside the picture. Above the picture a sizeable block of text tells us that diet and health go together. The text asserts that 'not only knowing how to make food and tasty dishes is important. The essential factor is to be familiar with nutrient values'.

As I see it, nutrition was not taught using the special idiom of nutritional science, but it is too simple to say that it was popularised or condensed: rather we may say it was translated. Messages about diets and health were translated into a 'visual language'. Nutritional values were transformed into concrete objects which in turn were given symbolic significance. Those things which were difficult, incomprehensible and abstract were made comprehensible and concrete via milk, cheese and butter. These three items became important symbols in the message nutritional science wanted to teach about diet and health, and when they are placed in a context, they also become tied to a concrete situation, the breakfast meal.

This advertisement also gives us the term 'protective foods', introduced by the American scientist Elmer V McCollum in 1918,[16] and its Norwegian translation *'vernekost'*. Both the English and Norwegian terms are mentioned and this is important. The words are not primarily used for their meaning. There is no attempt at explaining what they mean. They are used because their linguistic value lends a tone of 'professionalism' and 'English ness' to the text. This shows that even linguistic symbols have more 'meanings' than their context. In the article from 1960, Roland Barthes analyses an advertisement for pasta in France and says,

> . . . for the sign *Panzani* gives not simply the name of the firm but also, by its assonance, an additional 'flavour', that of 'Italianicity'. The linguistic message is thus twofold – 'denotational and connotational'.[17]

The word itself, the linguistic value and its visual appearance tell us that nutrition is a young science using new terms. In the text these words become symbols which offer associations to the world beyond Norway's borders, to something which is new and modern. In the magazine we may read that the term comes from the USA and means food that contains vitamins and salts which are vital to our health.

In an other advertisement there is a picture of the breakfast table (Fig 4). Here we find a bottle and a glass of milk, as well as a plate with some slices of bread and some raw carrots. 'The Oslo breakfast – the breakfast of the home' the text below the picture says, in this way referring to the above-mentioned breakfast served at Oslo schools. In 1932 it was decided that Oslo schools would serve breakfast, not the previously served midday meal. This breakfast, dubbed the 'Oslo breakfast', enjoyed a huge success not only in Oslo but also in other communities in the country. This meal certainly had nutritional significance, but probably even more importantly it also had a pedagogic purpose. Carl Schiøtz places most emphasis on the latter aspect. Breakfast at school was not only a social measure, it was a project of 'teaching the people'. From the cafeterias in Oslo schools the message

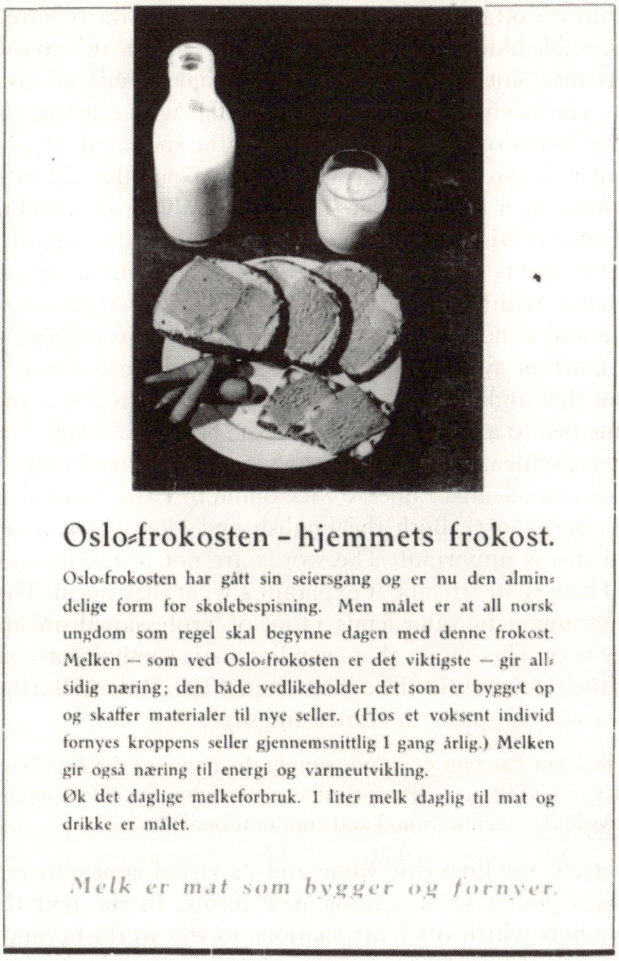

Fig 4. *Liv og Sundhet* [Life and Health] *(1936), 9.*

about a new diet, new eating habits and a new meal-time aesthetic would be spread to all the children in town.[18] The objective was to make the Oslo breakfast the morning meal of the home.

Our final advertisement tells us that this breakfast has won acclaim all over Europe (Fig 5). Here we are given the recipe for a 'luxury' version of this meal. Even here the linguistic aspect has 'meanings' beyond its content, as the recipes are given in English, Norwegian and German. The lady in the picture is seated at a table eating. She is wearing outdoor clothes – witness her hat. We sense the picture is taken at a restaurant. On the small, round café table there is a glass of milk, very bright and visible, and eggs, bread and half a grapefruit. Large letters beneath throw down the challenge, 'The Oslo breakfast is famous in this country and abroad. Have you introduced

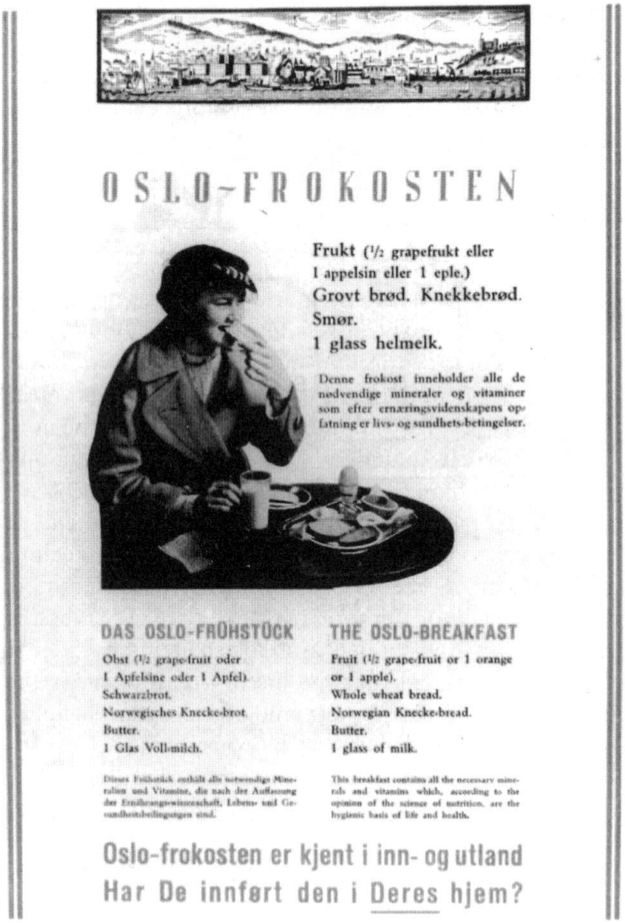

Fig 5. *Liv og Sundhet* [Life and Health] *(1936), 12.*

it in *your* home?' At the top of the page there is a sketch of Oslo seen from the waterfront. The advertisment gives connotations of big-city life and the world beyond us, something which is new and modern. But it is not merely foreign impulses which travel here, we also contribute something to the world out there. Norwegian nutrition experts are up there with the best of them. We have become modern too, Oslo is part of the world out there. The advertisement expresses faith in Norwegian nutritional expertise. Even the term 'Oslo breakfast' takes on special significance in this context.

The point of this examination is to demonstrate that more than dairy products are being advertised in these advertisements. We 'see' much more than milk, cheese and butter, we see a particular meal. By seeing this meal as a symbol, we will also be told about the ideology which it was part of. In this ideology breakfast has been given a new context and a new meaning. The pictures have told us what this meal should consist of: bread with cheese and butter and milk, preferably also fresh fruit or raw vegetables. Nevertheless, fresh milk as a drink is emphasised and given a special prominence in the pictures, possibly even more evident in the other 29 advertisements.

THE BREAKFAST

If we look to the old Norwegian 'agrarian community', there was no breakfast. In his book *Norsk Mat* [Norwegian Food] the Norwegian ethnologist Hilmar Stigum says that breakfast is a new term. Previously there were two main meals, called *dugurd* [the mid-morning meal] and *non* [the midday meal].[19] For the mid-morning meal, which was the second meal of the day, served around 9.30, porridge and milk were served, but the milk was rarely fresh. In traditional Norwegian diets milk had an important position. Diets were lacto-vegetal, based on cereals and potatoes supplemented by milk and dairy products. But fresh milk and indeed fresh food were not common in the old diet. Most items on the menu were cured by such techniques as salting, drying or smoking. Some food was boiled, but boiled food belongs to a more 'civilised diet'. Not without reason did Lévi-Strauss establish the culinary triangle with raw, boiled and rotten items each in their corner, and it has also been claimed that the history of cookery is the history of the civilisation of man. Using cookery and conservation techniques, food is processed so that prepared dishes may be consumed. Boiling and conservation techniques, however, are more than technical and chemical processes. They are also symbolic actions, in that they transform unsafe and dangerous nature into culture.

By nature man is omnivorous, but nonetheless does not eat everything that is edible – not everything that is edible is food. Food is a culturally defined category. In older times milk was included in the edible category, but it was still not a finished product. Fresh milk dwelt in a no-man's land between nature and culture. Through churning and cheese-making, milk was transformed into new products, into cheese and butter. Butter was nobler than anything else, as it could be sold in the marketplace or made into ornamental cookery for festive occasions, but milk might also be the lowest of the low, used as part of the daily diet of the poor – as skimmed milk – what was left after the butter had been processed. Milk was raw material, and as such it had an ambiguous status.

Fresh milk did not only have an ambiguous status, it might even be dangerous, extremely dangerous. Milk was shrouded in basic uncertainty as it might be the source of sickness and contamination. Even if this generally applies to any fresh food, milk was in a special position. 'Milk is thus a peculiar article of food, powerful and more beneficial than anything else, however, it also requires particular care'.[20] Transforming milk into new products means transforming raw and wild nature into culture, making the dangerous safe, bringing what was ambiguous under control. Working with milk was thus a process of cultural transformation, bringing uncertain nature itself under control. In order that fresh milk could have a separate place in the Norwegian diet, the requirements for hygiene had to be improved. The use of fresh milk grew out of the development of dairies which in turn depended on the great revolution taking place in the agrarian society. Important technological underpinnings such as the cream separator, dairy management, milk testing and refrigeration gradually enabled milk to become a totally safe product which could be used without worrying about hygiene.

In the nutritional science message about diets and health, milk was a source of health and strength. This was made possible by technological improvements, but these were not enough. Fresh milk would have to traverse a process of *cultural* change. In order that fresh milk should become a separate product, becoming something in itself, 'our most versatile food article' as the advertising claims, something had to be done with it. Fresh milk had to be given a new status, not as a potential source of contamination, nor as a raw material for new products, but as a thing in itself.

This is the milk we see in the pictures. The white, fresh milk in clean clear glasses acquires new status. The milk in the pictures has metamorphosed through a cultural process of transformation – not through boiling and preservation techniques, nor through being processed into new products, but through aesthetics. Through aesthetics fresh milk has been made pure. What was ambiguous has been brought under control. Nature has acquired a culturally formed naturalness. The eye-catching fresh milk in these pictures is a symbol, not only of something beyond itself, it also proves something about itself. It tells us that it is clean. The clean glass of milk is both a goal and a means.

THE RATIONAL MEAL

In nutritional science rhetoric on diets and health, fresh milk received not only a clean, new status, but also a special position. Being the most versatile of our foodstuffs, it was to be an essential part of the Norwegian diet. 'The essential means for improving the Norwegian diet is increased milk consumption', the advertising says. The reason why milk and not other dairy products such as cheese and butter attained this position is tied to economic concerns. Butter has always been a status item in Norway, thus it was also given decorative shapes, as when beautiful dishes holding butter were set on the table for parties. The butter was not to be consumed, it was to display status and skill. It was called 'ornamental cookery' by Roland Barthes, and 'trophy food' by the old farmers, thus giving it religious overtones. In the advertisements butter is also presented as ornamental cookery. In some ways all food in advertising is ornamental, at least that is what Roland Barthes claims. In advertisements for milk and dairy products, however, butter enjoys a different position from milk and cheese. Butter is not presented as cheese is, something has been done to the butter. The butter has been sculpted into small rippled pats, decoratively placed in a dish. It is more like trophy food in the old sense. It displays higher status. The small pats of butter say that butter is different.

There are many discussions about butter in the many articles on school breakfast in the magazine itself. Butter is expensive, and it was replaced with margarine in many places, which was not satisfactory from a nutritional point of view. Milk, however, was cheap. Hence economic concerns were the reason why such emphasis was given to milk. '25 litres of milk give 1 litre of butter', says one of the advertisements, the message being to use more milk. But are milk and butter the same thing? Is it at all possible to compare these two products? Even though milk is not butter, and butter is not milk, it is possible to compare them in this context. They contain the same nutritional values, and these, not the food itself, are what is most important. In the nutritional rhetoric food has become 'nutritional values', an abstract category which nevertheless can be weighed and measured.

In the various dietary plans which were formulated nutritional values and economy were balanced against each other. In this context milk is better than butter. Fresh milk became an essential part of the Norwegian diet because it was so inexpensive. *Anybody* could put milk on their breakfast table, which was also the objective. Nutritional rhetoric made *everybody* the target group. Everybody could change their diets for the better.

The League of Nations divided food into two groups, protective food and supplemental food, and the former category received much attention. Many names are found for the same thing here. In addition to 'protective food' there is talk of 'fundamental nutrients'. In Norway the 'fundamentals' were first and foremost milk fresh from the cow, some wholewheat bread, fresh fruit and vegetables. This brings us back to the pictures. What we see depicted in them is the protective food or fundamental nutrients. [21]

'The most important thing is to provide each person with a sufficient amount of what is called fundamental nutrients',[22] *Liv og Sundhet* says, and these should be part of your daily diet. This brings us back to breakfast. Breakfast as a meal is the same each and every day, with little variation. This meal is easy to control nutritionally. Carl Schiøtz underscores this argument.

One obvious question remains to be asked: why was such attention paid to breakfast? Why not carry on as before? To answer this issue, which is of a more ideology-critical nature, another essay would be required. It is evident that many ideological signposts would direct attention to general diets, for example, in relation to the work force. To have good workers, a healthy and strong population is needed. The right diet was required for this purpose. I have endeavoured to show why emphasis was laid on breakfast and not on other meals. When it is desirable that the entire population should enjoy the same meal, breakfast was the more viable alternative from a purely economic perspective. Nutritional science rhetoric on diets and health intended to change the diet of the whole population. To this end many interests joined forces, not necessarily with the same end in mind, but they nevertheless agreed to collaborate on this one issue. As such a breakfast is also a symbol, but of another type, and examining this aspect would also require another paper.

BIBLIOGRAPHY

Aarbog for norsk forening for sundhedspleie [Yearbook for the Norwegian Society for Health Care], Kristiania, 1885–1890.

Alsvik, Ola. '"Friskere, sterkere, større, renere". Om Carl Schiøtz og helsearbeidet for norske skolebarn' ["Healthier, more Wholesome, Stronger and Cleaner". On Carl Schiøtz and his work for Norwegian School Children], History Thesis University of Oslo, 1990.

Barnes, Barry and Shapin, Steven. *Natural Order. Historical Studies of Scientific Culture*, Beverly Hills, 1979.

Barthes, Roland. *Mytologier,* Uddevalla, 1969; Bildets Retorikk [Rhétorique de l'image (1960)], *I tegnets tid Utvalgte artikler og essays,* Oslo, 1994.

Drummond, Jack Cecil and Wilbraham, Anne. *The Englishman's Food. A history of five centuries of English diet*, London, 1939, 1994.

Erken, Henriette Schønberg and Schiøtz, Carl. *Trygg kost for norske hjem* [Safe Diet in Norwegian Homes], Oslo, 1939.

Espeland, Wigdis Jorunn and Riddervold, Astri. Mennesketsynet, med særlig vekt på kvinner, hjå Eilert Sundt og Peter Christen Asbjørnsen i modernisering-sprosessen [The conception of mankind, or more specifically womankind, as expressed by Eilert Sundt and Peter Christen Asbjørnsen in the process of modernisation], *Dugnad*, tidsskrift for etnologi, 2/3 (1993), 77–95.

Fürst, Elisabeth L'Orange. *Mat – et annet språk* [Food – Another Language], Oslo, 1995.

Goody, Jack. *Cooking, Cuisine and Class*, Cambridge, 1991.

Grøn, Fredrik. *Om kostholdet I Norge* [On Diet in Norway], Oslo, 1941.

Haave, Per. 'Ernæringsspørsmålet I norsk politikk fra 1930–årene til 1946' [The Question of Nutrition in Norwegian Policy 1930–1946], History Thesis, University of Oslo, 1990.

Hirdman, Yvonne. *Matfrågan Mat som mål och medel Stockholm 1870–1920* [The Question of Food. Food as aim and means. Stockholm 1870–1920], Stockholm, 1983.

Ihde, Aaron J. *The Development of Modern Chemistry*, New York, 1964.

Ihde, Aaron J and Becker Standley, L. Concepts in early vitamin studies, *Journal of the History of Biology* (1971), 1-33.

Levenstein, Harvey. *Revolution at the Table, the Transformation and the American Diet*, Oxford,1988.

Liv og Sundhet [Life and Health], 1934–38.

McCollum, E V and Simmond, Nina. *The Newer Knowledge of Nutrition. The use of foods for the preservation of vitality and health*, New York, 1929.

National Health Insurance Medical Research Committee Special Report. Series no 38: *Om vitaminerne. Hvad man officielt kjender til deres karakter og virkemaate* [Present State of Knowledge Concerning Accessory Food Factors], Kristiania, 1919, 1923.

Poulsson, Edvard. *Om vitaminer spesielt om vitamin A og torskelever tran* [On Vitamins, Especially Vitamin A and Cod-liver Oil], Copenhagen, 1923.

Ropeid, Andreas. Fornuftigt Madstel [Sensible cookery], *By og Bygd* (1975), 77–113.

Schmidt, Lars-Henrik and Kristensen, Jens Erik. *Lys, luft og renlighed. Den moderne socialhygienes fødsel* [Light, Air and Cleanliness. The birth of modern social hygiene], Copenhagen, 1986.

Todhunter, E Neige. Some aspects of the history of dietetics. *World Review of Nutrition and Dietetics,* 18 (1973), 1–46.

Wold, Knut Gezt. *Kosthold of levestandard. En økonomisk undersøkelse* [Dietetic and Living-standards. A study of economics], Oslo, 1941.

NOTES

1 Erken and Schiøtz, 1939, 7.
2 Drummond and Wilbraham, 1939; ibid, 1991; Ihde, 1964; Idhe and Becker, 1971; Levenstein, 1988; Todhunter, 1971.
3 Ropeid, 1972; Espeland and Riddervold, 1993.
4 This was taken from Ola Alsvik's history thesis on Carl Schiøtz.
5 Erken and Schiøtz, 1939, 7.
6 ibid, 23.
7 ibid.
8 Wold, 1941.
9 Haave, 1990.
10 *Liv og Sundhet* (1935), 179.
11 Erken and Schiøtz, 1939, preface.
12 ibid, 10.
13 ibid. My underlining.
14 Barthes, 1964; ibid, 1994, 22.
15 The advertisements do not succeed each other in the order presented here.
16 Todhunter, 1973, 26.
17 Barthes, 1994, 24.
18 Alsvik,1991,161.
19 Stigum, 1965, 15.
20 *Aarbok for den norske forening for sundhedspleie*, 1889, 15.
21 Alsvik, 1991, 162.
22 *Liv og Sundhet* (1935), 11.

11 'Keep fit and slim!' Alternative ways of nutrition as aspects of the German health movement, 1880–1930

Sabine Merta

'The Germans eat too much and too fat,'[1] according to the latest scientific findings of the 'German Institute for Food Research'.[2] Statistically, every third German suffers from being overweight. Major health problems, such as obesity, cardiovascular diseases, diabetes mellitus and cancer, are caused by overnutrition.[3] Excess weight is health risk factor number one in our modern state of prosperity. According to the 'German Minister of Health' over 83 billion DM, one third of Public Health funds, are probably spent on diseases which are sequels to being overweight.[4] However, there are not only health reasons for the enormous boom in the diet, health and fitness industry.[5] There is also the beauty standard of a 'young, athletic and slim body' represented by models in the mass media. The result of a representative inquiry by the 'Society for Market Research'[6] shows that the actual BMI (body mass index = weight [kg]/divided by the square of the height [m^2]) is around 18 and 20, which corresponds to the lowest extremity of standard weight.[7] Women, especially, want to achieve this by 'dieting'.[8] Meanwhile, 'diets' belong to our everyday life.[9] But what is known about their historical origins and connections?

Most people nowadays consider modern diet to be just a consequence of our scientific knowledge about nutrition and a response to the current 'slenderness-model', which at most goes back to the time of the extreme slender figure of the 1960s, embodied by the famous British mannequin 'Twiggy'.[10] But in reality the roots of diets and the slimness fashion reach deeper. Thus, the two main questions of this paper are: when do we find the earliest forerunners of our modern dietary, which has developed more and more under the influence of a 'new' fashionable body, fitness and slimness cult, into a 'reducing diet', and why did it also never lose its initial hygienic meaning as therapy, health maintenance and/or health improvement? And how closely are the senses of health, nutrition and body connected with one another?

The word 'Diät' [diet], from the Greek 'díaita' (regimen), can be recovered in its original significance and in dominance in the recent period of the German health movement (1880–1930).[11] At the beginning of the German health movement 'Diät' was initially a synonym for nutrition, but

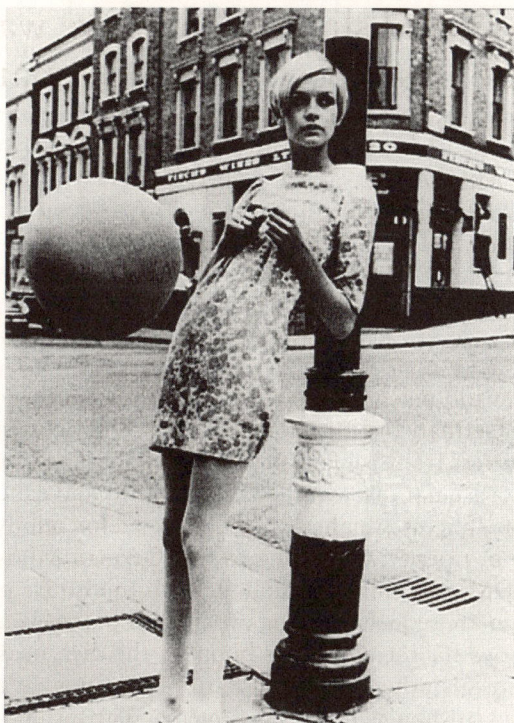

Fig. 1. *The extreme slenderness standard of the 1960s embodied by Leslie Horn-bey, better known under the name 'Twiggy'.*

the common restriction today to low-calorie food was first introduced later in the 1920s.[12]

NATURISM AS MENTAL SUPERSTRUCTURE

Following the call of the French Philosopher Jean Jacques Rousseau (1712–1778) of 'back to nature', and perhaps also influenced by American Puritanism and British and French vegetarianism movements, nature-cure practitioners were the first to rediscover the ancient concept of dietetics, which had fallen into oblivion. They developed diets further using them as a natural way of healing.[13]

THE GERMAN NATUROPATHY MOVEMENT

The German physician Christoph Wilhelm Hufeland (1762–1836), in his book *Macrobiotics* (1796),[14] already suggested temperance as a necessity of life, particularly with regard to food. His idea and those of the whole German health movement was a novel concept of pathology and a view of the entire human being consisting of body and soul. Civilization was criti-

cized for estranging man from nature. Correspondingly, disease was interpreted as a result of a constant 'unnatural' way of life, as an accumulation
of contagious matter. The purpose of the treatment by natural remedies was
to awake the vital forces in the body by using natural elements like water,
earth, light, food and air.[15] In contrast to medicine not only the symptoms
but also the cause of the diseases was to be attacked.

In the 1880s the German health movement became a mass movement,
emerging from dissatisfaction with academic medicine. This phenomenon
can be interpreted as a common reaction of the public towards the deficiencies, failures and false developments of medical research, which kept
becoming more professional and scientific. As a consequence, the gap
between patient and doctor grew and questions of public health services
were neglected. Suddenly, the supporters of this hygienic 'laymen movement' entered into competition with scientific medicine and a vehement,
public conflict followed. The nature-cure practitioners were defamed by
the physicians as 'Kurpfuscher' (quacks) and they demanded specific laws
to be promulgated against it. As a consequence, they advanced the term
'Schulmedizin' (scholastic medicine) to differentiate themselves from the
'Giftmischer' (poisoners) and 'Allopathen' (allopaths). This altercation continued in the so called 'Eiweissdiskussion' (discussion about the right quantity of proteins in everyday fare) and later in the discussion about the
correct slimming methods. Journals like *Der Naturarzt* (Nature-doctor),
medical reviews, public newspapers and meetings became battlefields of
disputes.[16]

Hydrotherapy brought the German health movement to a climax. In this
context Vincenz Priessnitz (1799–1851), an expert on cold-water therapy,
and Sebastian Kneipp (1821–1897), still renowned worldwide for his special water-cures, have to be mentioned. The hydrotherapeutics prescribed
individually for every patient involved water drinking cures, cold or warm
gushes, wet compresses, showers and other bathing methods to stimulate
the excretion of poisonous matter out of the body via the skin pores.[17]

SCHROTH'S TREATMENT, OR, FROM HYDROTHERAPY
TO TROPHOTHERAPY

Johannes Schroth (1798–1856) was the first hygienist to combine wet and
hot sweating-packs with strict hunger and thirst cures. He tried to stimulate
excretion as an auxiliary with the help of diet via the kidneys and intestines.
He had already defined 'overeating' as a major health problem, and established a sanatorium in Linderwiese-Freiwaldau (Bohemia). Patients disap-
pointed by hydrotherapy came there to be healed through abstinence. For
his slimming method he let his patients sweat in wet heat, withdrew fluids
from them for days and limited their food intake. During this phase of
therapy, on *Trockentage* (dry days), the patient was only allowed to drink
small amounts of light wine and eat dry bread rolls. At intervals, there were

normal eating and drinking days, but even during these 'Trinktagen' (drinking days) only the quantity of home-grown wine chosen for the individual's perceived diseased state was allowed. Hence, his principle of fasting used to be based on a personalized series of dry and drinking days. From ancient times diet was known as an universal remedy, but at this time during the first half of the nineteenth century it was rarely used as therapy. Although Schroth's treatment was often criticized by other naturopaths, because of his use of alcoholic wine, his merit was to have rediscovered and revived fasting and diet as healing.[18]

THE GERMAN VEGETARIAN MOVEMENT

The final turning-point in the direction of dietary regimens introduced the former pharmacist and naturopath Theodor Hahn (1824–1883). The curative effect of his therapy was mainly based on vegetarian diet. He continued the tradition of the old dietetics by believing in normal and abnormal *Lebensreize* (stimulants of life). He considered normal stimulants to be food and drink, air, heat, light, electricity, exercise and recreation. Abnormal stimulants had an alimentary or toxic character. His maxim was to heal by means of wholesome food. From his point of view only the vegetarian diet could be the right regimen and healthy permanent fare in the sense of Rousseau's naturism. 1852 Theodor Hahn started to live as a vegetarian and defended vegetarianism during his life-time. In his book '*Die naturgemässe Diät, die Diät der Zukunft*,' he presented historical, anatomical, physiological and ethical arguments for vegetarianism.[19] This 'nature doctor' laid the foundation of the German vegetarian movement.

The German vegetarian movement was not only concerned with a pure vegetable diet, but also carried a whole ideology with it, though this was a heterogeneous construct influenced by many individuals. The designation 'vegetarianism' has nothing to do with the main food, vegetables, as often believed. It comes from the Latin *vegetus* and means fresh, alive, 'fit as a fiddle'. The core of vegetarianism was and still is abstinence from animal meat, without (vegan vegetarianism) or with the addition of eggs (ovo-vegetable vegetarianism) or milk (lacto-vegetable vegetarianism) or both (ovo-lacto-vegetable vegetarianism). The three main theses of vegetarianism were:

1. Killing animals leads to killing humans. Meat makes aggression!
2. A natural vegetable diet influences the soul.
3. The human body is only made for vegetable food. Only to live 'frugivorously' is natural and healthy!

These theses always formed the main arguments of the vegetarians against the physicians in the discussion about the right quantity of foodstuffs in the diet.

The initiators of the German vegetarianism movement were the German revolutionary of the year 1848/49, lawyer and publicist Gustav Struve

(1805–1870) and Wilhelm Zimmermann (1819–1882). The theoretical foundation of German vegetarianism was based on Struve's '*Pflanzenkost. Eine Grundlage einer neuen Weltanschauung*' (Vegetable diet. The basis of a new philosophy of life).[20] In 1868 Struve together with twenty other vegetarians registered and promoted the 'Vegetarische Gesellschaft Stuttgart eV' (Stuttgart Vegetarian Society).[21] The title of Wilhelm Zimmermann's book[22] shows that for the vegetarians the German social question was a question of the right diet.[23]

THE GERMAN LIFE REFORM MOVEMENT

The Protestant theologian Eduard Baltzer (1814–1887) developed the ideological concept still further to an all-embracing idea of a reform of all living conditions. Baltzer's contribution to the German vegetarianism movement was to proceed from a literary, theoretically oriented approach to an active approach of practical agitation. He created an ideology to reform health problems through a new ethical way of life. To promulgate his central concept, he published a book in four volumes between 1867 and 1871, '*Die natürliche Lebensweise*' (The natural way of life) with a universal reform programme.[24]

The name of this programme was 'Lebensreform' (life reform). Its first use can be traced to the year 1896. Around 1900 it suddenly emerged into public usage. Previously synonyms such as 'Diätreform' (diet reform), 'Reform der Lebensweise' (reform of the way of life), 'Hygienische Reform' (hygienic reform), 'allseitige Reform' (universal reform) or 'Reform der gesamten Lebensweise' (reform of the whole way of life) were used. The oldest expression 'Diätreform' (diet reform) shows that its origin goes back to the first phase of the German health movement, the naturopathy movement or even earlier to the influence of American Puritanism, and English or French vegetarian movements, although in historical research it is still unclear to which of them it owes more.[25]

However, under Baltzer's influence, the first vegetarian organization with the more common name 'Verein für natürliche Lebensweise' (Association for a natural way of life) was formed on 27 April 1867. Later it changed its name to 'Deutscher Verein für naturgemässe Lebensweise (Vegetarianer) (German Association for a natural way of life (vegetarians)).[26] In this lively period club activities, literature, affiliated companies, lectures and touring groups flourished.

'Life reform' was the name and programme of a movement which wanted a fundamental renewal of all life's functions. Eating, drinking, moving, breathing, sleeping, relaxing, working and living should be brought back to their natural condition by following sanitary regulations, observing moderation in each of them, especially abstemiousness in eating.[27] The intention was to work against the progressive decline of health due to the ailments of civilization. The elements of the German health movement are: naturopathy, vegetarianism, nudism, reform of land-owning, of dwellings and of clothing, utopian colonies, hygiene, total abstinence, antivivisection and antivaccination, sport and gymnastics, youth movement, art nouveau and environmental concerns, to mention just some of them. All these can be subsumed under the idea of a natural life.[28] However, its aims still cause an after-effect: the current awareness of health, food, environment and body.

On one hand life reform meant a reform of the individual, by changing everyday habits in the direction of a more natural life style. The individual aim of bringing the people closer to nature should also achieve greater self-knowledge. On the other hand life reform meant the wish to change the whole life style of modern German society. It was a new philosophy of life, that arose from dissatisfaction with the socio-economic and socio-cultural changes at the end of the nineteenth century. Thus, in historical research the life reform notion is not only interpreted as a health movement, but also as a movement to reform civilization, although it never achieved this ulterior purpose, perhaps because it remained politically unorganized and passive.[29] Among their contemporaries they were seen, because of their ideas (which today seem very progressive), as strange 'sectarians' and in public newspapers and journals negatively labelled as 'Naturaposteln' (nature apostles), 'Körnerfresser' (granivorous feeders) or 'Hungerleider' (starvelings).[30]

The practical transformation of their ideas took place in the new branch of the production of health foods. The first health food shop is documented for the year 1887 in Berlin.[31]

The first health food producers were life reformers, too. Natural ways of food production and consumption were practised in the luxury settlements as for example in Ascona at Monte Verità (Italy)[32] or in the fruit-growing settlement (Eden) around Berlin.[33]

The historical development of the German health movement originates in the first half of the nineteenth century in diverse phases. Until World War I a complex of various movements had developed and reached their climax in the 1920s and 1930s. There are three historical phases of the German health movement:

1. Health movement based on naturopathy.
2. Health movement based on a natural life style, especially on a natural diet (diet reform movements) and a natural form of life (natural farming; notions of utopian communities).
3. Health movement based on the rediscovery of the natural beauty of the human body (body reform movements).[34]

The emphasis of this paper will be on the second and the third phases, which are particularly interesting for the historical reconstruction of the development of the modern regimen.

GERMAN DIET REFORM MOVEMENTS

The diet reform idea was the central point of the programme from the very beginning and it remained constant. Many diet reformers defended a vegan or lacto-vegetable form of nutrition. In contrast to the German vegetarianism movement, which was an independent organization, not everybody was obliged to be a vegetarian, because one was allowed to live on mixed food.[35] To find alternative ways of nutrition expressed and demonstrated some kind of protest. The ordinary fare and the excessive gluttony of modern civilization were censured in public. There were mainly ecological motives for a universal diet reform, which means that for diet reformers only food produced by biological-dynamical agriculture and by ways of production favourable to the environment was healthy. The diet system of the 'full of value' food may be traced to this idea. In addition, there were economic incentives to choose a vegetarian diet, and alternative nutrition was analysed, under the aspect of saving of expense, as a solution to the social question in Germany. The diet reformers wanted to update the diet. Their wide-ranging aim of a universal diet reform could never be reached. One reason might be that too many different ideas about the right diet existed alongside each other, so that no collective agreement could be found. However, their diets can be specified in main diet-groups, which still exist today.[36]

HAIG'S THEORY AS THE BASIS OF THE GERMAN DIET REFORM MOVEMENTS

Haig's theory is the basis for the development of most diet systems. The English physician Alexander Haig (*1853) was himself a vegetarian and an important member of the English vegetarian movement.[37] His theory on uric acid waste products in the blood and in the histological cells as the main reason for diseases fundamentally influenced the pathological interpretation of the naturopaths and still does today. By intensive experimental research he discovered that uric acid and analogous substances, a result of eating too much meat, were the reason for most illnesses. Accordingly, he supported the vegetarian diet, which is low in protein and uric acid. Haig developed a system for determining uric acid in the blood, which is still known in modern medicine as the 'Haycraft method'. In 1884 he published his findings in a book, which was translated into German by the Swiss diet reformer Max Bircher-Benner in 1902.[38] In this book he warned against immoderate consumption of meat, alcohol, coffee and tea, which could increase the concentration of uric acid in the blood many times over. This diseased state of the blood substance, the result of disturbed solubility of uric acid salts, he called 'Collämie', the consequences of which are eg migraine, hysteria or depression etc. Chronic 'Collämie' would lead to the so-called 'Rentention', which means, after a while, the uric acid salts could be pushed aside in the surrounding cells. 'Rentention' diseases are gout, rheumatism, cardiac disorders etc.[39] Haig's theory formed the main argument of diet reformers.

'FULL OF VALUE' DIET MOVEMENT

The first step towards a 'full of value' diet was made by Gustav Schlickeysen (1843–1893), who proclaimed his idea in 1875 in the book *Obst und Brot* (Fruit and Bread).[40] It is very surprising that the question of full value food in connection with natural diet was asked at such a late date, because, before the discovery of fire, the natural food of human beings used to be uncooked; cooking was developed as a result of the process of civilization.[41] Schlickeysen's diet system was based on Cuvier's theory of the original frugivorous human. It expressed already the main maxim of this movement: food is health only if it derives directly from nature. From his point of view, natural nutriments were pure fruit (fruit, cereals, tuberous plants, root vegetables and wholemeal bread).[42] As a breakfast he created a fresh cereals porridge, made of grain wheat and apple.[43] It was a forerunner of 'Müsli'. His treatment was a pure fruit diet. Schlickeysen called it 'sunlight food',[44] already anticipating the ideas of Max Bircher-Benner. However, Gustav Schlickeysen laid the basis for the 'full of value' diet movement, which can be subdivided into a raw vegetarian diet movement and into a whole wheat diet movement.

RAW VEGETARIAN DIET MOVEMENT

Today the Swiss physician Maximilian Bircher-Benner (1867–1939) is accepted as the founder of the modern uncooked vegetarian diet. Bircher-Benner was the first person who tried to formulate a scientific argument for its healing effect by means of the so-called 'light quantum theory'.[45] Because of him a raw vegetarian diet was integrated into modern dietetics. He is the 'inventor' of the world famous 'Müsli'[46] which is now an everyday food.

A profound experience made the doctor switch from medical treatment to a treatment by natural remedies: one day a woman with a chronic gastric disorder, of some 30 years duration, came to his practice in Zürich, searching for help. He tried every possible medical therapy without success. Then he did something which was quite unusual for his time and from the point of view of modern medicine strictly forbidden. He prescribed an uncooked vegetarian diet, containing just fruit, nuts, salads, wholemeal bread and uncooked and stewed vegetables. The woman was cured. Bircher-Benner decided to employ a raw vegetarian diet. In 1897 he opened his sanatorium. There he did research work to discover a scientific explanation for his observation.[47] Eventually, he found a solution by means of the two physical energy laws, when he applied the second law, the entropy law to nature. The result was his 'light quantum theory' which says: 'Wir werden nicht durch Kalorien, sondern durch Lichtquanten ernährt' (Not calories nourish us, but the sunlight quanta).[48] He based on this theory his order of nutriment which differentiates three main levels:

1. Accumulators of the first order are all uncooked edible parts of plants (leaf, fruit, seed, cereals, tuberous plant and root).
2. Accumulators of the second order are cooked food or food prepared in any other way.
3. Accumulators of the third order are meat, mushrooms, stimulants (coffee, tea, cocoa, tobacco), chocolate, preserved food, strongly heated and very spicy food.[49]

Today Bircher-Benner's 'light quantum theory' is untenable in its original form. Nevertheless, he promoted a diet rich in vitamins a long time before the 'vitamin-revolution'.[50]

The director of the Institute for Hygiene in Rostock, the bacteriologist Professor Werner Kollath (1892–1970) advanced in 1941 a theory explaining the curative effect of raw vegetarian food, the so-called 'theory of mesotrophy', which is still valid. It was the result of twenty years of experimental work (vitamin experiments with rats). The word 'mesotrophy' is Greek and means translated 'half nourished'.[51] The 'theory of mesotrophy' described also a diseased state of a chronic half-nourishment which maybe made a long life possible, but which also was responsible for the development of chronic diseases, because of the absence of growth substances in the plants. The expressions 'full of value food' and 'fragment value food' go back to Kollath's findings.[52] In his dietetic order only the unchanged food, was 'full of value'. Kollath evolved a special test method to show the degree of full value in the nourishment by means of the growth and the increase of vegetable cells. His rule was: the higher the degree of variation by human techniques the less is the worth of the food and the more the food has lost value. Thus, Kollath's order of nutriment states:

1. Food of the first order: seeds and fruit.
2. Food of the second order: tubers and roots.
3. Food of the third order: leaves and stems.[53]

Kollath's maxim was: 'Leave the food as natural as possible!' He distinguished between 'vital and non-vital foodstuffs'. A 'vital foodstuff' was defined as a food rich in supplies for living, in the form of vitamins, minerals and integral growth substances. Food which was changed in any way was 'non-vital'.[54] He recommended a fresh whole grain porridge, which is still called 'Kollath-breakfast' today.[55] His present followers are Karl von Koerber, Claus Leitzmann and Thomas Männle, a team of nutritionists from Giessen.[56]

The first school for diet 'full of value' was opened 1908 by Emil Drebber (1873–1943).[57]

WHOLE WHEAT MOVEMENT

An American pioneer of the whole wheat movement was the former parson of a Presbyterian parish and strict total abstainer Sylvester Graham

(1794–1851). Graham propagated a wheat bran bread which was made from raw milled wheat, prepared and baked with fresh milk, without any yeast. After a bad cholera epidemic in 1832 the famous 'Graham-bread' spread quickly in America. He preached a general reform of diet and even maintained that his bread could heal diseases. Graham's bread became famous all over the world.[58] The first German supporter of this movement was Gustav Schlickeysen, who had already recognized the importance of whole wheat for digestion, before science confirmed it later.[59]

Another famous reformer of bread was Gustav Simons (1861–1914). Simons took over a Russian processing technique for his bread. The bread was made only of steeped rye-grains.[60] In this way 'whole wheat bread' came to Germany and was sold in health food shops under the name 'Simon's bread'.[61] Around 1870 Simons promoted an 'Association for Improvement of Bread' in Berlin-Charlottenburg.[62]

The diet reformer Stefan Steinmetz (1861–1914) in 1890 invented a special method of wet peeling grain to improve the bread. Two years later he took out a patent. Steinmetz designated white, industrial fine milled flour as 'luxury flour' and whole wheat flour as 'bread flour'.[63]

NUTRIENT SALT MOVEMENT

The creator of the theory of the importance of nutrient salt in the diet was Heinrich Lahmann (1860–1905). The central starting point of his research about the correct diet was the metabolism of minerals in the human body. During his medical studies he produced a 'vegetable milk', which played an important part in baby nourishment at that time.[64] He commercialized also other processed foodstuffs (nutrient salt products),[65] while he was still studying. Thus Heinrich Lahmann was amongst the important producers of health articles.[66]

At first Lahmann worked as a nature-cure practitioner in Stuttgart. Then he opened his sanatorium 'Weisser Hirsch' in Dresden-Loschwitz.[67] Finally, he published in 1891 his book *Die diätetische Blutentmischung als Grundursache der Krankheiten*' (The dietetic blood-decomposing as primary cause for diseases)[68] in which he gave reasons for his theory of the 'Dysämie', according to which an incorrect diet introduces false ingredients into blood, leading to a faulty composition of body substance. In his opinion only the nutrient salts and minerals in the food would be able to avoid this, because of their positive 'vitality'. These vitality compounds would be used up after a while and have to be added constantly via food. His diet advice was to live on a lacto-vegetable diet. Today Lahmann's theory is no longer tenable. Although Lahmann criticized Haig's theory, he had the same idea about pathology.[69] An extraordinary contribution of Dr Lahmann was the idea to take the determination of the 'particular weight' as a measure for the physical condition of a human being. He used an arithmetical method, similar to the body mass index of today. The 'particular weight' of a healthy person should vary between 1,065 and 1,072. All valences lying above he interpreted as 'Hydrämie' (obesity and dropsy) and lower valences as too great a thinness.[70]

Two other diet reformers, who promulgated lacto-vegetable food, were the German dentist and dietician Carl Röse (1864–1947) and the Swedish chemist and nutritionist Ragnar Berg (1873–1956). Röse had dedicated himself to research in nutriment since 1894. He studied the influence of basic nutrient salts on human health. Röse discovered two things: firstly that an augmented consumption of proteins leads to malnutrition and secondly that a protein minimum of between 30g and 50g per day is enough to stay alive and to keep fit. Thus, he also supported a lacto-vegetable diet rich in basics and poor in acids, consisting of calcareous milk, fruit and vegetables (especially potatoes and tomatoes).[71]

Ragnar Berg for twelve years led the physiological-chemical laboratory at Lahmann's sanatorium and made experiments with both ill and healthy patients, his so-called 'Nährsalzbilanzversuche' (nutrient salt balance experiments),[72] with the result that a basic diet should be mainly responsible for the healthy effect of food. He developed a method of analysis for most victuals, subdivided them according to their acidity or basicity and summarized the results in tables.[73] Berg's maxim was: 'Eat five or seven times more potatoes, vegetables and fruit than all other foodstuffs together, except for milk. Eat half of it raw!'.[74]

LOW IN PROTEIN AND RICH IN CARBOHYDRATE COUNTRY FARE, OR, MIKKEL HINDHEDE IN THE FOCUS OF THE 'PROTEIN-DISCUSSION'

The Danish physician Mikkel Hindhede (1862–1945) defended ordinary country fare, such as farmers in Denmark used to eat, chiefly based on coarse-grained bread, potatoes, groats supplemented with milk, fruit and vegetables. Hindhede formed an opinion about the correct diet from experiences of his childhood.[75] His main idea was to bring city-dwellers back to a simple life and to frugal food. Mikkel Hindhede already lost his belief in the legal 'protein dogma' in 1895, when he demonstrated in an experiment on himself that it is possible to live on a diet low in protein and to stay healthy.[76] In 1909 Hindhede organized an experimental laboratory in Copenhagen and showed by scientific experiments, that a human being can easily live on a protein minimum of around 30g, instead of the 118g per day prescribed by nutritionists at this time (Voit's protein dogma)[77] and still be in a healthy condition. The nutritionists were wrong, and had to revise their opinion. An impetuous quarrel between leading nutritionists Justus Liebig (1803–1873), Carl Voit (1831–1898), Max Rubner (1854–1932) and diet reformers which had started the German vegetarian movement went on.[78] The life-reformers set an example for a life based on a vegetarian diet which was, according to the latest findings of the nutritionists, impossible.

The answer to the 'protein question' was the central issue of German health movements. It was the only possibility for a general appreciation and ratification of the vegetarian life-style. Hindhede published numerous treatises about nutrition.[79] His aim was to fight the predominantly false doctrine of the high nutritive value of meat, which still existed as a result of Liebig's 'meat gives meat' thesis.[80] He saw in this belief the main problem for the undernourishment amongst the poorer working-class population. Thus, one of his main arguments for a lacto-vegetable diet was one of economy. In 1917, during World War I, when a fodder blockade was imposed on Denmark, Hindhede could demonstrate in public a major experiment of the healthy and economic aspects of his diet system. The surprising effect of this huge experiment was that firstly nobody had to starve in Denmark, and, secondly, in the last years of the war, when the people there lived mainly on vegetarian food, the death rate was statistically reduced.[81] The Danish doctor had finally found evidence for the economic and healthy effects of his vegetarian diet.

Two very progressive recommendations by Hindhede were:
1. To consume the vegetable cooking water as well; to use roughly ground flour and to eat whole wheat bread.[82]
2. A 'brain' worker should eat less than a 'physical' worker.[83]

FASTING MOVEMENT

Fasting has a long, traditional history. Fasting has always been a religious technique (eg in Buddhism, Islam and Christian faiths), succinctly defined by the word 'asceticism'.[84] In addition, it always used to be and still is a medical therapy.[85]

Next to vegetarian and a 'full of value' diet the starvation cure took shape as a low diet system at the turn of the century. It seems illogical that in the second half of the nineteenth century the fasting cure was reintroduced by the naturopaths. In medical treatment starvation cures were not normally used because of the influence of the scientific reading of diseases: on the contrary, it was conventional to fight against the instinctive wish of any patient to starve himself as an 'error of nature'.[86] At the very beginning of the German modern fasting movement stood the American doctor Edward Hooker Dewey (1840–1904). He re-established the starvation cure as an independent systematic natural remedy. The American carried out fasting experiments on himself to perfect his therapy and developed two ways of fasting:
1. Morning fasting is a good therapy for dyspeptic people; only breakfast is left out and eating consists of two meals, which have to be eaten slowly and to be chewed well to prevent the patient from eating too much.
2. During full fasting one is only allowed to drink fresh water, until a distinct feeling of starvation appears.

It is due to the influence of Dewey that fasting was able to gain a foothold in Germany, where Adolf Just (1859–1939), Gustav Riedlin (1861–1949) and Otto Buchinger (1878–1966) were the most famous doctors employing fasting cures.[87] Under the influence of a friend, who heard about the healing successes of the American doctors Dewey and Henry Tanner, Gustav Riedlin developed his system of starving.[88] Riedlin's fasting therapy was designed to heal by activating the natural vitality, which exists in every body.[89] He defined the terms of fasting more precisely. For him fasting was not only treatment by natural remedies, but also the meditative way of obtaining self-knowledge. Thus, he defined it not only as a limited food intake, but also as a mental attitude. In this theosophical point of view Riedlin differed from other fasting doctors.[90]

Today the naturopath Buchinger is the most famous representative of fasting cures and the term 'Buchinger-fasting' found its acceptance in academic medicine.[91] Buchinger's fasting starts with so-called 'relief-days' in the form of pure fruit-, rice- and a 'full of value' diet, the food intake is reduced step by step, until just fruit and vegetable juices, warm vegetarian soup and herbal teas, which contain essential vitamins and minerals, are still allowed. The length and the curative effect of fasting is dependent on the severity of a sickness. When the fasting period is finished, so-called 'building-up-days' can follow.[92] Otto Buchinger cured overweight as well as underweight patients with his fasting-system. During his life-time, especially during the 1920s, he was critical that his fasting-method was used more and more to obtain the modern, slender, ideal shape.[93] The fasting doctor Eugen Heun (*1898) should also be mentioned. He created his own raw fruit- and vegetable juices fasting cure.[94]

FLETCHERISM OR THE 'CHEW CHEW FAD'

The motto of the American diet reformer Horace Fletcher was: 'Wir leben nicht von dem was wir essen, sondern von dem was wir verdauen und assimilieren'. (We do not live on what we eat, but we live on that what we digest and assimilate.)[95] Horace Fletcher (1849–1919) started his second career as diet reformer with the publication of his book '*What Sense? Or economic nutrition*'[96] Fletcher created a philosophy of chewing as a diet therapy for people who were overweight or underweight. He became interested in malnutritional diseases as a result of his own problem of being overweight. With the help of his special chewing programme he was able to lose 25 kilos within six months and won back his vitality and health. In Fletcher's diet it was not so important what you ate, but how you ate it.[97] The so-called 'Fletcherism'[98] was a changed eating method, which guaranteed a better utilization of victuals and made quicker satiation possible, which meant at the same time better nutrition and a more healthy life. Fletcher also saw his diet of better chewing as an economic aspect, as an opportunity to solve the social question. But he never got the chance to demonstrate this in public.[99] His idea was that the digestion process should start in the mouth by good chewing and salivation. He described this act as 'Ausschmecken' (tasting out),[100] until instinctively a natural swallowing reflex follows; tasteless food should be spat out again. He maintained that exact information about the physical and nutritional condition can be found in an examination of the excretions. In addition, you should only eat if you feel distinct hunger-pangs, what he called 'Instinktessen' (instinct eating).[101] Horace Fletcher tried to introduce his diet reform system around 1900 into the United States of America, when the health movement was already at its climax there. However, his plan at first failed. Fletcher found the first supporters of his extraordinary chewing diet in England, after he had the chance to study human metabolism at the 'Sir Michael Foster Laboratory' in Cambridge in 1902, where he found encouragement from famous nutritionists. As a result of his increasing popularity the Fletcherism wave flooded America too. The fashionable 'munching-parties' became popular in America. Fletcher was at his zenith from 1904 until 1910, when his chewing idea expanded all over Europe, too.[102] The expression 'Fletcherism' and the name 'Fletcher' are synonyms for his diet of intensive chewing even today.[103]

The so-called 'vitamin-revolution' of the 1920s and 1930s brought the German diet reform movements to a climax.[104]

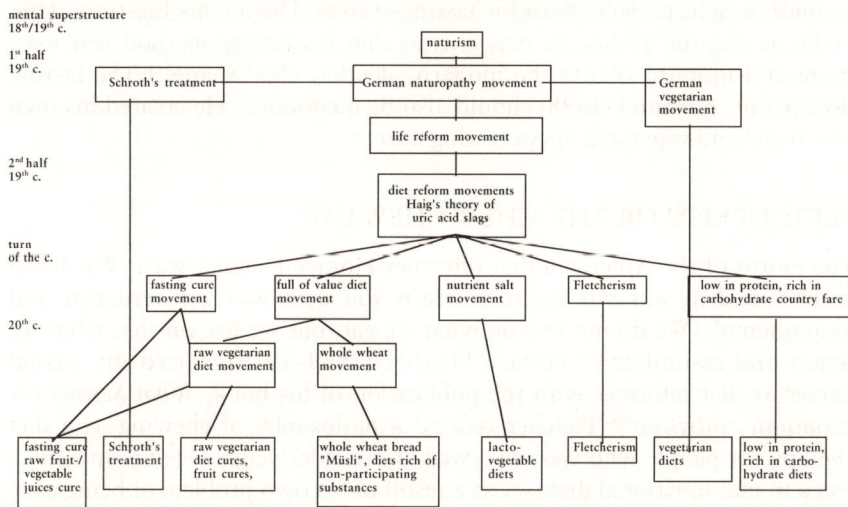

mental superstructure
18th/19th c.

1st half
19th c.

	naturism	
Schroth's treatment	German naturopathy movement	German vegetarian movement

life reform movement

2nd half
19th c.

diet reform movements
Haig's theory of
uric acid slags

turn
of the c.

fasting cure movement	full of value diet movement	nutrient salt movement	Fletcherism	low in protein, rich in carbohydrate country fare

20th c.

raw vegetarian diet movement	whole wheat movement

fasting cure raw fruit-/ vegetable juices cure	Schroth's treatment	raw vegetarian diet cures, fruit cures,	whole wheat bread "Müsli", diets rich of non-participating substances	lacto-vegetable diets	Fletcherism	vegetarian diets	low in protein, rich in carbohydrate diets

Fig. 2. *'Instead of corsets – lean cheese and celery.' The reconstructed phases of the modern slimming diet. The first impulses for a changed consciousness of the body.*

THE REDISCOVERY OF THE BEAUTY OF THE NATURAL HUMAN BODY OR THE NEW BODY CULT

At the turn of the century the German health movement had become a complicated conglomeration of different reform efforts when the third historical phase of the rediscovery of the beauty of the natural human body started.[105] The German health movement also included a revolution of an individual's attitude towards the body and sexuality in its programme.[106] The health reformers not only fought an antiquated social order, but also its rules and morals. They aimed at a change in the consciousness of people. Taboo topics which were restrained by a sense of shame as a result of education were to become public themes.[107] A German historian has said: 'Die Wiederentdeckung des Körpers im ganzheitlichen Sinne ist die eigentliche Leistung der Lebensreformbewegung.' (The rediscovery of the body in an all-embracing sense is the essential achievement of the German health movement.)[108]

The different German body reform movements were: nudism (including sexual reform efforts), the clothing reform movement (including emancipating reform efforts), the gymnastic/sport and fitness movement (including educational, aesthetical and dancing reform efforts) and the youth movement (including artistic reform efforts).[109] A pre-condition for the planned 'thought revolution', respectively 'revolution in the mental attitude of the people towards their body',[110] was a new definition of health and beauty.

The starting point of the thematic actualization of the body were hygienic interests. The interest in the body started with atmospheric therapy (light air bathing cure) and gymnastic and exercise therapy (fresh air exercises) during the first phase of the German health movement (treatment by natural remedies).[111] The initiator of the German nudism movement, Karl Wilhelm Diefenbach (1851–1913), came under the influence of the naturopath Arnold Rikli (1823–1906), the inventor of the so-called 'Lufthütten' (airhuts),[112] to the atmospheric bath. Diefenbach conceived the ideology of the new body cult by uniting art and an ideal natural life-style . His outward appearance was reminiscent of an original Christian. He abstained from owning property and from excess consumption, wore long hair, long robes designed by himself, and sandals and lived on vegetarian, organically grown food.[113]

His student Hugo Höppener (1869–1948), better known as 'Fidus', became a renowned art nouveau artist at the turn of the century. With the help of art Fidus expressed the ideological feeling for the body. The young, slender, naked body became a leading element in his art of the outgoing nineteenth century.[114] Many members of the youth movement saw the symbols for the epoch of a new, liberated and natural way of life in the art of Fidus.[115]

The German word 'Nacktkultur' (nudism) was coined by the sociologist, social hygienist and body-propagandist Heinrich Pudor (1865–1943), better known under his pseudonym 'Heinrich Scham'.[116] He published in 1893 his first book *'Nackende Menschen Jauchzen der Zukunft'* (Naked People – exult in the future)[117] and said in it: '. . . ein nackender Mensch ist für die Menschen unserer Zeit eine Geschmacklosigkeit und wirkt wie ein Schlag ins Gesicht - so unnatürlich sind wir geworden.' (. . . a naked human is a tasteless thing for people of our time and has the effect of a slap in the

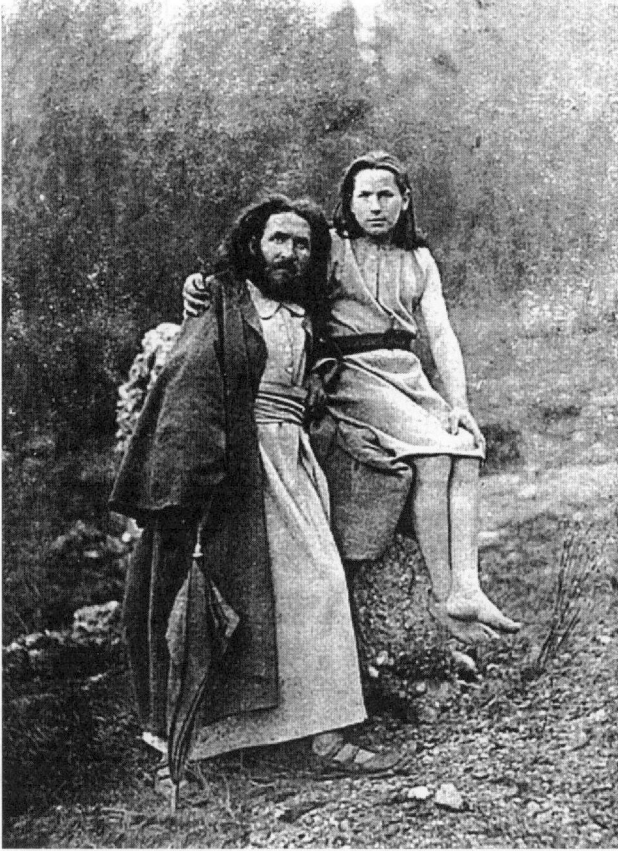

Fig. 2. *The 'nature-apostle' Karl Wilhelm Diefenbach and his pupil, the art nouveau artist 'Fidus'.*

face, we have become so unnatural.)[118] When the term nudism was tinged with negative associations, because of scandals, the expression 'Lichtbewegung' (light-movement) was introduced instead. Later in the 1920s the term 'Freikörperkultur' (nudism), which is still used today, came into use.[119]

Another representative was Richard Ungewitter (1868–1958). He found his way to nudism by an atmospheric cure, too, but his interpretation ended up in thoughts about race, which foreshadowed the fanatical racial ideas of the Third Reich.[120]

The German nudism movement had an enormously scandalising effect in public. Many legal proceedings against nudists were instituted, because of disorderly conduct. Fines, arrest and spells in asylums were the consequences,[121] although the nudists always declared emphatically the morality of their naked bathing. From their point of view air-bathing in the sun was a liberated act of building a unity with nature and a way of self-knowledge and had nothing to do with sexuality, although they had sexual reform ambitions.[122] Some historians see the main reason for the miscarriage of their aim for social reform in this ambivalent character of the German health movement, in the hesitant waving between revolt and regression.[123]

Their thesis was that shame of the human body was a result of the civilizing process, like the cooking of food: 'Die Natur kennt keine Kleider.' (Nature knows no clothes.)[124] With the beginning of modern psychoanalysis at the end of the nineteenth century this statement found attestation and the naked human became a popular motive in the modern art of this epoch.[125]

THE NEW SPORT AND FITNESS CULT

The roots of a German sports movement[126] were already detectable when in the second half of the nineteenth century the English sports wave flowed over Germany. Many sports journals and books support the initial, direct connection between nudism and sport with documentary evidence.[127] The first journal for physical training was published in 1901 under the title *Physical Strength and Beauty*[128] and showed the origin of what is today summarized under the more general term 'fitness'. At the end of the nineteenth century light air baths were combined with gymnastic or sport institutions or swimming-pools and became very popular. The sun-bathing cult had started. To be pale was not 'in' anymore.[129] To have a tan was evidence of health. The life reformers had started with sun-bathing. Suddenly gymnastics, sports, dancing and body-building also became means of obtaining 'body beauty'.[130] Thus, after the liberation of the body from clothes, another idea was that of body styling by means of sports and special diets. While training programmes for the men were mainly developed to enhance physical strength,[131] how to get muscles, the training programmes for women[132] had as their aim physical attraction, how to keep fit, young and in good shape.

A new feeling for the body also needed a new fashion of clothes, which allowed more physical activities than the crinoline and the wasp-waist-corset.[133] The leading forerunner of the clothes reform idea was the physician Thomas Samuel Soemmering (1755–1830). He had already at the end of the eighteenth century criticized the injuries to health of a pair of stays.[134] But as happened so often, the first real impulses came from America. The Puritan Marie M Jones fought against the crinoline in a lecture at a conference of the 'New York Health Association'. Her speech was eventually published in 1870 in Berlin.[135] She set the German clothes reform efforts in motion. The aim of the German health movement was for clothing that fitted the natural body anatomy and did not deform and mark the body.[136]

The main idea was, like all other ideas, based on hygienic considerations. There were two groups of clothing reformers. One group looked to reform underwear, and wanted to change the materials clothes were made from. Starting from nature-cure pathology, they developed underclothes of spe-

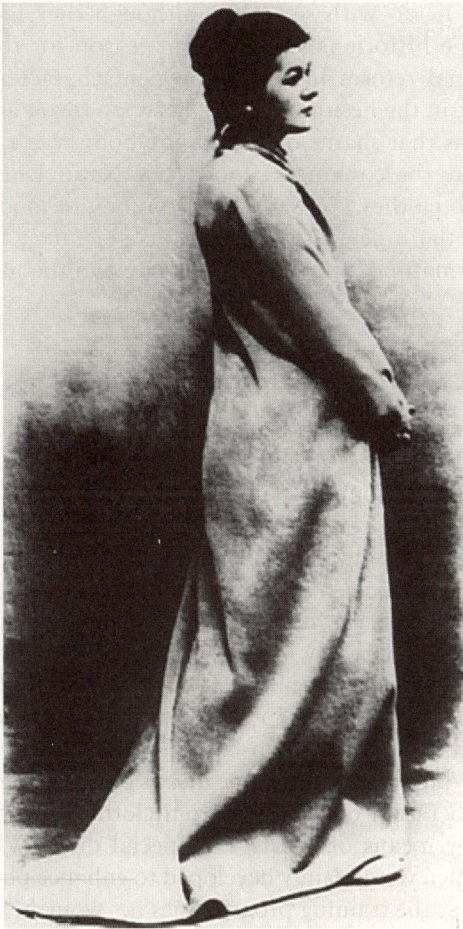

Fig. 3. Typical reform dress designed by 'Fidus' for his wife Elsa Höppener.

cial materials with the task of freeing the body from dangerous waste products produced by sweating and breathing. To this group belonged Gustav Jaeger (1832–1917), Heinrich Lahman and Sebastian Kneipp.[137] The other group were the clothing reformers, who wanted to change the whole fashion of dresses. The reform-clothes should be made of lighter, breathing-active materials and should only be carried by the shoulders, to be more birth-, organ- and motion-friendly. Their style was reminiscent of dresses from ancient times.[138]

Art nouveau artists, like Henry van de Velde and Fidus, designed special patterns and cuts to make the dresses more attractive.[139] The main propagandist of this group of clothing reformers was Paul Schultze-Naumburg (1869–1949). In his '*Die Kultur des weiblichen Körpers als Grundlage der Frauenkleidung*' (The Culture of the Female Body as a Basis for Dress)[140]

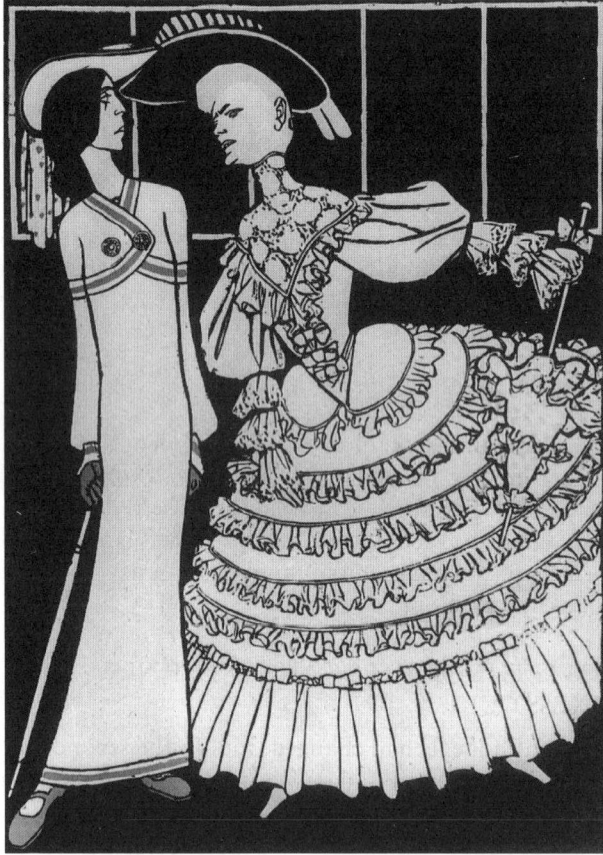

Fig. 5. *The Caricature 'Quarrel about fashions' shows impressively this confrontation.*

he articulated a new consciousness for health and body. He looked for inspiration to the beauty of the natural human body, especially of the female body without bone and organ deformations. First Schultze-Naum-burg (1869–1949) censured the wasp-waist ideal dictated by fashion and said that the mistake of the fashion designer was that the silhouette was dictated by the dressed body and not by the normal figure of a naked body, which should be 'slender, vital and beautiful'.[141] The health reformer, Else Wirming-haus, combined emancipatory reform efforts with the idea of clothing reform. She designed special dresses for the working woman of modern times.[142] The German youth movement, which cultivated walking in nature and many rec-reational activities, also demanded a new more sporty kind of clothes.[143]

Clothing reformers were the first to make the public attentive to the need of a more motion friendly style in fashion and forced traditional fashion to be confronted by it.[144]

The Parisian fashion designer Paul Poiret responded to this new demand and developed more mobile two-part costumes.[145] Special sports costumes and leisure wear followed. Corsets could not be hidden as well as before under the clothing and the individual shape of the body was increasingly the centre of interest. This trend is described as the introduction of 'slender line' in the history of fashion.[146]

The turn of the century was the time of radical changes and it was characterized by immense medical, scientific and technical progress, by the discovery of modern psychoanalysis, by new publicly discussed taboo topics, such as body and sexuality, by the discovery of youth and by the rediscovery of the beauty of the body.[147]

THE NEW YOUTH CULT

Youth became the time symbol of this new epoch.[148] The young, slender body became a leading motive in art nouveau. The girlish, virginal type of woman was a new erotical beau ideal, because it demonstrated positive social virtues, like moral self-control in eating and sexuality.[149] The German health reformers had given the first impulses for a new feeling for the body, which was unknown before.

TO BE SLIM IS THE NEW SLOGAN OR THE NEW SLENDERNESS CULT

Additionally, health ideals had changed, too. In the second half of the nineteenth century the misconception still existed that it would be more healthy to be fat, because fatter people would be more resistant to diseases. Nevertheless, at the turn of the century the latest findings in nutritional science confirmed more and more that a fat-, carbohydrate- and sugar-poor form of nutrition was better in order to keep fit. In parallel, as a result of this new knowledge of eating, the beau ideals changed towards becoming more and more slender.[150]

While at the end of the nineteenth century a woman with a full figure was a reigning beauty,[151] the first extreme slenderness ideal of the 'garçonette'[152] the so-called 'Linealfigur' (straight-edge-shape),[153] became the new fashion in the 1920s. Hence dieting and fasting became fashionable too, in order to fit into this new slender ideal. After the privations of World War II a 'more female' body ideal followed, again, but this time more perfected with the correct proportions in the right places.[154] The most extreme body ideal came along in the 1960s and led to an increasing rate of eating disorders and deaths.[155]

Thus, health and beauty were newly defined after a long historical process of changing mentalities. The new slogan in the advertisement of the modern performance-orientated society of the twentieth century was: 'sporting, dynamic, young and productive.'[156] And to fulfil these social standards, you have to 'keep fit and slim!'[157]

Fig. 6. This advertisement says: 'Gute Figur schafft Erfolg' (A good figure provides success).

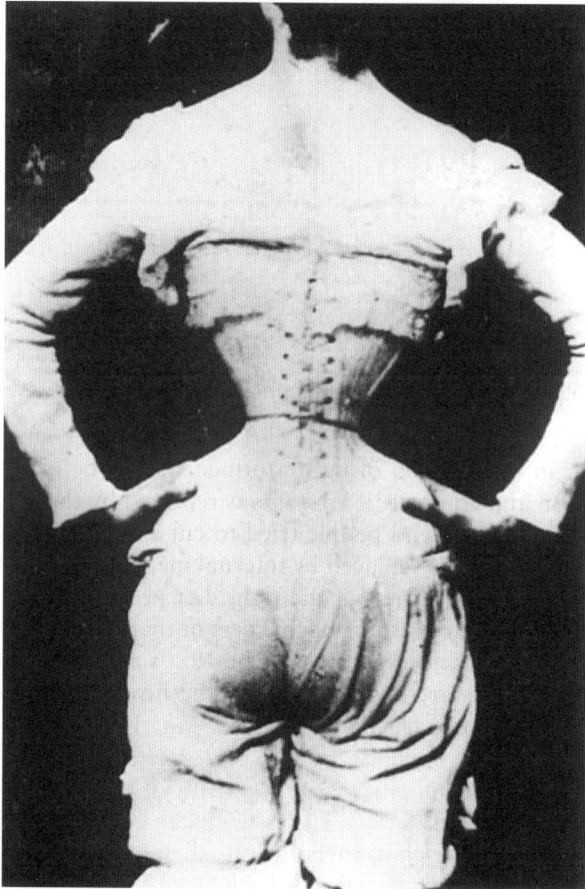

Fig. 7. The 'lacing mania' of the nineteenth century.

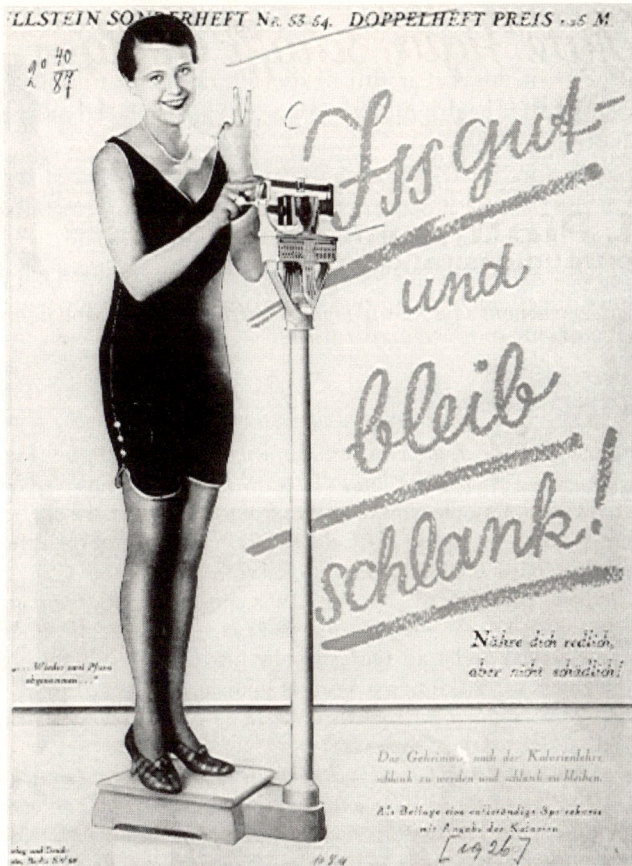

Fig. 8. *The 'dieting mania' of the twentieth century.*

The corset, in its function of figure former, had to be given up for reasons of function and comfort.[158] First it was replaced by the shape-forming hip-supporter and in the end people tried to cut a fine figure by means of diet. External means were replaced by internal means to maintain a slender outward appearance. In search of the right diet people discovered the secondary slimming effect of reform diets. Diets of the German health reformers celebrated a comeback, especially in the 1920s and 30s.[159] Most of our modern reducing diets are descended from the historical tradition of the German health movement, such as:

1. vegetarian diets,
2. 'full of value' diets,
3. lacto-vegetable diets,
4. low in protein and rich in carbohydrate diets,
5. Schroth's treatment,
6. Fletcherism,

7. mineral water cures and
8. fasting-cures.[160]

Nowadays the book market is full of diet literature. An analysis of these diet books shows that health motives for a diet are replaced more and more by beauty motives.

The 'lacing mania' of the nineteenth century was replaced by the 'dieting mania' of the twentieth century.[161] Outwards control was taken over by eating control: 'Instead of corsets, lean cheese and celery.'[162]

Meanwhile the slenderness ideal has been exaggerated to such an extent, that eating disorders, such as anorexia nervosa and bulimia nervosa are the other extreme of our modern civilization.[163]

BIBLIOGRAPHY

Ackerknecht, Erwin H. *Therapie von den Primitiven bis zum 20. Jahrhundert. Mit einem Anhang: Geschichte der Diät* (Therapy from the Primitive People to the 20th century. With a supplement: history of diet), Stuttgart, 1970.

Altpeter, Werner. *Zur Geschichte der Lebensreform* (History of the Life Reform Movement), Berlin, Bad Homburg, Hamburg, 1964.

Andritzky, Michael, Rautenberg, Thomas. *'Wir sind nackt und nennen uns Du': Von Lichtfreunden und Sonnenkämpfern: Eine Geschichte der Freikörperkultur* ('We Are Naked and Call Ourselves by our Christian Name': Friends of Light and Fighters for the Sun: a history of nudism), Giessen, 1989.

Baltzer, Eduard. *Die natürliche Lebensweise* (The Natural Way of Life), Nordhausen, 1867–1872.

Barnett, Margaret. *The Chew Chew Fad of the Edwardian Era: Horace Fletcher's remedy for both over and under eating*. Programme of the conference of the Society for the Social History of Medicine and the Glasgow Nutrition Group, 2–3 April 1993, Glasgow, 1993.

Baumgartner, Judith. *Ernährungsreform - Antwort auf Industrialisierung und Ernährungswandel: Ernährungsreform als Teil der Lebensreformbewegung am Beispiel der Siedlung und des Unternehmens Eden seit 1883* (Reform of Nutrition - Answer to industrialization and change of eating habits: diet reform as aspect of the life reform movement with reference to the settlement and firm Eden since 1883), (Europäische Hochschulschriften, Reihe 3, 535), Frankfurt a.M., Berlin, Bern, New York, Paris, Wien, 1992.

Berg, Ragnar. *Die Nahrungs- und Genussmittel* (Foodstuff and Luxury Foodstuffs), Dresden, 1913; *Die Grundlage einer richtigen Ernährung* (The basis of a right diet), Dresden[8], 1931.

Bircher-Benner, Max. *Ordnungsgesetze des Lebens als Wegweiser zur Gesundheit* (Order of Life as a Guide for Health), Zürich, Leipzig, Wien[4], 1945; *Vom Werden des neuen Arztes: Erkenntnisse und Bekenntnisse* (The Development of a New Physician: findings and confessions), Reutlingen[3], 1949.

Boehn, Max. *Die Mode: Eine Kulturgeschichte vom Barock zum Jugendstil* (Fashion: a cultural history from the baroque style to art nouveau), Minden, 1986.

Borosini, August von. *Das Fletchern: Ernährungs-ABC als Grundlage aller Körperkultur und Krankheitsbekämpfung* (Fletcherism: nutrition-ABC as basis for body cult and therapy), Dresden, 1913.

Brauchle, Alfred and Walter Groh, eds. *Zur Geschichte der Physiotherapie: Naturheilkunde in ärztlichen Lebensbildern* (History of Physiotherapy: treatment by natural remedies and its medical personalities), Heidelberg[4], 1971.

Buchinger, Otto. *Das Heilfasten und seine Hilfsmethoden* (The Fasting Cure and its Remedial Methods), Stuttgart, 1935; *Verfahren und Ergebnisse der Fastenbehandlung: Die natürliche Heilweise im Rahmen der Gesamtmedizin* (Methods and Results of the Fasting Cure: Natural remedies in universal medicine), Jena, 1938.

Conti, Christoph. *Abschied vom Bürgertum: Alternative Bewegungen in Deutschland von 1890 bis heute* (Farewell from the Middle Classes: alternative movements in Germany from 1890 until today), Reinbek bei Hamburg, 1984, 66–86.

Deutsche Gesellschaft für Ernährungsforschung, ed. *Ernährungsbericht 1992* (Nutrition report 1992), Frankfurt a.M., 1992, 30–45.

Dewey, Edward Hooker. *Die Fastenkur* (The Fasting Cure), Berlin, 1905.

Drebber, Emil. *Diätschule für Ernährungskunst, Atmungskunst und Gedankenschulung* (Diet School for Dietetics, Breathing Exercises and Thought Training), Elberfeld, 1912.

Engelhardt, Dietrich von. Hunger und Appetit: Essen und Trinken im System der

Diätetik - Kulturhistorische Perspektiven (Hunger and appetite: eating and drinking in the system of dietetic–cultural historical perspectives). In Alois Wierlacher, Gerhard Neumann and Hans-Jürgen Teuteberg, eds, *Kulturthema Essen: Ansichten und Problemfelder* (Cultural Topic – Eating: opinions and problems), Berlin, 1993, 137–49.

Fletcher, Horace. *What sense? or, economic nutrition*, Chicago, New York, 1898; *Die Esssucht und ihre Bekämpfung* (Original title: Gluttony or Epicure), Dresden[3], 1911.

Frecot, Janos. Die Lebensreformbewegung (The life reform movement). In Klaus Vondung, ed. *Das wilhelminische Bildungsbürgertum: Zur Sozialgeschichte seiner Ideen*, Göttingen, 1976, 138–52.

Frecot, Janos et al, eds. *Fidus 1869–1948. Zur ästhetischen Praxis bürgerliche Fluchtbewegungen* (Fidus 1869–1948. Aesthetical practice of escapism in the middle classes), München, 1972.

Giese, Fritz. *Körperseele: Gedanken über persönliche Gestaltung* (Body-soul: thoughts about individual shaping), München, 1924.

Gillis, John R. *Geschichte der Jugend: Traditionen und Wandel im Verhältnis der Altersgruppen und Generationen* (A History of Youth: traditions and change in the relationship between the age groups and generations), Basel, 1980.

Grauer, Angelika and Peter F Schlottke. *Muss der Speck weg? Der Kampf um das Idealgewicht im Wandel der Schönheitsideale* (Has the Fat to be Removed? The struggle for the ideal weight in the change of beauty standards), München, 1987.

Grob, Marion. *Das Kleidungsverhalten jugendlicher Protestgruppen in Deutschland* im 20. Jahrhundert am Beispiel des Wandervogels und der *Studentenbewegung* (The Way of Clothing as a form of Protest from Youth Groups in Germany in the 20th Century with Reference to the Movement of Ramblers and Students), *(Beiträge zur Volkskultur in Nordwestdeutschland, 47)*, Münster, 1985.

Habermas, Tilmann. *Heisshunger: Historische Bedingungen der Bulimia nervosa* (Ravenous Appetite: historical conditions of bulimia nervosa), Frankfurt a.M., 1990; *Zur Geschichte der Magersucht: Eine medizin-psychologische Rekon-*

struktion (History of Anorexia Nervosa: a medical-psychological reconstruction), Frankfurt a.M., 1994.

Hahn, Theodor. *Die naturgemäße Diät, die Diät der Zukunft* (The Natural Diet, Diet of the Future), Freiburg, Leipzig, 1871.

Haig, Alexander. *Harnsäure als ein Faktor bei der Entstehung von Krankheiten* (Uric Acid as a Factor in the Causation of Disease), Berlin[2], 1910.

Hermand, Jost, ed. *Jugendstil* (Art Nouveau), Darmstadt, 1971.

Heun, Eugen. *Die Rohsäfte-Kur: Grundlage, Methodik, Heilerfolge* (The Raw Fruit- and Vegetable-Juice Cure: basis, method and successful treatment), Stuttgart, 1951; *Das Fasten als Erlebnis und Geschehnis* (Fasting as an Experience and Event), Frankfurt aM, 1953.

Hindhede, Mikkel. *Eine Reform unserer Ernährung: Lebe gesund! Lebe kräftig! Lebe billig!* (A Reform of Our Diet: Live healthy! Live good! Live cheaply!), Kopenhagen, 1908; *Die neue Ernährungslehre* (The New Dietetic), Dresden, 1912; *Deutsche und dänische Ernährung während der Kriegszeit* (German and Danish Nourishment during World War I), Hamburg, 1919; *Moderne Ernährung* (Modern Nutrition), *Vol 2: Praktisches Kochbuch zu Hindhedes System* (Practical Cookery-Book for Hindhede's Diet System), Berlin, Leipzig, Wien, Zürich, 1915; Ernährungsfrage (The question of the right diet), *Berliner Klinische Wochenschrift, 53*, 1 (1916), 446–9, 471–5, 501–5, 534–41; *Moderne Ernährung* (Modern nutrition), *Vol 1: Theoretischer Teil* (Theoretical Part), Berlin, Leipzig, Wien, Zürich,[3] 1927.

Hoffmann, Heinrich, *Struwelpeter*, s.l., 1845.

Hufeland, Christoph Wilhelm. *Makrobiotik oder die Kunst, das menschliche Leben zu verlängern* (Macrobiotic or the Art of Lengthening Human Life), Jena, 1796. 'Iss gut und bleib schlank!' Nähre dich redlich, aber nicht schädlich: Das Geheimnis nach der Kalorienlehre schlank zu werden und zu bleiben ('Eat well and keep slim!' Eat enough, but not too much! The secret of becoming and keeping slim by the help of the caloric method), *Ullstein Sonderheft, 53*, 54 (1926).

Jäger, Gustav. *Mein System: Zugleich 4. völlig umgearbeitete Auflage von 'Die Normalkleidung als Gesundheitsschutz'* (My system: plus the fourth completely revised edition of 'The normal clothing as hygiene'), Stuttgart, 1885.

Jones, Marie M. *Die weibliche Kleidung und ihre sittlichen und leiblichen Beziehungen* (The Female Dress and its Ethical and Physical Connections), Berlin, 1870.

Junker, Almut and Eva Stille. *Zur Geschichte der Unterwäsche 1700-1960. Eine Ausstellung des Historischen Museums Frankfurt 28. April bis August 1988* (History of Underwear 1700-1960. An exhibition of the Historical Museum Frankfurt from the 28th April to August 1988), Frankfurt a.M., 1988.

Just, Adolf. *Kehrt zur Natur zurück! Die wahre naturgemässe Heil- und Lebensweise, Wasser, Licht, Luft, Erde, Früchte und wirkliches Christentum* (Back to Nature! The proper natural therapy and way of life, water, sun-light, air, earth and fruit and true Christian faith), Jungborn-Stapelberg,[7] 1910.

Kleinspehn, Thomas. *Warum sind wir so unersättlich? Über den Bedeutungswandel des Essens* (Why are We so Insatiable? The semantic change of eating habits), Frankfurt a.M., 1987.

Kles, Felix. *Die Schrothisch-diätetische Heilmethode auf Grund eigener ärztlich-praktischer Erfahrung populärwissenschaftlich dargestellt* (Schroth's Treatment Described on the Basis of own Medical and Practical Experience in a Popular Scientific Way), Dresden, 1871.

Köhler, Michael. 'Lebensreform durch Körperkultur' (Life reform by nudism). In Koerber, Karl et al. *Vollwert-Ernährung* ('Full of Value' Diet), Heidelberg⁴, 1985.

Michael Köhler and Gisela Brache, eds, *Das Aktphoto: Ansichten vom Körper im fotographischen Zeitalter* (Photo from the nude: Views of the Body in the photographic Age), München, 1985, 289–303.

Kollath, Elisabeth. *Werner Kollath. Forscher, Arzt und Künstler: Biographie und Werk* (Werner Kollath. Researcher, medician and artist: biography and opus), München, 1973.

Kollath, Werner. *Der Vollwert der Nahrung und seine Bedeutung für Wachstum und Zellersatz* (The Full of Value Diet and its Importance for the Growth and Replacement of Cells), Stuttgart, 1950–1960; *Die Ordnung unserer Nahrung* (The Order of our Nutriment), Stuttgart², 1951.

Krabbe, Wolfgang. *Gesellschaftsreform durch Lebensreform: Strukturmerkmale einer sozialreformerischen Bewegung im Deutschland der Industrialisierungsperiode* (Social Reform by Life Reform: structural characteristics of a social reformatory movement in Germany during the period of industrialization), (Studien zum Wandel von Gesellschaft und Bildung im 19 Jahrhundert, 9), Göttingen, 1974; 'Die Weltanschauung der deutschen Lebensreformbewegung ist der Nationalsozialismus': Zur Gleichschaltung einer Alternativströmung im Dritten Reich ('The ideology of the German life reform movement is the National Socialism': the co-ordination of an alternative movement in the Third Reich), *Archiv für Kulturgeschichte*, 71 (1989), 431–61.

Lahmann, Heinrich, *Die diätetische Blutentmischung als Grundursache der Krankheiten* (The Dietetic Blood-Decomposing as Primary Cause for Diseases), Leipzig 1894; *Die Reform der Kleidung* (The reform of clothing), Stuttgart,⁴ 1903; *Nährsalztheorie im Lichte praktischer Anwendung: Eine* gemeinverständliche Belehrung über das Wesen a. des Pflanzen-*Nährsalzextraktes, b. der vegetabilen Milch, c. des Nährsalzkakaos; d. der Nährsalzschokolade* (The Nutrient Salt Theory in the Light of Practical use: a popular lecture on the nature of a. vegetable nutrient salt extract; b vegetable milk; c. nutrient salt cocoa; d. nutrient salt chocolate), Köln, s.a.

Landmann, Robert. *Ascona. Monte Verità: Auf der Suche nach dem Paradies* (Ascona. Monte Verità: in search of paradise), Zürich, Köln, 1973.

Levenstein, Harvey. *Paradox of Plenty: a social history of eating in modern America*, New York, Oxford, 1993.

Liebig, Justus. *Über die Gärung und die Quelle der Muskelkraft* (The Zymosis and the Source of Muscular Strength), Leipzig, 1870.

Linse, Ulrich. *Barfüssige Propheten: Erlöser der zwanziger Jahre* (Barefoot prophets: redeemers of the twenties), Berlin, 1983.

Loschek, Ingrid. *Mode im 20. Jahrhundert: Eine Kulturgeschichte unserer Zeit* (Fashion in the 20th Century: a cultural history of our time), München², 1984.

Mar, Lisa and Friedrich Wolf. *Schlank und gesund: Ein natürlicher Weg zur Beseitigung des heutigen Kultursiechtums: Ein zuverlässiger Weg zur Beseitigung der Körperfülle* (Slender and Fit: a natural way to remove the ill-health of modern civilization: a reliable way to remove corpulence), Stuttgart, Weil der Stadt, 1928.

Meischel-Hess, Grete. *Die sexuelle Krise: Eine sozialpsychologische Untersuchung* (The Sexual Crisis: a social-psychological study), Jena, 1909–1917.

Mensendieck, Bess M. *Funktionelles Frauenturnen* (Functional Physical Exercises for Women), München, 1923.

Menzler, Dora. *Die Schönheit deines Körpers: Das Ziel unserer gesundheitlich-künstlerischen Körperschulung* (The Beauty of your Body: The aim of our healthy-artistic physical culture), Stuttgart[19], 1924.

Metzler, Franz G. *Körperkultur und Sittlichkeit* (Nudism and Morality), Wien, München, 1900.

Meyer-Camberg, Ernst. *Wenn du dich recht gesund befinden willst: Aus der Geschichte unserer Naturheilkunde* (If you Want to Keep Fit: history of our naturopathy) (Arzt und Arznei, 2), Berlin, 1957; *Das praktische Lexikon der Naturheilkunde* (The Practical Encyclopaedia of the Treatment by Natural Remedies), München, 1977.

Meyer-Renschausen, Elisabeth. The porridge debate: grain, nutrition, and forgotten food preparation techniques, *Food and Foodways*, 5, 1 (1991), 95–120.

Mohrbutter, Alfred. *Jugendstil: Das Kleid der Frau* (Art nouveau: women's dress), Darmstadt, Leipzig, 1904.

Müller, J P. *Mein Freilichtbuch* (My Open-Air Gymnastic book), Leipzig, Zürich, 1927.

Pudor, Heinrich. *Nackende Menschen – Jauchzen der Zukunft* (Naked People – exulting in the future), Dresden, 1893.

Reicher, K. *Die Korpulenz – eine Gefahr: Ein zuverlässiger Führer zu normalem Körpergewicht ohne Schädigung der Gesundheit* (Corpulence – as a health risk: a reliable guide to standard weight without damage to health), Stuttgart, 1931.

Riedlin, Gustav. *Faste Dich rein und iss Dich gesund!* (Fast Yourself Clean and Eat Yourself Healthy!), Pfullingen, 1921; *Fastenkuren und Lebenskraft: Ein Führer zum methodischen Gebrauch* (Starving Cures and Vitality: A guide for the methodical use of fasting), Berlin, 1921.

Rikli, Arnold. *Die Thermodiätetik oder das tägliche Luftbad in Verbindung mit naturgemässer Diät als zukünftige Heilmethode* (Thermodietetic or the Daily Air-Bath in Connection with a Natural Diet as a Method of Treatment for the Future), Wien, 1869.

Röse, Carl. Vierjährige Ernährung an der Grenze des Eiweißmindestbedarfes (Four years living at the edge of the protein-minimum), *Zeitschrift für die gesamte experimentelle Medizin* (1934); Zur Eiweissfrage (Protein question), *Zeitschrift für Volksernährung*, 12, 9 (1937), 126ff; *Eiweissüberfütterung und Basenunterfütterung* (Albumen-overfeeding and base-underfeeding), Dresden, s.a.

Rothschuh, Karl Eberhard. *Naturheilbewegung, Reformbewegung, Alternativbewegung* (Naturopathy Movement, Health Movement, Alternative Movement), Stuttgart, 1983.

Rousseau, Jean Jacques Rousseau. *Emil oder über die Erziehung* (Emile or About Education), Amsterdam, 1762.

Rubner, Max. *Wandlungen in der Volksernährung* (Changes in Public Nutrition), Leipzig, 1913.

Sandow, Eugen. *Kraft und wie man sie erlangt* (Strength and How to Get It), Berlin, 1903.

Schlickeysen, Gustav. *Obst und Brot: Die wissenschaftliche Diätetik des Menschen* (Fruit and Bread: the scientific dietetic for the man), Freiburg[3], 1875.

Schultz, Uwe. *Speisen, Schlemmen, Fasten: Eine Kulturgeschichte des Essens* (Eating, feasting, fasting: a cultural history of eating), Frankfurt aM, 1993.

Schultze-Naumburg, Paul. *Die Kultur des weiblichen Körpers als Grundlage der Frauenkleidung* (The Culture of the Female Body as Basis for Dress), Leipzig, 1902.

Simons, Gustav. *Die Brotfrage und die Brotantwort* (The Bread Question and the Bread Answer), Berlin, 1902.

Sömmering, Samuel Thomas. *Über die Wirkungen der Schnürbrüste* (Injuries to Health by Wearing Stays), Berlin, 1793.

Spohr, Wilhelm, *Fidus*, Minden, 1912.

Sportswear: Zur Geschichte und Entwicklung der Sportkleidung (Sportswear: history and development of sportswear), (Eine Ausstellung des Deutschen Textilmuseums in Krefeld, 10. Mai bis 30. August 1992), Krefeld, 1992.

Steiner, Rudolf. *Anthroposophie: Eine Einführung in die anthroposophische Weltanschauung* (Anthroposophy: an introduction in the anthroposophical ideology), Dornach⁵, 1959.

Steinmetz, Stefan. *Unser tägliches Brot, wie es ist, und wie es sein sollte!* (Our Daily Bread, the Way It Is and the Way it Should Be!), Leipzig, 1894; *Mobilmachung aller Brotesser gegen die Unvernunft in der Ernährung* (Mobilization of All Bread-Eaters Against the Absurdity in Nutrition), Freiburg i.B., 1914.

Stolz, A. *Mannesschönheit* (Men's Beauty), München, c 1900.

Stratz, C H. *Die Schönheit des weiblichen Körpers* (The Beauty of the Female Body), Stuttgart⁸, 1900.

Struve, Gustav. *Mandaras Wanderungen* (Mandara's wanderings), s.l., 1833; *Pflanzenkost: Eine Grundlage einer neuen Weltanschauung* (Vegetable Diet. The basis of a new philosophy of life), Stuttgart, 1869.

Teuteberg, Hans-Jürgen. Zur Sozialgeschichte und Soziologie des Vegetarismus (Social history and sociology of vegetarianism). In Sigrid Weggemann and Joachim Ziche, eds, *Soziologische und humanethologische Aspekte des Ernährungsverhaltens: Strategien und Maßnahmen* (Sociological and Human Ethnological Aspects of Nutritional Behaviour. Strategies and actions), (Schriftenreihe der Arbeitsgemeinschaft Ernährungsverhalten e.V., 9) Frankfurt a.M., 1993, 64–78.

Thiel, Erika. *Geschichte des Kostüms: Die europäische Mode von den Anfängen bis zur Gegenwart* (History of Costume: European fashion from its beginnings to the present), Berlin, 1980.

Velde, Henry van de. *Die künstlerische Hebung der Frauentracht* (The Artistic Encouragement of the Dress), Krefeld, 1900.

Voit, Carl. Physiologie des Stoffwechsels (The physiology of metabolism), *Zeitschrift für Biologie*, 1 (1865), 84ff.

Vossen, Arno. *Sonnenmenschen: Sechs Jahrzehnte Freikörperkultur in Deutschland* (People of the Sun: six decades of nudism in Germany), Hamburg, 1956.

Wangen, F L and Scheuer, O F. *Das üppige Weib: Sexualleben und Wirkung: Künstlerische und karikaturistische Darstellung der dicken Frau:* Vom Urbeginn bis heute (The Full Woman: sexual life and effect: artistic and caricature presentation of the stout woman. From the first beginnings until today), Wien, Leipzig, 1928.

Wildt, Dieter. *Sonnenkult: Von der vornehmen Blässe zum nahtlosen Braun* (Sun-Bathing Cult: from the noble paleness to seamless suntan), Düsseldorf, Wien, New York, 1987.

Wirminghaus, Else. *Das Kleid der arbeitenden Frau* (The Dress of the Working Woman), Karlsruhe, 1916.

Wirz, Albert. *Die Moral auf dem Teller, dargestellt am Leben und Werk von Max* Bircher-Benner und John Harvey Kellogg, zwei Pionieren der modernen

Ernährung in der Tradition der moralischen Physiologie (Morality on the Plate, Described by the Life and Opus of Max Bircher-Benner and John Harvey Kellogg, Two Pioneers of the Modern Diet in the Tradition of Moral Physiology), Zürich, 1993.

Wittern, Renate. *Natur contra Naturwissenschaft: Zur Auseinandersetzung zwischen Naturheilkunde und Schulmedizin im späten neunzehnten Jahrhundert* (Nature versus Natural Science: the argument between the naturopathy movement and academic medicine at the end of the 19th century), Erlanger Universitätsreden, 37, Erlangen, 1992.

Zimmermann, Wilhelm. *Der Weg zum Paradies. Oder: die einzigen und wahren Mittel, das physische und moralische Elend unserer Zeit im Keim zu ersticken und auszurotten* (The Way to Paradise. Or the only and real way to nip physical and moral distress in the bud and to wipe it out), Quedling, 1843.

NOTES

1 The headline of an article in the newspaper *Rheinische Post*, 24, 29.1.97.
2 Deutsches Institut für Ernährungsforschung in Potsdam.
3 Deutsche Gesellschaft für Ernährungsforschung (1992), 30–45.
4 *Zitty,* 14 (1994), 216.
5 eg in 1993 the annual sales in Germany were 23 billion DM, tendency increasing: cf *Wirtschaftswoche*, 12, 18.3.94.
6 Gesellschaft für Marktforschung in Hamburg.
7 A BMI from 20 to 25 for men and a BMI from 19 to 24 for women is standard weight. A BMI of about 30 means adiposity.
8 36 per cent of all women in Germany want to modify their 'figures'. 40 per cent are dissatisified with their weight. In addition, every second German woman has already tried a diet.
9 eg Kellogg's Cornflakes, 'Bircher-Müsli', whole-meal bread, 'light' products etc.
10 The German psychologist, Tilmann Habermas, also states this in his book. Habermas, 1990, 151. cf fig. 1. Loschek, 1984, 256.
11 Meyer-Camberg, 1977, 61–62.
12 Engelhardt, 1993, 137–149; Baumgartner, 1992, 70.
13 Rousseau, 1762; on the front page is written: Sanabilis aegrotamus malis; ipsaque nos in rectum natura genitos, si emendari velimus, juvat.
14 Hufeland, 1796.
15 Rothschuh, 1983.
16 Wittern, 1992.
17 Rothschuh, 1989, 68–89.
18 Kles,1871.
19 Hahn,1871.
20 Struve, 1869.
21 Vegetarische Gesellschaft Stuttgart He.V. still exists today.
22 Zimmerman, 1843.
23 Teuteberg, 1993, 64–78.
24 Baltzer, 1867– 1872.
25 Krabbe, 1974, 12.
26 Teuteberg, 1993, 69.

27 Meyer-Camberg, 1977, 173.

28 Rothschuh, 1983, 113, 133–40.

29 For information about political tendencies of the German life movement held by some individuals, see Krabbe, 1989 and Linse, 1983.

30 Krabbe, 1974, 159–66.

31 Altpeter, 1964, 12. The first health food store was owned by the textile businessman and life reformer Carl Braun (1858–1943). Later it was called 'Gesundheitscentrale'.

32 Landmann, 1973.

33 Baumgartner, 1992.

34 Frecot, 1976, 138–52.

35 Programme of the diet reform movement printed in the *Naturarzt* (Nature doctor), 25 (1897).

36 cf chart 1.

37 Brauchle and Groh, 1971.

38 Haig, 1910.

39 Brauchle and Groh, 1971, 85.

40 Schlickeysen, 1875.

41 Meyer-Camberg, 1957, 69.

42 Schlickeysen, 1875, 157.

43 ibid, 171.

44 ibid, 157ff; Rothschuh, 1983, 98.

45 Brauchle and Groh, 1971, 118. Meyer-Camberg, 1957, 74–75.

46 Wirz, 1993, 47, 72.

47 Bircher-Benner, 1949.

48 Wirz, 1993, 62.

49 Bircher-Benner, 1945.

50 Expression from Levenstein, 1993.

51 Kollath, 1973, 243.

52 Kollath, 1950–1960.

53 Kollath, 1951.

54 ibid, 53, 68.

55 Kollath, 1973, 183. First a health food owner from Frankfurt sold it under his name.

56 Koerber et al, 1985.

57 cf Drebber, 1912.

58 Wirz, 1993, 152ff.

59 Schlickeysen, 1875, 172.

60 Simons, 1902.

61 It is still available under this name in German health food shops.

62 Simons, 1902, 20–1.

63 Steinmetz, 1894; 1914.

64 Lahmann's vegetable milk can be found in nearly every journal at this time.

65 Lahmann, s.a.

66 Krabbe, 1974, 113.

67 Brauchle and Groh, 1971, 86; Meyer-Camberg, 1957, 72.

68 Lahmann, 1894.

69 ibid, 207–26.

70 Brauchle and Groh, 1971, 89.

71 Röse, s.a.
72 Berg observed the intake and excretion of nutrient salts by individual patients for weeks. He prepared a balance-sheet with the help of this collected data. Berg could then draw conclusions from this balance-sheet about the disorder of metabolism or malnutrition of the patient.
73 Berg, 1913.
74 Meyer-Camberg, 1957, 77; Berg, 1931.
75 Brauchle & Groh, 1971, 92–94.
76 Hindhede, 1912, 10. 'After these experiences I had lost all my belief in the old [protein] dogma!'.
77 Voit, 1865, 84ff. Voit's dogma said: An adult worker needs a minimum of 118g protein, 56g fat and 500g carbohydrate in his daily food to stay alive and fit.
78 cf key-word 'Volksernährung' (Public nutrition) in medical journals, such as *Blätter für Volksgesundheitspflege* (Weekly paper for hygiene), *Berliner Klinische Wochenschrift* (Clinical weekly paper from Berlin), *Münchner Medizinische Wochenschrift* (Medical weekly paper from Munich) and *Zeitschrift für Volksernährung und Diätkost* (Journal for public nutrition and diet) in his life-time.
79 cf bibliographical data under the name Mikkel Hindhede.
80 Liebig, 1870.
81 Hindhede, 1919.
82 Hindhede, 1915.
83 Hindhede, 1916, 535.
84 Schultz, 1993.
85 Dietetics in the ancient time, eg Hippocrates; dietetics of the Middle Ages, eg Paracelsus.
86 Brauchle and Groh, 1971, 81.
87 ibid.
88 Heun, 1953, 32–35.
89 Riedlin, 1921.
90 ibid.
91 Buchinger, 1938.
92 Buchinger, 1935.
93 ibid, 16.
94 Heun, 1951.
95 Fletcher, 1911, XV.
96 Fletcher, 1898.
97 Fletcher, 1911, 15–17
98 Definition of 'Fletcherism' in Fletcher, 1911, 15 or Borosini, 1913. Diet and body cult are already combined in this title.
99 Barnett, 1993, 8.
100 Fletcher, 1911, 23.
101 ibid, 8.
102 Barnett, 1993, 8. Wirz, 1993, 151–86.
103 Barnett, 1993, 8.
104 Levenstein, 1993. cf chart 1.
105 Frecot, 1976, 143.
106 Rothschuh, 1983, 119–132. With references to the now following body

reform movements, which developed under the influence of the German health movement.

107 Conti, 1984, 66–86. Conti added to the title of the chapter 'Lebensreform' (life reform), the addendum 'Die Sorge um den Körper' (the care of the body).

108 Andritzky and Rautenberg, 1989, 16–7. The German life reformers introduced the term 'Körperseele' (body-soul), which expressed not only a new feeling for the body, but also a new philosophy. Physical exercises were seen as a medium for expressing their own personality. 'Körperseele' meant a new physical feeling, culture experience and expression. cf Giese, 1924.

109 Rothschuh, 1983, 119–132; Krabbe, 1974, 93–111, 142–150.

110 Ulrich Linse used these expressions in his book, already mentioned.

111 Two important naturopaths of these methods were Arnold Rikli and Adolf Just. Rikli, 1869; Just, 1910.

112 Rothschuh, 1983, 95.

113 cf Fig. 2. Conti, 1984, 72.

114 Hermand, 1971.

115 Spohr, 1912.

116 Rothschuh, 1983, 128; Vossen, 1956, 6.

117 Pudor, 1893.

118 ibid; quote from Vossen, 1957, 6.

119 Krabbe, 1974, 95; Vossen, 1956, 17.

120 Andritzky and Rautenberg, 1989, 19.

121 Vossen, 1956, 8. eg a legal process against Richard Ungewitter, which lasted two years and which he finally won, had cost the German government 25,000 Reichsmarks.

122 Metzler, 1900. eg Karl Vanselow, the editor of the journal *Kraft und Schönheit* (Physical strength and beauty), formed with some readers of his journal the *Vereinigung für Sexualreform* (association for sexual reform). *Kraft und Schönheit*, III (1906), 359. Another German health reformer with sexual reform ambitions was Grete Meischel-Hess (1909–1917).

123 Andritzky and Rautenberg, 1989, 20–21.

124 Köler, 1985, 289–303, here 342.

125 Hermand, 1971.

126 The German gymnastic movement's educational and national tradition and German naturopathy with its open-air-gymnastics, following the Greek example, were important pre-conditions for the German sport movement.

127 eg *Kraft und Schönheit: Körperkultur: Künstlerische Monatsschrift für Hygiene und Sport* (Physical strength and beauty: nudism: artistic journal for hygiene and sport); or Müller, 1927.

128 Krabbe, 1974, 94. Later the journal was misused by the National Socialists for their propaganda.

129 Andritzky and Rautenberg, 1989, 17–18; cf Wildt, 1987.

130 Body-styling by excercises and dance, eg Menzler, 1924; or Stolz, 1900.

131 eg Sandow, 1903.

132 eg Mensendick, 1923.

133 *Sportswear,* 1992.

134 Sömmering, 1793.

135 Jones, 1870.

136 Rothschuh, 1984, 119–132.
137 Jäger, 1885; Lahmann, 1903. cf Kneipp's health articles in *Kneipps Kalender* (Kneipp's Calendar) (1909).
138 cf Fig. 4. Frecot et al, 1972.
139 Velde, 1900; Mohrbutter, 1904.
140 Schultze-Naumburg, 1902.
141 ibid, 59.
142 Wirminghaus, 1916.
143 Grob, 1985.
144 cf Fig. 5. Caricature 'Streit der Moden' (Quarrel about fashions) from Bruno Paul, *Simplicissimus*, 1904/5.
145 Boehn, 1986, 168.
146 Thiel, 1980, 354.
147 Andritzky and Rautenberg, 1989, 21: 'Die Körperkultur der Jahrhundert-wende fand ihren revolutionären Ausdruck in der öffentlichen Inszenierung des <schönen> nackten Körpers' (The body cult at the turn of the century found its revolutionary expression in the public staging of the <beautiful> naked body).
148 Gillis, 1980.
149 Schultze-Naumburg, 1902, 49ff.
150 Habermas, 1990, 163. At the turn of the century health was newly defined. Suddenly 'slim' was associated with 'healthy'. Mar and Wolf, 1928, 10. 'Schlankheit ist also keine Modesache! Schlankheit ist eine Gesund-heitssache! . . . Schlank sein heisst gesund sein, gesund sein heisst schlank sein!' (Thus, slenderness is not a question of fashion! Slenderness is a ques-tion of health! ... To be slender means to be fit, means to be slender!)
151 Stratz, 1900, 201–2.
152 Habermas, 1990, 153.
153 *Modespiegel* (Fashion Mirror), (1923): 'Die Mode verlangt jetzt, dass die Frau wie ein Lineal aussieht' (Fashion demands that the woman has to look like a straight-edge, now).
154 Habermas, 1990, 153. A good example of this are famous filmstars from the 1950s such as Marilyn Monroe.
155 cf Fig. 1.
156 Is to be found in nearly every journal of the time.
157 cf Fig. 6. *Berliner illustrierte Zeitung* 37, (1927/8).
158 Habermas, 1990, 170.
159 Reicher, 1931, 12: 'Der Rohkost speziell kommt bei Entfettungskuren eine besondere Bedeutung zu ... und ist für viele Menschen geradezu ein Evan-gelium geworden.' (The raw vegetarian diet is of particular importance for slimming-cures ... and has for some people become some kind of religion).
160 eg Reicher, 1931.
161 cf Fig. 8. Junker and Stille, 1988, 199. cf Fig. 8. Cover of *Ullstein Sonderheft* 53–54 (1926).
162 Grauer and Schlotte, 1987, 50.
163 cf note 10 and Habermas, 1994. cf chart 2.

12 Vegetarianism in fin-de-siècle France: the social determinants of vegetarians' misfortune in pre-World War I France

Arouna P Ouédraogo

From 1870 to 1914, under the auspices of rationalism and hygienism, doctors form the main trend in spreading vegetarianism in France.[1] As opposed to the veganism advocated by Jean-Antoine Gleïzès,[2] the French precursor, these physicians recommend an ovo-lacto vegetarianism which prohibits meat and fish, but allows the consumption of some foods of animal origin, such as eggs, cheese and milk. The theosophist founders-to-be of the Société Végétarienne de France (SVF) start to meet in Paris about 1875 at the *Lotus Bleu*, the French meeting place of Eastern vegetarians. But the establishment and then the rapid expansion of a vegetarian movement in France are directly related to the successive and cumulative influences of the Swiss, English and Belgian vegetarians on the *Lotus Bleu* sectarians. Nevertheless, French vegetarianism has never been able to reach the level of development expected by its promoters. While, with the aid of their diet, the vegetarians want to ensure the physical, moral and social regeneration of their contemporaries, the latter do not seem to be very receptive to their arguments. French vegetarianism, constantly born and reborn, constantly expanding and disappearing, is all the time looking for an unattainable identity.

It is my purpose here to investigate the main problems encountered by the vegetarians while spreading the ideas and practices associated with their diet in fin-de-siècle France. I will point out the main characteristics of French vegetarianism through its institutions and topics, by distinguishing three phases in its evolution. During the first phase (1878–80), Swiss and then English proselytes come to France in great numbers, in order to help the French followers in their anti-meat campaign. Real awakeners of vegetarian awareness at the end of the nineteenth century, these indignant groups are minorities composed of members of the medical intelligentsia, intellectuals who believe that the solution to the social issue lies in abstinence, so that in their speeches they mainly deplore the life conditions of the working classes.

A second phase (1880–90) on which I will spend more time, because of its importance in the vegetarian trend, corresponds with the creation of French vegetarian societies and with the rise of national proselytes whose action is very significant. A third phase (1899–1914) corresponds with the rebirth of the SVF. I will analyse its expansion in relation to the particular problems concerning the diffusion of vegetarianism.

FROM AGITATORS TO THE PIONEERS OF FRENCH VEGETARIANISM: BEWAILING THE POOR'S FATE

A Swiss physician's speech on vegetarianism, delivered in July 1878, at the Trocadero in Paris, did more than start off vegetarian propaganda in France. It is true that the public had almost never heard about vegetarianism. The novelty of the topic reinforces the evangelical character of Dr Dock's speech. A member of the Society for the Prevention of Cruelty to Animals in German-speaking Switzerland, Dr Dock is the Director of a hygienic establishment in Saint Gall. A Protestant, he is an animal lover, a partisan of non-violence, and the impact of his sermon is all the more powerful since it is based on workers' life conditions. Since there is no specialised press, and since most vegetarian literature is in English or German, verbal expression is the main instrument of propaganda in France, and will remain so until about 1884:

> Vegetarianism fights against poverty and destitution as well as luxury, dissoluteness, celibacy, prostitution, in short, it is one of the surest safeguards of human existence, and one of the best guarantees of its prosperity. Vegetarianism constitutes one of our best moral laws; it gives its widest sense to the holy commandment, Thou shalt not kill, it seeks to achieve peace as much as possible, on earth, it wants to stop unnecessary war: between man and animal, and especially between man and man, these fratricidal wars which, for the most part, are caused by our passions, our lust, our cruelty. Vegetarianism is one of the surest means of ensuring the lot of workers, of reaching the least degree of inequality between the different classes. And in fact, isn't leading a more simple, cheaper life, a way of fighting against destitution and its inevitable consequences: crises, strikes, revolts and revolution? Today, we fear the socialist tendencies; well, the return to a simpler, more moral life, would be one of the means of solving the social problem. Yes, let us give a home, property to the working classes, and revolutions will stop of their own accord. Let us show them how to live a good and healthy life, how to succeed in saving, and we will not need strict laws to stifle aspirations, some of which are well founded. Those who are well-off must set the example of a normal life and a return to simplicity.[3]

Delivered barely two years after the first Working Classes' Congress held at Paris (1876), one year after Jules Guesde has introduced marxism in France, and not long before the Socialist Congress in Marseille (1879) has ratified the setting-up of the Parti Ouvrier Français, Dr Dock's speech reveals that the vegetarians find in their diet the best way to solve the then hotly debated social issue. After all, the social question in Switzerland is still dominated by the traumatism caused by the massacre of the workers boring the Saint-Gothard tunnel, who had gone on strike to ask for higher

wages and for a cut in working hours.[4] The intentions and strategic voca-
tion of Dr Dock's speech are well reflected by his conciliatory tone, which
is all the more moderated since it is delivered in public. Vegetarians are
more impetuous when they write. For instance, one of Dr Dock's friends,
Edouard Raoux, a Swiss clergyman, journalist and moral philosopher, who
is also engaged in the anti-meat campaign in France, demands a firm discipline against the immorality of those who spread disorder with their strikes.
For him, the workers are mainly victims of the ignorance, prejudice, vice,
tradition, whims and fashion perpetuated by necrophagous practices (or
ingestion of animal carcases).

Arguably, in the period of industrial expansion, when peasants, continu-
ously swarming into towns, are increasing the numbers of uprooted people
not adapted to factory discipline, working classes represent for the dominant classes the dangerous classes, impossible to control, who have the
knack of breaking the law, of violating all codes, especially those of work
and morality. Raoux is eager to see moral tranquillity restored. Prostitution,
the uncontrolled sexual life of the poor people, heralds an imminent catas-
trophe, and something must be done to prevent this before it is too late.[5]
How can self-control and regularity, asks Raoux, be introduced into the
habits of these new working classes whose 'coarse habits' only match their
instincts?[6]

> Physical health is degenerating: nervousness and anaemia are overcoming: intel-
> lectual disorder, fanaticism, superstitions, blind passions are increasing. Medi-
> cal, psychological and criminal statistics, everywhere reveal the existence and
> spread of this double evil which mainly accounts for all those afflicting our con-
> temporary society. Faced with all these disorders, it was appropriate to *ring the
> alarm* for the two kinds of health (of body and soul), in its two main centres:
> the marital home and school, and to show how *hygiene* and *education* can effi-
> ciently fight against these disorders.[7]

Vegetarianism will allow the tendency to be reversed, since it is the very
school of health and moral education. Its hygiene (or alternative medicine),
as well as dietary education, are instrumental in the metamorphosis of carnivorous barbarians into civilised beings that are vegetarians. Since the carnivorous prejudice has had a hold on man because he had deemed it good to
set aside the laws of Nature, whose harmony and innocence ensured a peace-
ful life and abundant vegetables, coming back to a simple life could redeem
him, first saving him from physical degeneration. Country people symbolise
body and mind purity as opposed to the fleshless town dwellers:

> Apart from the country people who still have muscles on their bones and blood
> in their veins, says Raoux, modern man is a skeleton wrapped in nerves, that is
> to say, a permanent passion, under the double influence of pleasure and pain.[8]

Peasants, who still live more or less in nature, are relatively safe from
the danger of over-indulgence in meat consumption. The vegetarians urge

them to resist the love of meat, with the hope that by adopting fundamental reforms at family and school levels, they will be more inclined to despise town life and enhance the value of their country life. That is where the rousseauistic ideas of the vegetarian agitators end. Unlike Jean-Jacques Rousseau, the author of *Emile*, who wanted to turn his pupil into a town savage, the nostalgia felt by vegetarian philanthropists gives proof of their love for rustic life. This leads them to praise peasants in the countryside. In fact, the vegetarians fear the peasants, once they have settled in towns. Here, they are crammed into insalubrious lodgings, surrender to sensuality and superstition, eat canned and adulterated foods, and thus become brutal, lecherous, idle, careless beings, and therefore parasites.[9]

This vision of vegetarianism as a remedy to the social issue is also shared by Anna Kingsford, an English theosophist and feminist vegetarian who emigrates about 1874. Dr Dock and Mr Raoux's main arguments are to be found in the medical thesis about vegetarianism, which Mrs Kingsford defends in 1880 at Paris, and which greatly encourages the French physicians to create a vegetarian movement.[10]

The example of Dr Anna Kingsford (1846–88) illustrates the predominance of England as the epicentre of European vegetarianism, and the relationship which unites the sectarian and feminist minorities with the diffusion of vegetarianism, in particular through the intermediary of emigration. From 1873 to 1880 the English Vegetarian Society is flourishing. Under the auspices of hygienism, it federates various theosophic and utopian sects, whose members are mostly from the middle-classes of London. A member of the English Theosophic Society, Mrs Kingsford is an exemplary representative of the English Vegetarian Society of which she is the Vice-President. The *Lotus Bleu* theosophists are among Mrs Kingsford's first Parisian contacts, to whom she communicates her vegetarian regeneration gospel.

These vegetarians' discourses aim at arousing the French public interest in vegetarianism, and make up the doctrinaire basis from which the French pioneers of the diet draw. They are composed of *Lotus Bleu* elders, who gather around Dr Hureau de Villeneuve, the founder of the Vegetarian Society of Paris in 1880 who also provides it with a monthly journal, the *Réforme alimentaire*. Among the new Society's well-known members one can find, besides Dr De Villeneuve, Dr Bonnejoy and Dr Goyart, who also praise the healing virtues of the vegetarian diet

Dr Hureau de Villeneuve, one of the *Lotus Bleu* members, who gets physicians to come there, is the typical vegetarian proselyte, who, having been cured of rheumatoid arthritis thanks to the diet, cannot stop speaking about it. After a long stay in Burma, where the efficiency of alternative medicine (a frugal diet, temperance, medicinal plants) on the natives had particularly appealed to him, he becomes Secretary General of the French Eastern Society, and is a member of several learned societies. His autobiographical narrative, in which he tells about his conversion to the vegetarian diet and makes proposals for its diffusion in France, is the reference point for French vegetarians until the end of the century. Dr Goyart, the author of a handbook about dosimetric medicine, praising Graham bread (after the famous American reformer of hygienic vegetarianism), replaces Dr De Villeneuve at the head of the Society, while Dr Bonnejoy is the most eloquent spokesman of French vegetarianism.

If in 1880 French vegetarianism does not seem to have a past, this is not due to a lack of followers, but, according to these pioneers, to the lack of a suitable organisation able to train and advise the vegetarians who, although numbering quite a few, remain isolated, and do not dare to flaunt themselves because of the prevailing carnivorous prejudice. Proselytes are very pleased to see that, at the practical and literary levels in Germany, England and Switzerland, vegetarianism is dynamic and has numerous companies, hotels, restaurants, journals, books, etc, devoted to its propagation.[11] They deplore the French lateness, which justifies all the more the need to create a Vegetarian Society. From their point of view, the lack of such a structure also accounts for the fact that the works of Jean-Antoine Gleïzès (1773–1843) have not had proper recognition in France, while the English and the Germans were inspired by them. The thing they have to do is to break the images and symbols of virility, strength and well-being associated with meat and, simultaneously, destroy the dreams it gives rise to in the poor people, in short, bring discredit on the taste of meat so as to persuade people not to eat it, and replace it by the virtues of vegetables.

Undoubtedly the vegetarian arguments take place in the context of the development of social crisis, linked with intense rural emigration and workers' unrest and the spread of agricultural crisis related to the import of cheap cereals from America. The creation of national vegetarian societies on the continent, in Germany in 1868, in Switzerland in 1878, and in Belgium and France in 1880, seems to be closely linked with social problems and account for the vegetarians' ambitions to reform. In most of the continental countries, the years 1878–80 witness the spreading out of towns and unhygienic conditions. Lack of town planning and destitution worsened the workers' situation in the big towns, and especially that of people working in big industry. As a result of phthisis, congestion of the lungs and rachitis, the infantile death rate remains important.[12] But if massive import of frozen meat contributes to the increase of average consumption, there is an important disparity in the types of meat the different social classes can afford. The poor people buy salted American meat and pork, essentially. And in the second half of the nineteenth century, food expenses remain by far the most important household expenditures in poor families, particularly in the big towns. It accounts for more than 50 per cent of the income of most workers, and physiological needs dominate in big families. For instance, an unskilled worker, head of a family of eleven, spends 22 per cent of his earnings on bread and 6 per cent on meat, whereas a railmender at the head of a family of four will spend 15 per cent on bread, and 33 per cent on meat.[13]

Moreover, the meat and other foodstuffs are sometimes unhealthy. Much of them come from the remains put out on a parallel and very active market, hawked by private and public sales, and also being sold on the black-market. Damaged, rotten foodstuffs constitute the dangerous consumption denounced by many hygienists.[14]

Whereas for the middle-classes, frugal clothing and food are the means of ensuring social success for their children, the working classes, with no such ambition, invest their earnings in things which are immediately satisfying and useful. Each category, aiming at something different, has its own morality concerning efforts. Eating meat and drinking wine were very important in those years, firstly because the dietary ideal of long undernourished populations tends to valorise energising foods. The vegetarian proselytes are the most extreme among the hygienists.[15] The meat consumption they unceasingly denounce among the poor does not reach, until about 1904, the levels recommended by the employers' hygienists, even if the latter are quite close to the vegetarians. It can therefore be easily understood that the ascetic message, which is essentially negative, is ignored by the poor, whose attitude towards food is wholly positive. Unable to win over the poor classes, Dr De Villeneuve, who is well received in the Parisian fashionable circles, decides to attract members of this milieu, who are not only the biggest meat consumers but are also familiar with the ideas of dietary hygiene. De Villeneuve is convinced that the upgrading of a vegetarian gastronomic cooking, with the names of the dishes imitating those of conventional gastronomy, will gradually revitalise the model which the élite is used to:

> One can, with vegetarian cooking alone, imitate the most refined dishes. I had a cepe pâté garnished with truffles made. It looks very much like a liver pâté, and is not less delicious, but with a different taste. As you can see, I have tried to transform the vegetarian diet into luxury food.[16]

In 1880, 1881, and 1882, the Parisian vegetarians organise big dinner banquets in the Lemardeley restaurant (100 Richelieu Street), where physicians, artists and journalists are invited. The menus proposed at these banquets exhibit the very demonstrative will and the gastronomic ambition of the Vegetarian Society. For example, the menu of the first banquet in 1880 consists of:

> *Soups*: Lentils, spring soup.
> *Hors-d'oeuvres*: Butter, radishes, olives.
> *Starters*: Soft-boiled eggs, asparagus branches.
> *Quaternians*: Macaroni with chicken white meat, garden peas.
> *Saccharines*: Vanilla cream, amygdaline hives, savarin.
> *Dessert*: Swiss cheese, compote of apples, strawberry jam, dates, oranges, wafers.
> *Wines*: Mâcon vieux, Saint-Emilion.
> Graham bread.[17]

But confronted with the indifference of the medical, scientific and literary elite, and with the absence of new members, the Vegetarian Society of Paris decide to disband and stop publishing its journal in 1882.

THE FRENCH VEGETARIAN SOCIETY OR THE
NEW MORAL CRUSADERS

In 1882, Dr Goyart immediately starts the anti-meat campaign. For this purpose, he founds the French Vegetarian Society (the SVF), determined to enlarge its social range. The longstanding followers, elders of the *Lotus Bleu*, form part of the SVF. Most of them are physicians, and can be classified as hospital consulting physicians, or academics who are amongst the so-called 'princes de la médecine', the 'gránds patrons'. Most of them are devoted to social medicine, and they represent the new clerks of the secular society.[18]

Dr Bonnejoy (1833–96), who will prove to be one of the greatest propagators of French vegetarianism, is a doctor at the hospice of Chars-en-Vexin in Seine-et-Oise. Dr Marcel Legrain is amongst the physicians who are the founders of the SVF. He is a leader of the French temperance movement, and becomes a fierce partisan of vegan raw diet. He publishes many works on alcoholism, namely *Hygiène et prophylaxie. Dégénérescence sociale et alcoolisme* (1895). He is the President of the Anti-Alcohol Association, while his wife is the Assistant Secretary General. Mrs Legrain is also the President of the French Women's Association for Temperance. We find there Dr Edmond Pivion, physician at the Health and Social Security, author of *Etude sur le régime de Pythagore et ses avantages* (1885), Dr E Contet, physician of the Health and Social Security at the Furtado Heine Dispensary in Paris, who publishes *Le végétarisme. Etude critique. Indications thérapeutiques* (1902), and lastly, E Tanneguy de Wogan, President of the National Encouragement Society for Prevention.

These proselytes foreshadow the modern style militants. Whether they write for the medical corps, or as popularisers, they are all prompted by the same spirit of missionary conquest. Besides their temperament and exceptional conviction, these followers enjoy financial independence and security which, unquestionably, determines their proselytism. Physicians are most prominently those who remain militants for an exceptionally long time. Having a militant career is all the more exciting for them, since they have the feeling of being pioneers and the inventors of a new cult. Dr De Villeneuve, Dr Goyart and Dr Bonnejoy militate until the end of their lives.

The SVF's proselytes seem to be less concerned with the poor's lot than with the proper praise of the beneficial action of vegetarianism. Their very purpose is to reform society as a whole. The popularity of hygienism in European vegetarianism, plus the fact that most of the SVF initiators belong to the medical corps, account for the latter's tendency to ground their diet on physiological arguments. Dr Bonnejoy, one of the greatest interpreters of French vegetarianism, sets the tone:

> What are said to be the reasons for adherence to the principles of vegetarianism vary a little in foreign countries, but most of them can be summarized as the association of religious feelings with love for animals, or pity for their sufferings.

> Philosophy only comes second. The one I refer to for my doctrine, is scientific
> Reason supported by medical and physiological deductions, whence the name
> rational, that I add to it. It is much more appropriate to the French character.[19]

The French vegetarians' action which informs and expresses at the same
time what is being done in the Vegetarian Society, is determined by a sci-
entistic and hygienic ideology, so that it is impossible to separate the two
levels of analysis. Idealising the virtues of talent, personal effort, intelli-
gence, energy and self-control, the proselytes do not hesitate to present their
own social positions and their probable longevity as the direct consequences
of their sober and frugal diet. Vegetarianism thus appears as the self-made
man's diet, *par excellence*, by means of which the individual, who never
has to worry about his health, is capable of competing, of always being the
strongest.[20] The idea of an association of economic success in business and
a vegetarian diet dawns, and will continually be reinforced. Always ready
to make the most of scientific knowledge to illustrate their arguments, the
precursors of the SVF use all the major scientific innovations in zootechnics,
anthropometry, natural selection, food chemistry, pasteurian microbics, etc.
With their hyper rationalism, they come to consider the trend of abstinence
founded on pity and love for animals as sentimentalism. They also come
to consider the trend of vegetarianism derived from the rejection of all
products of animal origin (veganism) as diet sophism. According to the
French vegetarians, vegetarianism is *the* rational diet which, when associated with natural hygiene (refraining from alcohol and tobacco, practising
regular exercise, breathing fresh air) is not only the best way to guarantee
good physical condition and restore good health when needed, but is also in
accordance with the French character,[21] owing to the scientific arguments
on which it is based. Such a definition which, moreover, shows the split
with Gleïzès's vegetarian trend, is characteristic of the medical sectarianism, which will tend to increase as the role of members of the medical corps
becomes more and more important in the vegetarian movement.

Helped on by physiological optimism, vegetarians develop a broad con-
ception of man's perfectibility through the medium of hygiene, which seems
to correspond with the liberal aspirations of members of the upper social
classes, to whom the virtues of diet are now addressed. The groups nearer
to the learned élite are also those who are the most likely to adopt vegetarianism, because they can best understand its principles. Owing to their high
level of education and knowledge, members of these groups are supposed to
know about the composition and nutritive value of different kinds of foods.
Consequently, they can be receptive to a campaign about debunking meat.

Arguably, the Manichean view which prevails until about 1884 among
the vegetarian leaders is characteristic of the youthfulness of French vegetarianism. It brings the leaders to repeat again and again the religious,
romantic and utilitarian arguments of justification of the diet, and then to
consider that the success of the diet is all the more logical since, according

to them, it is the very symbol of God. The promoters of French vegetarianism agree that illness and death, which inevitably lie in wait for the careless meat eater, are almost divine punishments, showing the falsehood of the former's choice of his diet. Through the medium of transposition or direct loan words, vegetarian proselytes' arguments in this period echo religious discourses to a large extent. In all their written work, they constantly insist on the fact that the rational vegetarian diet they propose is compatible with the Christian moral requirements of temperance and moderation, and that this accounts for its compliance with social norms and justifies its widespread acceptance. In most cases, the precursors of the SVF were born between 1830 and 1850, so that their aesthetic and moral awareness seems to have developed during the 1870s. These are years of great hardships, and hence provide other grounds for justifying the validity of the diet, dedicated in a way to the happiness of humanity. With their references to the population's anthropophagous stench, the physicians want to show that food reform pedagogy has equally got prospective virtues. The great impression produced by the Manichean vision accounts for the importance of moral qualities in the discourse, and of voluntarism in the action of the pioneers of French vegetarianism, represented by Dr Bonnejoy up to 1896. He is the first leader of the new Society to publish a book about the diet, in 1884. In this book, he advocates:

> The restoration of simple, natural diet, as close as possible to what is the least expensive, to what requires the least preparation . . . Eat little, and you will be your own doctor, says he to his readers. Feeding on very little, choosing natural substances free from every kind of alteration, preparing them in the simplest and best way possible. This is where, together with pure and healthy air, the secret of health lies.[22]

Bonnejoy's reference point is the simple peasant way of life in the South of France, a real paradise on earth. The predominance of home production economy in the Southern French diet, where people consume mainly vegetables (including oil), bread, milk and eggs, marked the peasants as those living closest to nature, as the less debased, as those who have the most kept out of the ugliness caused by the ill effects of the town. Life in the open air, adjusted to the rhythm of the seasons, manual work, regular exercise, vegetables, etc . . . , are the favourite norms of the vegetarians of Bonnejoy's generation. The latter, also a typical representative of the SVF, devotes his time to spreading its ideas. Being a traditionalist, he rises up against the decline of the moral values of the past, marriage, family. Being austere, he advocates asceticism in food, drinks, clothing as well as in all aspects of life. As from 1884, the Vegetarian Society functions informally, and through the intermediary of dinner banquets organised in his castle at Chars-en-Vexin, in 1884 and 1886, Bonnejoy maintains the social interactions between the present or potential followers, thus animating the life of the Society. Bonnejoy invites several members of the medical corps and of the scientific press to these banquets because he wants to give vegetarianism the social strength of a collective representation, especially since at the beginning of 1884 (19 January), brewers and other restaurant owners who organised a splendid culinary exhibition showed commercial aggressiveness.

The 4 July banquet menu, considered by Bonnejoy as representing the sublime French vegetarian cooking, underlines vegetarians' fondness for fresh foods. For starters, they had a freshly churned butter from Brittany, and that morning's fresh eggs. The dishes are composed of wild hops cut with their morning dew, artichokes from the valley picked early in the morning, boiled in spring water from the park, sauce made from freshly whipped cream. They also ate local wild cherries picked that morning. The banquet is also an occasion to show the vegetarians' preference for the domestic mode of production and preparation of food. The vegetarian wheat and rye bread eaten is made according to an ancient home recipe, composed of fresh grains, harvested and ground in Chars-en-Vexin, kneaded and cooked the day before in the home oven. For drinks, they have the choice between pure source water from the park, buttermilk which comes from the Breton cow milked the same morning ; the cider proposed is made from local apples from the last harvest. There is also some famous great Bordeaux wine, which had matured thirty-five years in the Megalithe house cellars.[23]

The purpose of the different operations which intersperse the banquet programme, is to bring the guests to accept, then share, the virtues of a universe of beliefs which, according to M Mauss, is at the basis of the efficacy of magic.[24] Before being elements of propaganda due to publicity and formality, the Society banquets are above all educational and symbolic moments for the vegetarians. In addition to the great care taken in the composition of menus which must be simple, frugal, but original, many efforts are made to create a natural, warm atmosphere during the meal. And, deliberately organised in July, the banquet takes place in the open air, in the shade of the tall elms of the Megalithe property, and cheerfulness and liveliness of the mind seem to dominate there.[25]

The vegetarians reverse the prevailing order of values and reveal through their diet a specific view of the world. They urge their contemporaries to prefer living food to dead food, because the proteins needed by the animal body are immediately available in plants, and have only to be absorbed, whereas flesh comes from the corpse of animals, and therefore from a life cycle which came to an end much earlier. Their rejection of bourgeois cooking goes together with that of the life style of the upper classes. According to the vegetarians, the sensuality, immorality of the rich people account for the economic crisis, social collapse, shown for instance, by the decrease in birth rate. The harshness of vegetarians against the infertility of the bourgeoisie confirmed by a statistician like Bertillon, is all the more obvious since they do not consider the fertility of the poor classes as beneficial to society. The vegetarians are sensitive to growing eugenism, and, like the previous century nobles, tend to be seriously concerned with genealogy and heredity. Consequently, they fear that the decline of families with better education to the benefit of the lower classes would transfer the sovereignty of the world to the less dignified races.[26] This fear is reflected many times in their discourse. With the imagery abundantly used by the vegetarians, which shows how sour they are, they denounce meat eating, this octopus that infects and kills. They also have recourse to a vocabulary related to beasts to condemn the ill-effects of meat which devours, exterminates, catches its prey. Withered by orgies, weakened by its immoderate taste for flesh, the bourgeoisie, as well as the rich people in the towns, bear the marks of their life style. They have become so ugly in their physical appearances that the influence of necrophagous practices on the beauty of the figure is clearly not misleading.[27]

Suspicion of the State is associated with the condemnation of the bourgeois life style. While the former is responsible for leading the people towards what is just and good, the Tax Department, says Bonnejoy, lives on alcohol, and the alcoholic is a good taxpayer. Since the State fails in its duty to protect the citizens from danger, the only solution to disorder is the casuistry recommended by vegetarian physicians, who, as visceral individualists, have never believed in any other government than that of people's health. Natural dietetics and those who represent it are the natural leaders in this government.

The vegetarian discourse conveys dissatisfaction, which brings the vegetarians closer to other groups, and as a result they associate other causes with theirs. Such are their relations with the pacifists, feminists and anti-colonialists. At the end of the nineteenth century, the anarchists who want to oppose the ideal of a natural life to the ugliness, corruption and tyranny of the capitalist system refer to the same principles of rejection of the SVF vegetarians. However, the consequences of the individualism which characterises these two trends of vegetarianism are quite different, so that they will tend to exclude each other. Represented by naturian and savagist groups consisting of progressive, libertarian intellectuals, the anarchist trend requires the institution of naturian communities, in which vegetable consumption associated with nakedness, free love, and protection of nature against the effects of industrial mechanisation would found the ideal of freedom.[28] On the contrary, the hygienic regeneration doctrines spread by the SVF proselytes remain very normative. They nurture a fierce hatred for the trouble-makers in society, and moreover consider order, discipline and purity, in short, the conservative values, as the most praiseworthy. For the vegetarian hygienists, family stability and cohesion, marriage blessing, respect for hierarchy, are the signs of a virtuous life. The importance they give to sexual hygiene, after Tissot and Graham, shows how closely they link moral order and the diet they recommend.

A comparative study of the social history of the different trends of social reform then on the increase would easily show that in spite of many common features between the pioneers of vegetarianism and their philanthropic counterparts, their idea of the individual (body and soul) as the only stronghold which matters at the end of the nineteenth-century agitated world, leads them to outbid the reform conditions which move them away from the others. This gap is obvious when we consider for instance that whereas for the freethinkers of the temperance movement vegetarian anti-alcoholism is a motive for union, the latter believe that human suffering is not only due to bad food habits and alcohol consumption but also to all the other violations of natural physiological laws, such as lack of sexual hygiene.[29] And the vegetarians' concern for the moral reform of the individual distinguishes them more particularly from the social economy followers like the founders of the Musée social (1894) such as the engineer Emile Cheysson, the Minister Jules Siegfried, or Charles Gide, who are trying to guarantee social peace by developing macroeconomic structures like cooperatives, popular banks, or patronage committees,[30] etc . . . For instance, although like De Villeneuve and De Wogan who, in 1870, join the Union de la Paix sociale[31] – a materialisation of the social economic doctrine, in a way – many vegetarians join the Comité de défense et de progrès social, created not long after the Musée social, and, according to their different specialities, participate in its public conferences on temperance, social lodgings, diet, etc ..., they cannot believe in the efficiency of collective reform structures.[32] The vegetarians tend to claim that their marginality in the field of social reform is a proof of the soundness of the cause they defend, and which is destined to prevail one day. In many ways, this sectarian attitude expresses the youthfulness of French vegetarianism. English vegetarianism was remodelled, especially from the 1860s, at the expense of a greater opening on to society and a greater number of reforming movements.[33]

The vegetarians do not believe in the institutional physicians' skills, any more than in the government of politicians, and in this they are faithful to M Rousseau's teachings. Their distrust for the State goes together with their rejection of classical medicine, and they denounce its complicities with the pharmaceutical industry, with the necrophagous social order. In their request that vegetarians should be put forward as candidates in the Academy of Medicine or at least in universities, the vegetarian physicians are aiming at the restoration of a new medical order. They want to impose on the medical institutions the teaching of vegetarian medicine, or physiatrics, since they are convinced that this is the first step towards wider diffusion of the vegetarian diet in society. Anyway, how can one have such unshakeable faith in the *vis medicatrix naturae*, without a coherent system of reference? Vegetarians want a simplified type of medicine which would emancipate the individual from the conservative medical corporations of the Faculty. Their physiological individualism leads them to prefer non-orthodox medicine, and they are already attracted by hydrotherapy and homeopathy, and are full of praise for their natural virtues.

Although they claim to be followers of traditional medicine and reject the prevailing medical system, the vegetarian physicians constantly seek the acknowledgement of hygiene and physiatrics as branches of medicine. For them, the medical institution is the only society with the moral authority essential for imposing certain values on people, and they hope that the practices of vegetarianism, certified as belonging to the medical field, will have a social status, a scientific legitimacy and thus a permanent authority. Convinced that they are right, the vegetarians consider themselves as martyrs, as victims of misunderstanding. This feeling is especially reinforced since they have the impression that the official therapeutics constantly append their arguments. It is true that, converted to the vegetarian diet because he was cured thanks to it, Dr Dujardin Beaumetz, the famous Professor of Therapeutics at Cochin Hospital (Paris), recommends it in cases of constipation and disturbances. However, if he fully agrees with the therapeutic influence of the ovo-lacto vegetarian diet, he contests the social role of vegetarianism, and its so-called effects on moral and intellectual faculties, and claims that one can eat meat and still be virtuous.[34] Dujardin-Beaumetz, Armand Gautier and Bouchard are diet hygiene therapists at Cochin and Saint-Antoine hospitals in Paris, teach at the Faculties of Medicine in Paris and Montpellier, and are members of the Academy of Medicine. Dr Bouchard and Dr Gautier also think that vegetarianism is a rational diet. Gautier, who is credited with the invention of modern dietetics, shows that vegetarianism has got the many advantages of a normal diet and the disadvantages of veganism, which, according to him, is harmful. If he does not see the dietetic relevance of a daily vegetarian diet, he nevertheless recommends it in a few pathological cases. For these dieticians, vegetarians are fanatics, hotheads, who are trying to justify through science a type of diet which is socially unacceptable.[35]

The Academicians' arguments are closely related to the progress made in the fields of hygiene, physiology of nutrition and pharmacology, as well as of agriculture and stock farming.[36] In the background, there is an evolution in the diet trend, and it is expressed amongst the bourgeoisie particularly by changes in tastes, related to the increasing popularity of diets, of dietetics. Being well off, this social class enjoys the advantages of dietary education, inculcated in fact by the conventional hygienists. As from the beginning of the 1880s, there is a more and more important decrease in bread, cereal products, meat, alcohol and liqueur consumption, while fresh fruits and vegetables, which are now more and more available, are in greater demand.[37] Among the working class, the consumption of proteins of animal origin, such as milk, eggs, butter, cream, cheese and fat, which appears clearly at the end of the century, is equally also a consequence of recent efforts of the dominant institutional diet hygienists, who also show the close link between food content and the strength required for such and such an activity. Through their Trade Unions and papers, the workers themselves take up and claim the theory of energising food, while the employers' hygienists put forward the role of a cheap rational diet, which also takes into account the combination of different foods and their nutritive value.

In such a context, vegetarianism seems to have dubious prospects. Reasonably speaking, the groups aimed at by the diet do not have any motive for adhering to it. Moreover, the vegetarians' arguments about refraining from eating meat and drinking alcohol as a way of fighting against illness and keeping in good health become outmoded. The hippocratic character of their health conceptions becomes outdated. Medical aetiology develops increasing sanitary controls in markets which tend to limit illnesses provoked by food. Hygienists and physicians seize the towns and wage war on dirtiness and illness, the enemies of a rational and productive society. Epidemiologists travel to every corner of the country, sit in hygiene committees and make out severe diagnoses.

Undoubtedly, the predominance of conventional hygienists in the field of diet reform strongly challenges the legitimacy of vegetarian physicians, and accounts for the fact that they are marginals even in the medical hierarchy, which is all the more detrimental to them since apart from a Vegetarian Society, these vegetarians have no other point of reference. The Vegetarian Society fails to be reconstituted in 1889.

REVIVAL AND SOCIAL DIFFUSION OF VEGETARIANISM (1899–1913)

A real millenary quivering is to be found in all the vegetarian societies as the end of the century draws near. For the French followers, 1900 is a fateful date which will see the revival of French vegetarianism or confirm its death. In 1899, thanks to the support of their Belgian counterparts, Bonnejoy's disciples found the SVF again, in the hope of perpetuating it once and for all.[38] Planned in Paris for 1900, the Universal Exhibition offers the French people an opportunity that they cannot ignore, without taking the risk of the regrettable isolation ... of all those who have acknowledged the beneficial action of vegetarianism, or who want to experiment with it.[39] The Vegetarian International Congress which takes place from 21–23 June 1900, in Paris, within the framework of the Universal Exhibition, is the real baptism for the French vegetarians of the new generation. In his opening speech, Dr Jules Grand, the President of the new SVF, gives an outline of the definition of the French vegetarianism of 1900, which confirms Bonnejoy's rationalism and resolutely unfurls its flag under the aegis of physiology:

> Although the means of spreading vegetarianism are almost the same everywhere, there is however a difference in the ways of putting them into practice, which are specific to each country, and better suited to its temperament. In some, the vegetarian societies ask their members to sign a formal engagement, stating that they will strictly observe the vegetarian diet. Other countries mainly or only base their vegetarian rules on pity for animals, and condemn and fight against vivisection. We do not think that it would be a good thing to follow this example, and we are convinced that such demands would be hateful in this country, and

far from favouring our propaganda, would move away from us many people who are friendly to us.[40]

That respect for animals should be the main topic of a great debate in the Society as soon as it is founded again, reveals its importance for the supporters as well as for the leaders. Georges Guillaumin, the supporter who introduces the debate, summarises the SVF anthropocentric doctrine in a long text.[41] He points out that respect for animal life cannot be given as a determining motive for making anyone adopt the diet, since this idea comes mainly within feelings, aesthetics, in brief, within morality, and does not constitute a strong enough argument to force conviction. Inviting the vegetarians to pay attention to the methods used, Guillaumin adds:

> The diet question is essentially physiological; from this connection draw precise, direct arguments liable to be experimentally demonstrated. Produce facts – a fact is all powerful – and arguments to counter precisely what is being put forward.[42]

In reply to the moralists, Guillaumin takes up the main arguments which, throughout the nineteenth century, were spread by protectors of animals in France, and which are mainly structured round the refusal of ill-treatment of domestic animals in public:[43]

> It is certainly very true that animals are protected against unecessary cruelty, says Guillemin. Man has *some duties* towards them, and speeches about these duties find their place in a treaty on morality. Talking about . . . the *rights of animals* seems a more debatable issue to me, since then you will not be able to prevent someone from claiming, in his turn – with nearly as much logic – the rights of plants to take them away from man's ascendancy over them, and then, what will you live on?[44]

This argument undoubtedly echoes the conceptions then developed by Henry Salt and Edward Carpenter, the English vegetarians who founded in 1891 the Humanitarian League, in order to claim animal rights similar to human rights. Guillaumin recommends not to follow these people who, being under the influence of an untimely sentimentalism, misjudge the hierarchy of beings, as it results not from a pre-established order, but from the facts and very show of the world. The facts to which M Guillaumin is alluding are mainly recorded by Buffon and supported by the dominant clergy, according to whom man has dominated the world and imposed his supremacy on all the other beings.[45] Guillaumin adds accordingly:

> We have to acknowledge that in order to reach his goals, he has the right to use the inferior beings populating the planet with him, the right to reduce them to slavery to make them work for his profit, and even to eat their flesh, if necessary. I wouldn't be surprised if recalling the personality or dignity of an ox which is more or less gored, would prevent people from eating their daily steak, if they like it, and think it is necessary or even simply useful for their strength or brains. Give them other reasons, and if they are still convinced about it, you can then

point out that, amongst other consequences, the vegetarian diet is good for can-
celling many unnecessary cruelties and bloodshed, often hateful.[46]

Such a vision which reflects the influence of scienticism on the SVF,
accounts for the absence of its members from the Society for Prevention of
Cruelty to Animals (SPA), and from anti-vivisection and anti-vaccination
associations and, eventually, of SVF's ostracism of animal lovers. The latter
gathered around M Jacques de Marquette, a dental surgeon, who set up
the Trait d'Union in 1912. Foreshadowing the new structures for the diffusion of French vegetarianism after World War I, this Society is not only
vegetarian, but also naturist, and it attaches some importance to the moral,
philosophical and social aspects of the diet reform. It starts a journal, *Le
Végétarien*, and has more than one hundred members in 1914.

By distrusting the reasons of the heart on behalf of the reasons of
reason,[47] the vegetarians are extending Bonnejoy's enterprise which consisted in bringing vegetarianism to the altar of Science. The lunch banquet
offered to 35 guests, on 20 June 1890 at the Congress Restaurant, is composed of hors-d'œuvres, radishes with Isigny butter, garden peas prepared
in the French way, with scrambled eggs with mushrooms, asparagus in
white sauce, of desserts, strawberry with cream, and of water for drinks.[48]
If this menu does not display any significant changes in the composition of
the French vegetarian menu, the account given by the different representatives about their activities shows that, like the other exhibitors, the 1900
vegetarians belong fundamentally to the century spirit. They talk about the
rapid development of a vegetarian cuisine, rich in recipes whose essential
properties are their heterogeneous and cosmopolitan character. Anderson
Hanson, the American Vice-President of the Vegetarian Congress, in particular, constantly underlines the miracles produced by the vegetarian food
industry in his country. In 1900, Kellogg's represent the main vegetarian
food company, producing breakfast cereals as well as cooking ingredients,
soups, cream, butter, etc, subsidising distribution networks and preparing
to control, particularly through the intermediary of vegetarian sects set-
tling and developing in Europe, and especially in England, Germany, Switzerland, important channels of distribution of milk, eggs, sugar, etc . . .
This is particularly the period when Dr Kellogg creates the Sanitas Nut food
company which in addition to vegetable meat, produces *protose*, *nuttose*
and *nuttolene*, which are groundnut-based products, and provide vegetable
fat and proteins ready for consumption.[49]

For the 1900 vegetarian, man's natural diet, which like cane sugar, pow-
dered almonds, lemon, imported products, or like butter, ceravene (roast
oatmeal used for preparing soups, creams, baby's cereals, croquettes, etc),
canned foods from industries, is not defined by the usual criteria: local
products, unconditional freshness. Most of all, industry is not equivalent to
chemistry and artifice. Distrust of artificial foods is dispelled by the advantages they present – nutritional value, hygiene, high degree of concentration,

convenience in preparation, ease of carrying (especially suitable for tourists, walkers, alpinists, many of whom are vegetarians), etc. From then on, vegetarian books increase in number and, like those of Carlotto Schulz, the green cuisine chef, reveal vegetarians' acceptance of industrial foods.[50]

The particular importance attached by the 1900 vegetarian to his table, associated with book publication, recipe exchanges and circulation, appears as the innovating factor that most contributed to a better understanding of the diet by the population. Whether he has been formerly ill, or simply wants to stop eating meat, the 1900 vegetarian seems to be a faithful disciple of De Villeneuve and Bonnefoy. He is well aware of the chemical composition of food, and knows how to compare their different calorie and protein contents to feed himself. And while refusing to yield to traditional cooking, he wants to be a real chef, capable of cleverly copying the dishes (and their names), and of classical (including gastronomic) presentation. For hygiene reasons, undoubtedly, but also because he is a gourmet, Carlotto Schulz answers to the imaginary investigator. Thus, the hedonist dimension is not absent from vegetarianism, and it is with the aid of a culinary creativity that the vegetarian must fight against the vegetable and cereal prejudice which, together with the meat prejudice, is firmly rooted in tradition:

> Taste itself finds complete satisfaction in vegetarianism, which is far from imposing austerity. Get rid of present culinary habits and adopt faithfully the rules of vegetarian cooking ; although simple, they are not less essential for success, from the point of view of hygiene and pleasantness. And soon, with the revival of taste sensation, you will discover a nice surprise in vegetables, cereals and fruits, the flavour whose mellowness and nutritional value have been preserved by a judicious mode of preparation. Even when they are simply steamed, you can appreciate them, but if we hold on to a more flattering than healthy variety, there are plenty of skilful recipes.[51]

The vegetarian assures those who would object that he yields to necrophagous sensuality by accepting industrial products, that he is faithful to his values and contemptuous of necrophagous practices. He is all the more obstinate in his fight against bourgeois cuisine, since he does it scientifically. Papers written by vegetarians to urge industries to manufacture healthy products which retain their nutritive values can be found in the very first issues of the *Réforme alimentaire*. Until after the War, and even in the popularising works on the farm-produce industry, Jules Morand, the SVF Secretary General continues to show that vegetarians ask for industrial products. Saving the leftovers, measuring the exact quantities required for his meals, the 1900 vegetarian is like the good housewife, taking special care to avoid waste. Is that not the very foundation of canned food?

> We do not eat all the vegetables and fruits produced on earth at the moment Nature offers them to us. An important amount is wasted. We could use it by preserving it *naturally* by means of the appropriate processes, or by drying it. Our industry . . . should not neglect anything . . . Let's use everything that our

rich soil of France offers to us, let's not waste anything, but strive to preserve what we cannot eat immediately, and offer it for consumption, *in as near a natural state as possible, and at prices that everyone can afford.* We have to study carefully the possibility of delivering the preserved foods in glass jars with a practical system, so that jars, lids, sealing material can be given back and used again. With proper industrialization, this process would offer amongst other advantages, choice products, which are perfectly healthy, and can be controlled by the buyers themselves.[52]

However, vegetarian arguments show that they do not feel less guilty about the looseness of the values of purity and freshness which make up the ideological heritage they have to transmit. They feel very bad about it. Thus, as if to redeem themselves, they try to compensate for what they are abandoning in practice, by excessive mannerisms and moral outbidding. Thus in their written works, vegetarians strive to show that they contribute to the enhancement of the value of endangered culinary traditions, by integrating in their own cooking cereals and legumes which are less and less used in the different regions. Added to diet, in these years of excessive modernisation, this moral value acts as a foil to opposing arguments. Inviting all those who are used to considering fruits and vegetables as being of secondary importance to discover the numerous riches of the vegetable world, Carlotto Schulz puts forward the culinary and cultural revitalisation undertaken by vegetarianism:

> Oats given to animals in our country, but so much appreciated by the English, the Germans, and especially by the strong Scots; maize on which our Southern French fellowmen as well as Italians feed almost exclusively; rice which feeds so many eastern peoples, barley which is relegated so stupidly at our chemists'; and at last sarrasin and millet, whose taste is not as fine as that of the above mentioned, but whose nutritive value is still important.[53]

The vegetarian's duties are: temperance, the only thing that avoids the overworking of digestive organs harmful to digestion, and simplicity which requires that foods be consumed as much as possible in the state they are offered to us by nature, so as to preserve the precious substances it has elaborated.[54] Together with refinement, they are the key words of modern vegetarian cooking, which from comparative tables about the nutritive value of foods to detailed menus for different professions (for hard physical work, intellectual activity or sedentary people), for each day (morning, noon, evening), for each season, give emphasis to the proselytes' recommendations.[55]

In an increasingly urbanised context, the changes in the vegetarians' conceptions refer to the changes in the social composition of the Vegetarian Society, more than to the problems linked with the availability of fresh products with home production possibilities. The new French vegetarians, more concerned with health reforms than with academic applications, try to be more pragmatic, and are more sensitive to the dominant tendencies of hygienism. They are more open-minded about industry as well as about classical medicine. The management Committee elected by the SVF in 1905 reflects its new professional trends. Ten persons make up the Committee: a physician (Dr Jules Grand) as President, a merchant (M Jules Morand) as Secretary General, an economist (M Géré) as Treasurer, a pensioned captain, a biologist, Professor Jules Lefèvre, and other physicians. Being for order and management, these men want first of all to increase the social respectability of vegetarianism. They consider the Society as a privileged means of education. In 1907, Jules Morand, for example, starts *Hygie, the Practical Hygiene and Rational Diet Magazine*, which will survive the SVF and the *Réforme alimentaire*. From April 1908 onwards, he runs the very first vegetarian and Kneippist grocery store in Paris, the Naturo Vigor. Dr Lahmann's clothes made of rational material (or cotton), hand-made artificial leather shoes, hats, sports equipment, cooking pots for steamed food, or double boilers, cereals, as well as various other food products from many countries can be found there.[56] Morand simultaneously opens a vegetarian restaurant near the store in the fashionable neighbourhood of Saint-Germain des Prés. But the vegetarian restaurant is more expensive than equivalent restaurants, and this limits the number of customers. Does this not pose, in a general manner, the problem of the diffusion of vegetarianism? A minority of the size of the SVF cannot impose its laws on the market, although this does not constitute a real explanation. Faced with competition from butchers, grocers and other restaurant owners, vegetarianism with its characteristic individual diet is all the more expensive since it requires a strict selection of foodstuffs and since its commercial range is limited.

In 1900, the French vegetarians, anxious to reform, are forced, so to speak, to break with the rigorism to which their predecessors had accustomed their contemporaries. They have to be even more pragmatic since an evolution in diet awareness in the first quarter of the century leads the conventional gastronomes to use a language similar to theirs. For instance the first International Congress of Groceries, held in Paris on 13–15 June 1900, gives rise to a display of a conquering French gastronomy which was sponsored by Martel and Marie Brizard's corporations. Trustful of the future of their occupation, the grocers agree to lay stress on the study and the choice of the products, on the invention of new blendings, on pure fabrication of products, and especially on the knowledge of the nutritive, gustative or digestive peculiarities of the products.[57] Thus apart from active members practising vegetarianism, associates who are interested in spreading it, but cannot match their conduct to its principles,[58] are admitted into the midst of the SVF. From then on, vegetarians can set themselves precise tasks:

> Fight against the idea that meat is essential for health and life; denounce the falsification of foodstuffs, point out the inconveniences of a meat diet, as well as the *unnecessary* cruelties it gives rise to; study the principles of human nutrition; set the rules for a rational diet; look for a simple, healthy and strength-giving diet.[59]

The progression in the number of memberships which is reported in the *Réforme alimentaire* every month shows the main characteristics of followers of vegetarianism. The membership increases rapidly. From 1899 to 1913, it is mainly the lower and upper middle classes who join the SVF as active members as well as mere associates. In its first years, the SVF mostly recruits in the 6th, 7th, 8th, 9th and 17th Parisian districts. The main social categories who register at the SVF live in these zones and consist of physicians, surgeons, medical students, nurses (male and female), members of paramedical professions such as masseurs, manufacturers of hygienic food products, veterinary surgeons, midwives, college, high school – and primary school teachers, civil engineers, painters, booksellers, photographers, architects, solicitors, judges, army lieutenants and garrison majors. These categories which, like the SVF Management Committee, are dominated by medical and paramedical professions, seem to form the hard core of French vegetarianism.

Family memberships predominate, but they are irregular and precarious. Paris is the main vegetarian recruitment centre. But the close link between the areas of activity of the main national leaders and the numbers of memberships shows that the diffusion campaign is mainly a personalised and commercial one, limited to the promoters' geographical spheres. The commercial character of the campaign is all the more obvious since they are proposed by physicians, priests, teachers or magistrates.

In 1913, during the International Vegetarian Union Congress, created in 1900 – in relation with the celebration of Esperanto, another credo of vegetarianism – to favour contacts between national vegetarian societies, the SVF secretary shows that the small progress made by vegetarianism in France is due on the one hand to the medical corps conservatism and on the other to the French rationalist requirements:

> Serious arguments were essential to show to the world that vegetarianism is fully justified, and to present it in its real light. Without these arguments, vegetarianism would not have appeared as man's rational diet, but, to most people, it would have remained a doctrine, the idea of a few hotheads, a whim, snobbery, a fashionable item, a diet . . . In France, it is the scientific idea which has prevailed and which has up to now guided our steps, activities, works, and it is precisely because we have worked more particularly on these grounds that we have not been able to win over a great number of members, as opposed to what happened in countries where vegetarianism didn't need to be discussed and was naturally accepted because it amounts to an intimate feeling, an aspiration, a deep pity.[60]

Whereas with World War I the SVF activity is eclipsed, M Morand's opinion reveals the difficulties encountered by those spreading vegetarianism in France. Urged on by the health argument, the adherents first tend to register as active members, and then as associates, so that, in 1914, more than half of the 1736 SVF members are sympathisers, who do not, or no longer, practise vegetarianism. The SVF does not manage to widen its social basis.

This history of French vegetarianism presents one of the least known aspects of the intellectual history of health and moral reform in Europe: that of the marginal groups who do their utmost across the countries to succeed in the diffusion of their ideals. In all respects (ideologies, doctrinarian culture, organisational strategy, social composition, etc) French fin-de-siècle vegetarianism is a pure result of the European vegetarian connection. As the main features of their ideological youthfulness, the physician vegetarians have not been able to overcome their own certitudes to take into account the diversity and the complexity of the determinants which could lead a wide range of people from the different sections of society to adopt the diet. A medical sectarianism added to a class ethnocentrism have systematically held the French promoters of vegetarianism aloof from a sound appreciation of the social and dietetic realities and consequently have progressively led them to miss their targets. At all events, the principles these pioneers adopted and sought to propagate have in very fact anticipated and influenced the opinions of succeeding generations. After World War I, the rise of associations which advocate especially hygienic vegetarianism is a relevant sign of the impact of this trend of vegetarianism in France. But if the absence of a structured vegetarian society makes the analysis of the social reception of the diet very hard, the new data which are now being collected on decrease in meat consumption as well as on health practices, should contribute to a better knowledge of French vegetarianism and its relationships with the European trends.

BIBLIOGRAPHY

Agulhon, M. Le sang des bêtes. Le problème de la protection des animaux en France au XIXè siècle, *Romantisme*, 31 (1981), 81–109.

Aron, J P. Sur les consommations avariées à Paris dans la deuxième moitié du XIXè siècle, *Annales ESC*, 23 (Mars-Juin 1975), 553–61.

Bariety, M and Coury, Ch. *Histoire de la médecine*, Paris, 1963.

Bastié, A. *La croissance de la banlieue parisienne*, Paris, 1964.

Bonnejoy, Dr E (du Vexin). *Principes d'alimentation rationnelle et de cuisine végétarienne*, Paris, Berthier, 1884 (1896 2nd edition).

Carson, G. *Cornflake Crusade*, New York, 1957.

Dauphin, C and Pezerat, P. Les consommations populaires dans la seconde moitié du XIXè siècle à travers les monographies de l'école de Le Play, *Annales ESC*, 23 (Mars-Juin 1975), 537-49.

Dock, Dr F W. In Zollikofer, ed, *Du végétarisme ou de la manière de vivre selon les lois de la nature*, St Gall, 1878.

Dujardin-Beaumetz, Dr E. Du régime végétarien au point de vue thérapeutique, *Bulletin général de thérapeutique*, 4th conference (1890), 97–112; Du traitement de la diarrhée et de la constipation, *Bulletin général de thérapeutique*, 5th conference (1890), 289–300.

Gautier, Dr A. *L'alimentation et les régimes chez l'homme sain et chez les malades*, Paris, 1904 (2è éd).

Gide, Ch. L'idée de solidarité en tant que programme économique, *Revue internationale de sociologie*, I (1893), 253–65.

Gouraud, Dr F X. *Que faut-il manger? Manuel d'alimentation rationnelle*, Paris, 1910.

Grand, Dr J. Allocution au Congrès international végétarien, *Réforme alimentaire*, 4: 7 (1900), 1–3.

Groupe de travail pour l'histoire du mouvement ouvrier, *Le mouvement ouvrier suisse. Documents de 1800 à nos jours*, Genève, 1978.

Guillaumin, G. Sur la question du respect de la vie animale, *La Réforme alimentaire*, 5: 1 (1901), 1–6

James, W. *The Varieties of Religious Experience. A study in human nature*, London, 1902.

Kingsford, Dr A. *De l'alimentation végétale chez l'homme (Végétarisme)*, Paris, 1880.

Mauss, M. *Oeuvres*, 1, Paris, 1906.

Morand, J. Des conserves pour les végétariens, *L'industrie française de la conserve*, 22, (1918), 145–9.

Ouédraogo, A P. *Le végétarisme. Esquisse d'histoire sociale*, Ivry/Seine, 1994; The Sect and the Cenacle. A social genesis of western Vegetarianism to 1859. In Dare, Robert, ed, *Food, Power and Community: Essays in the History of Food and Drink*, Adelaide, S.A. 2000, 154–56; La viande ou le salut. Genèse sociale du végétarisme occidental, *Annales*, Juillet-Août 2000.

Perrot, M. *Le mode de vie des familles bourgeoises, 1873–1953*, Paris, 1961 (2è éd 1982).

Premier Congrès international de l'épicerie, à Paris les 13, 14 et 15 Juin, Paris, 1900.

Raoux, E. *Le tocsin des deux santés. Fragments sur l'hygiène et l'éducation du corps et de l'âme*, Lausanne and Paris, 1878.

Robert, Ch. *La suppression des grèves par l'association aux bénéfices*, Paris, 1870.

Schulz, C. *La table du végétarien: choix, préparation et usage rationnels des aliments conformément aux principes de la diététique naturelle (suivi de 700 recettes et règles d'hygiène)*, Paris, 1904; *La table du végétarien* (4ᵉ édition), *contenant 953 recettes*, Paris, 1910.

Siegfried, J. *La misère, son histoire, ses causes, ses remèdes*, Paris, 1879.

SVF, *Discours et toasts prononcés au Congrès international végétarien*, Paris, 1900.

de Villeneuve, Dr. Autobiographie. In Dr Bonnejoy, E. *Le végétarisme et le régime végétarien rationnel. Dogme, histoire, pratique*, Paris, 1891.

Teuteberg, H-J. Zur Socialgeschichte des Vegetarismus, *Vierteljaarschrift für Sozial- und Wirtschaftsgeschichte*, 81 (1994), 33–65.

Toutain, J C. *La consommation alimentaire en France de 1789 à 1964*, Cahiers de l'ISEA, t 5, 11 (1971), 2013–18.

Twigg, J. *The Vegetarian Movement In England, 1847–1981: With particular reference to its ideology*, London, 1981.

Worms, R. L'économie sociale, *Revue internationale de sociologie*, VI (1898), 452–68.

NOTES

1 Another trend, consisting mainly of anarchists, also promotes a vegetable diet, especially from 1895. This is a periodic trend which is in a minority in the midst of the French Anarchist Movement, and its irregular actions remain residual until 1914.

2 Ouédraogo (forthcoming article). Unlike the proselytes of the hygienic trend, Gleïzès advocated a strict vegetable diet grounded on ethical considerations which led him to become a famous crusader of respect for animal life.

3 Dock, 1878, 7–9.

4 *Groupe de travail pour l'histoire du mouvement ouvrier*, 1978, 58–66.

5 Raoux, 1878, VI, 25–6.

6 Ibid, 25.

7 Ibid, VI.

8 Ibid, 40.

9 Ibid, 42.

10 Kingsford, 1880.

11 About the vitality of British and German vegetarian trends, see respectively Twigg, 1981 and Teuteberg, 1994, 33–65.

12 Bastié, 1964.

13 Dauphin and Pezerat, 1975, 537–549.

14 Aron, 1975, 553–61.

15 Ouédraogo, 1994, 94.

16 Dr De Villeneuve, in Dr Bonnejoy, 1891, 247.

17 *Réforme alimentaire*, 2 (May 1881); Dr Dujardin-Beaumetz, 1890, 97–112. Quaternians are dishes composed mainly of food said to be quaternaries, ie eggs and milk; saccharins are sweet desserts.

18 Bariety and Coury, 1963, 788–9.

19 Dr Bonnejoy, 1891, 6.

20 James, 1902.

21 Dr Bonnejoy, 1891, 2. Most of the authors of this period also hold the same view.

22 Dr Bonnejoy (du Vexin), 1884, (1896 2nd edition), 12–13.

23 *Journal de la Santé*, 33 (1886).

24 Mauss, 1906, 17–26.

25 Dr Bonnejoy, 1891, 322–5.

26 Kingsford, 1880, 40–5. The same expressions are used by Bonnejoy and all the other vegetarian authors of the period.

27 Dr Bonnejoy, 1891, 33.

28 Two periodicals, *L'Age d'or* and *La Nouvelle Humanité*, are circulated by the 'naturian' and 'savagists'.

29 *La Tempérance*, 5 (1874), 53.

30 Robert, 1870; Sigfried, 1879.

31 It gathers together Catholic businessmen, priests, big landowners, and while gradually getting rid of its confessional character, it has the support of the liberal members of the bourgeoisie.

32 Worms, 1898, 453–61; Gide, 1893, 353–69.

33 Ouédraogo (forthcoming article).

34 Dr Dujardin-Beaumetz, 1890, 289–300.

35 Dr Gautier, 1904 (2nd edn); Dr Gouraud, 1910.
36 Toutain, 1971, 2013–18.
37 Perrot, 1961 (1982), 286–92.
38 The new French Vegetarian Society, together with the Belgian Vegetarian Society, distributes the *Réforme alimentaire*. This journal is published every month, on the 15th, until 1914. The sub-editor's secretariat is in Brussels, and the director of the journal until 1914, is Ernest Nyssens, from Brussels. Jules Morand, a Parisian merchant, is the Secretary General of the SVF for 15 years.
39 Grand, 1900, 1.
40 Ibid, 131.
41 Guillaumin, 1901, 1–6.
42 Ibid, 1.
43 For the social history of animal protection in nineteenth-century France, see Agulhon 1981, 81–109.
44 Guillaumin, 1901, 3.
45 Ibid, 3.
46 Ibid, 3–4.
47 Ibid, 6.
48 SVF (1900).
49 Carson, 1957, 80.
50 Schulz, 1910, 7.
51 Ibid.
52 Morand, 1918, 145–9.
53 Schulz, 1910, 10.
54 Ibid, 19–20.
55 Ouédraogo, 1994, 109–15.
56 *Réforme alimentaire*, 12: 5 (1908), 143.
57 Congrès, 1900.
58 Ibid, 1–2.
59 *Réforme alimentaire*, 3: 3 (1899), 2.
60 *Réforme alimentaire* (1913), 16–17.

13   The medical discourse and the drunkard's stereotyping in Belgium, 1840–1919

Peter Scholliers

1919: 'L'ALCOOLISME, DONT LE PROCÈS N'EST PLUS À FAIRE' [1]

Three days after coming into power in November 1918, the socialist minister of Justice, E Vandervelde, banned by decree virtually all consumption of alcoholic beverages in Belgium. On 29 August 1919, the *Loi sur le régime de l'alcool* abated something of the impact of the 1918 decree, but the drinking of alcohol in public remained prohibited, while taxes on alcohol import quadrupled, consumption duties rose drastically, and infringements by both tradesmen and consumers were heavily penalised. The consequence was that the (officially registered) consumption of alcoholic drinks halved between 1910–14 and 1919–24, to reach 2.2 litres (at 50°) per head and per year, a quantity that was considered to be acceptable. After decades of assiduous combats, half-hearted enactments, and intensive campaigns, the long-awaited goal had finally been reached. The *Enemy* had been beaten.

The government had not considered it necessary to motivate the law at length when it was submitted to Parliament in 1919. The only elaborated argument related to the need for the population to utilise all resources for rebuilding the country after the war, and heavy drinking would certainly impede this. Before 1914 alcohol drinking had diminished, and the government hoped to extend this shrinkage by using the conditions of the moment, ie the enforced 'de-alcoholisation' of the war years. No direct argument against drinking was advanced. Seemingly, all members of Parliament were convinced of the manifold nuisances of alcohol drinking. [2] Apparently, the idea that alcohol was highly damaging had become part of a 'common sense'.

The medical profession contributed tremendously to the forming of this 'common sense' about alcohol drinking. This paper aims at investigating when, how and why physicians started to view alcohol drinking as a medical problem, and if, when and how this view was accepted by the anti-alcohol movement.

CREATING A SOCIAL TRAUMA, c 1840–80

For long, *jenever* (the *eau-de-vie* of grain) has been part of the everyday life of all social layers in the Southern Netherlands. At the beginning of the nineteenth century, the production process was industrialised, and cheap materials were used. After the independence of 1830, the young Belgian state prohibited the import of Dutch gin, and at the same time lowered the *accijns* (consumption tax), which allowed local producers to develop swiftly.[3] The consequence was that more, and cheaper, good-quality gin was produced. Consumption rose, the more so since the price of beer and wine had augmented somewhat. Tax statistics indicate that 5.8 litres (of 50°) per year and per head were consumed in 1810, 7.5 litres in 1828 and 8.3 litres in 1835.[4]

This increase was not viewed as a major problem by contemporaries up to the early 1840s. Of course, public drunkenness was radically combated just as it had been in previous centuries. In 1843 Ducpétiaux, the director of the Belgian prisons, lamented over the occasionally heavy drinking by both men and women of the urban working classes; he denounced the augmented intake, and pointed to the danger of alcoholic heredity. At the same time, however, he could understand why workers drank: it was their only leisure occupation and social activity.[5] A quite similar view was given in 1845 in another reputable publication. The authors, two physicians, stressed that only a little measure of gin was bought in the morning or evening, that especially better-off workers could afford this, and that gin was a necessary stimulant. Naturally they too blamed the abuse of gin, but they saw it as a consequence of poverty and ignorance. Medical comments with regard to abusive drinking were absent.[6] Drinking was perceived as a personal affair involving only the drunkard's family.

This view changed during the economic crises of 1847 and 1853–5. Searching to explain the brutal social consequences of both crises, many observers pointed to the widespread misuse of the wage: if workers would drink less, their pay would suffice for acquiring the necessities of life. Thus, it was certainly not poverty that led workers to drink, but the drinking that led to poverty. This view associated alcohol with the (industrial and urban) working class as a whole. The 'bad' worker (as opposed to the 'good', non-drinking worker) was stereotyped as a drunkard (*le buveur*), and in former years the number of 'bad' workers had greatly increased. Gin drinking was put within the context of class struggle: it branded the *whole* of the working class as potential drinkers.

Once the crisis of 1855 was over, this radical perception softened: the totality of the workers were no longer perceived as likely drunkards, although the social dimension of drinking remained, and the whole of the working class was considered as vulnerable. A well-documented text submitted to Parliament in 1868 by the minister of Finance, Frère-Orban, synthesised the contemporaries' perception, as well as the state's position on public drunkenness.[7] The minister related heavy drinking to disease, poverty, crime and mortality, thus emphasising the public dimension of drinking. He referred to the general agreement among the *autorités médicales*, quoting that 'l'alcool est un poison qui pénètre le sang et les os'. Yet, medical objections to alcohol were limited to very general observations of the kind 'l'usage détermine parfois la mort'. However, he stressed the restorative qualities of gin, and demonstrated that gin consumption had decreased in past years. He asked that the problem should not be exaggerated. His hidden agenda was that, being a firm believer in economic liberalism, he discarded the idea of state interference. He concluded that the *abuse* of gin ought to be stopped, but that nothing could be done for the moment, except to instruct and moralise.

In the 1870s, this moralist discourse on drunkenness prevailed: drunkards were pictured as weak characters causing great public disorder and degrading themselves, their family and the community. However, the discourse lacked a well-defined, consistent logic and goal, and, hence, it remained without practical impact. The only measure in Belgium consisted of the increase of the consumption tax, which was applied only hesitatingly.[8] This contrasted strongly with some surrounding countries where more or less radical measures were then being introduced.

FROM IVROGNERIE TO ALCOOLISME, 1878–85: PHYSICIANS ON THE ASSAULT

Around 1800 the confidence in what medicine might achieve was immense. However, in the subsequent decades some shocks beset this: doctors quarrelled constantly among themselves, 'illegal' medicine challenged their skills, they found themselves dependent on a limited clientèle, their income was threatened, and, particularly, doctors did not stand a chance against the cholera epidemic of 1832 and 1849. An identity crisis was imminent.[9] Around 1850, Belgian doctors perceived their situation as quite unfavourable. They tried to overcome this. The *Académie royale de médecine* was created (1841), journals were launched (eg *Le Scalpel*, 1848), and higher medical education was re-organised (1849). Preventive medicine played a prominent role in these initiatives. This implied a large involvement by doctors in public matters such as housing, hygiene, nutrition, sexuality or education. Predominant was the concern with alcoholic beverages. Naturally, doctors had for long shown interest in drunkenness but much more than economists or jurists, they had considered it on the individual's level. Around 1880, they wished to lay claim to a public problem that awaited, according to them, a professional and specialised approach.

In 1878, Dr Barella, a member of the *Académie royale de médecine*, published *De l'abus des spiritueux. Maladie des buveurs*. This book may be seen as a transition between 'old' and 'new' attitudes towards alcohol drinking. 'Old' was the indulgence towards moderate alcohol drinking, the characterisation of the problem as an *abuse*, the proposing of modest measures, and the accusation of the urban working class. What was new was Barella's broad attention to clinical consequences of gin abuse, its chemical analysis, the *scientific* identification of drunkenness, and the outspoken wish to introduce the medical voice in the public debate on drinking, invoking emphatically the clinical authority.

This 'outing' had practical implications. Barella became the secretary of the Catholic-inspired *Association belge contre l'abus des boissons alcooliques*, set up in 1879. He was not the only physician: out of 174 members 79 were doctors. The *Association*'s motto, *Uti, sed non abuti* (use, but don't abuse), reflected the idea that total abstinence was considered impossible in Belgium, and that too-radical views would put people off. In 1880 the society sent a petition to Parliament, referring to Frère-Orban's 1868 position and affirming that since then the question has matured. Yet, nothing more than an inquiry into alcohol drinking was asked for.[10] Some doctors wished to take a more radical stance, though. On the occasion of the anti-alcohol congress held in Brussels in 1880, Dr Carpentier produced startling statistics on the rate of intoxication of the Brussels working class. This caused a genuine shock, and it incited participants to demand severe measures such as the right to lock up the alcoholic whose condition is recognised as a medical problem.[11]

A crucial initiative of the medical world to put itself into the heart of the anti-alcohol movement was made in 1881 when the *Académie de médecine* organised a contest about the question 'What are the effects of alcoholism on material and physical matters of the individual, as well as on his offspring?'. This question implied that *alcoholism* (note the use of this new, clinical word) was perceived as 'une véritable maladie organique', and thus as the pre-eminent field of medicine. The medical world wished to designate the drunkard not as a morally reprehensible person but primarily as an *ill* person.[12] The contest's winner was Dr Lentz, director of the *Asile des aliénés* at Tournai. He stressed that a little intake of alcohol is not only harmless but necessary; it is the abuse that causes *alcoholism*, disorder, decay and misery. Lentz described at length the clinical implications of drunkenness, and in his condemnation of overconsumption he was quite frank when he wrote 'C'est ainsi que l'alcool tue le corps'.[13] The *Académie de médecine* was delighted with the social dimension of Lentz's work, thus applauding the combination of a clinical with a more general approach.

This turning of the *Académie* towards the identification of *alcoholism* as a medical problem seems to have invigorated the anti-alcohol movement. New journals were launched (1884, *Le Mouvement Hygiénique*, directed by physicians and devoting much attention to gin drinking), many books were published, the *Ligue patriotique contre l'alcoolisme* was established (1884), and an international meeting was organised (1885). The *Ligue* succeeded to the *Association*, doubling its membership.[14] The *Ligue* was somewhat more radical though it did not favour prohibition. It believed strongly in propaganda to stop the *fléau* of gin.

This renewed attention cannot be understood without a reference to statistics of gin consumption. These figures were criticised, but it is not the aim, here, to evaluate them. It should only be stressed that official statistics were widely used in the anti-alcohol discourse and, especially, that these statistics registered a level in the 1880s that lay some 25 per cent higher than in the 1860s (see Appendix). Together with the economic crisis, this caused the greatest distress as well as new enthusiasm in the anti-alcohol camp.

On the occasion of the 1885 world exhibition in Antwerp an international meeting was organised. It wished to inform the Belgians about anti-alcoholic measures in the surrounding countries. All 560 participants agreed on the nuisance of alcohol abuse, but they could not compromise on one set of measures. There were two tendencies. One preferred total abstinence, the other was in favour of moderation. The meeting concluded that much time was needed before even a modest goal could be reached.[15] The harrowing picture of drunkards presented by the doctors at the congress could not arouse unity. Doctors themselves were divided according to the aforementioned tendencies. Despite their discord, however, physicians had succeeded within a few years in appointing themselves as the specialists on alcohol drinking, adding surplus-value to the gamut of anti-alcohol arguments, and 'rectifying' other points of view.

THE DOCTORS TEMPORARILY FALLING ASTERN, 1886 AND 1887

In March 1886 Belgium witnessed workers' demonstrations, strikes, meetings and riots. The establishment was profoundly upset, and it brutally repressed the movement. Inspired by Leplaysian ideas on social reform, the government set up an investigation committee into the living conditions of the working class. The aim was to introduce some urgent measures. A comprehensive questionnaire, interviews, meetings and reports were supposed to help in shaping a new social policy. The committee had 37 members among whom were lawyers, entrepreneurs, clergymen and professors but, surprisingly, no doctors.[16]

Alcohol abuse held a prominent position in the committee's activity. The questionnaire contained questions on alcohol drinking, and among the many diverse respondents there were only three doctors. The latter emphasised the clinical consequences of drinking, but two of them replied rather phlegmatically. Dr Kuborn, for example, started off with a brief narration on gin but went on about the nuisance of tobacco![17] Neither in quantity nor quality, could the medical *authority* equate the opinion of clergymen, local politicians or civil servants. These hardly picked up elements of the medical discourse. Tolerance vis-à-vis moderate gin drinking came into view, and many respondents observed that alcoholism was not as widespread as one might expect.[18] The final *Rapport sur la question de l'intempérance* (note the use of the word 'intempérance', and not 'alcoolisme') was written by a professor of law who immediately started off by considering the possible remedies without identifying the 'gravité du mal'.[19] This report proposed many repressive measures which were hardly discussed at the committee's meeting.[20] Cauderlier, one of its 37 members, a *publiciste* and the secretary of the *Ligue patriotique contre l'alcoolisme*, was absent when the report was debated: *specialists* were either 'eliminated' or showed only feeble interest. The medical profession held an insignificant position in the committee's work which suggests that in the mid-1880s physicians were not *incontournable*.

The *Mouvement Hygiénique* reported on the committee's activity. It was pleased with the fact that workers themselves had demanded measures but it was less satisfied with the propositions that, up to the journal, indicated that the committee undervalued the importance of the matter.[21] Surely, the repression of public drunkenness or the control of the pubs' opening hours were steps in the right direction but many more resolute measures were needed, such as gigantic moralising campaigns or the opening of special asylums.

The rather moderate view on drinking of the *Commission du Travail* may be retraced in the *Loi concernant l'ivresse publique* of August 1887. Indeed, the only measure the government proposed was the punishment of drunkenness that caused disorder, scandal or danger. Drunkenness in itself was not penalised. The inferior role that the medical discourse had played during the activities of the *Commission du Travail*, endured in the Parliamentary debates. Only two representatives referred to the 'maîtres distingués de l'art médical', but de Mérode who presented the law in Parliament, made fun of the *specialists*, arguing that imprisonment of the *alcoolisés* would lead to the incarceration of a lot of their honourable colleagues.[22] The law passed with 83 against 10 votes and 10 abstentions in Chambers, and with 43 votes and 3 abstentions in Senate. In 1889, a law was voted on the *droit de licence*: a sum of money had to be paid before starting a pub, in order to restrict the number of tiny businesses.

The 1887 law prompted some doctors to radicalise. In *Le Mouvement Hygiénique*, Dr Belval fiercely attacked the 'esprits superficiels' regarding moderate drinking as harmless: 'who can say if this jolly drunkard of today will not be a wretched murderer tomorrow?'. Moderation would not suffice, total abstinence was the sole solution. However, this could not be achieved by a single law but by a cascade of measures of which the imprisonment was the final stage.[23] In a subsequent issue of the *Mouvement Hygiénique*, Dr Moeller pleaded for the immediate introduction of two measures, the interdiction for *alcoolisés* to administer financial matters, and the detention of *dangerous* drunkards.[24]

THE OVERPOWERING MEDICALISATION, 1895-1914

The reaction by some doctors to the 1887 legislation coincided with the publication of many books and brochures, both by doctors and non-doctors. Physicians stressed their perception of drunkenness as a disease, picturing with great imagination the physical consequences of heavy drinking. Other authors put the emphasis on vulnerable groups such as women or children, regularly referring to medical findings.[25] Also, the membership of the *Ligue patriotique contre l'alcoolisme* increased from 700 in 1888 to nearly 2,000 in 1895, while new organisations were started up all over the country.

Physicians played a prominent role in these new societies and in the anti-alcohol movement in general. They had become very visible, choosing clear, radicalised positions. A consequence of this was their manifest presence in the official *Commission d'études relatives à la question de l'alcoolisme*, set up in April 1895 and chaired by the Catholic Senator Lejeune. Out of fifteen members, seven were doctors. The government legitimated this committee by the belief that measures up to then had been inadequate, as demonstrated by the increase of official consumption statistics between 1890 and 1894 (see Appendix), as well as of statistics on crime, health and poverty. It wished to apply new regulations. This was to admit that the 1887 legislation had failed. Together it was conceded that doctors were necessary to provide expert advice.

The medical profession dominated the committee, not least by the production of well-documented, specialised reports. The final report contained two sections, the first primarily devoted to clinical matters related to alcohol drinking, the second dealing with new, radical measures. The first section aimed at elucidating some points that were still more or less controversial, and at rectifying some errors raised in certain publications. Moreover, this part of the report warned against a too weak an attitude vis-à-vis moderate gin drinking. Temperate, daily drinking was seen as more dangerous than acute drunkenness: it was a creeping poison.[26] It was argued that science was not (yet) in a position to provide definite answers, although a growing number of researchers maintained that alcohol in any quantity was a nuisance.[27] Did one sip not suffice to stumble into the arms of King Alcohol? With this view, doctors took up an entirely new and indeed radical position.

The committee proposed a doubling of the *accijns*, an augmentation of the tax on pubs, intense propaganda especially in schools, financial support of temperance societies, and the incarceration of dangerous drunkards. Influenced by these propositions, the *accijns* was increased in 1896, while Lejeune added the category of *alcoolisés* to the list of the *aliénés*, in his renewed presentation to Parliament of a law on special asylums.[28]

The vigour of the medical profession unfolded in 1898 when the *Société médicale belge de tempérance* was set up (note: a moderation movement). The aim of this society was to underpin scientifically the medical view with regard to alcohol drinking, as well as to propagate this. The society's journal simply stated that the doctors were in the best position to block the heavy drinking, and that they had a duty to inform the general public: 'Without the help of medicine nothing can be seriously tried against the alcohol deluge'.[29] Their systematic study of human life authorised them not just to give advice but also to guide, judge and condemn: doctors perceived themselves as the absolute leaders of the anti-alcohol movement. This approach was successful: the society started with 46 members, it doubled its membership within a year, and had 170 members in 1902. At the start, its members were not expected to be teetotallers, but in 1910 an abstinence section was set up within the society.

A central component in the *Bulletin*'s discourse was the shaping of a *common sense* with regard to drinking. Phrases such as 'Is it necessary to go into this further?', 'It is evident that . . .' or 'It is enough for us to . . .' suggested a commonly shared opinion. This, however, contributed primarily to the construction of a specialised, patronising medical view on alcohol drinking. The authoritarian reference to *incontestable facts* ('Une poignée de faits', 1898), the *scientificity* of the articles ('De l'action physiologique de l'alcool', 1899), the reference to statistics ('La consommation réelle de l'alcool', 1911) and the use of expressive graphs ('L'alcool et la mortalité', 1898) helped to forge and spread the doctors' view on alcohol drinking.

In attempting to definitely get hold of the anti-alcohol movement, the *Société* decided to concentrate on one strategic goal, ie the prohibition of absinthe. In December 1901 the *Bulletin* published no fewer than three articles on absinthe, and, in January 1903, Dr Bienfait – the secretary of the society – wrote 'L'absinthe et la prohibition' that may serve as a genuine example of an invention of a problem! Absinthe was hardly drunk in Belgium, something the doctor was well aware of, but he sensed great danger coming from France: 'The people have not yet touched it [. . .] but we must stop this invading flood before it drowns us' (424). It was *commonly known*, he argued, that absinthe was a far more toxic liquor than gin, leading to extreme drunkenness, instant intellectual and physical degradation, and all kinds of horrible diseases; thus, the evil should be nipped in the bud. This construct coincided with the presentation of a law to prohibit the production, the transport and the selling of absinthe in Belgium.

The *Société* concentrated fully on the absinthe question. Several articles were published on the matter in the course of 1903 and 1904. However, the largest public impact related to the organisation of a referendum among the medical profession on the desirability of prohibiting absinthe. No fewer than 2,300 signed the petition, of whom the great majority were doctors, the remaining being pharmacists. This represents one half of all medical doctors in Belgium, assuming that 2,000 doctors signed.[30]

The *Société*'s propaganda and referendum had a large impact. During the debate in Chambers, Carton de Wiart, who presented the law, referred to articles by Dr Bienfait, Dr de Vaucleroy and other physicians. Particularly, he emphasised the success of the referendum. In short, 'les autorités les plus sérieuses' were acclaimed in Parliament, which contrasted highly with the 1887 discussion. Carton de Wiart was very persuasive, or – more likely – no representative had to be convinced of the danger of absinthe. Indeed, no one wished to discuss the drastic law that was passed unanimously (except three nays and two abstentions).[31] The *Société* was satisfied with the result, stressing its own role in the continuing propaganda.[32] After so many years, this was seen as a sign that the mentality had finally changed. However, a few months later the extent of the law was restricted, and some liquors with particular flavours were authorised. Of course, the *Société* deplored this. For Dr Bienfait, this meant an incentive to intensify the association's efforts.

The *Société médicale belge de tempérance* continued to exert its (scientific) propaganda up to 1914. A medical library was set up, congresses were organised, and brochures published. In 1909 a *Fédération internationale des médecins abstinents* was launched, while in 1910 the *Société* organised a second petition (containing a general condemnation of alcohol drinking), signed by 35 per cent of all Belgian physicians. The society, as well as other temperance organisations, obtained important governmental funds.[33]

The persisting actions of the anti-alcohol movement from the early 1880s onwards persuaded the government to increase the consumption tax on alcohol. Increases were systematically asked for, but it was commonly accepted that only severe rises would prove effective.[34] Up to 1880, tax increases were mainly motivated by budgetary needs. From the 1880s on, however, explicit reference was made to the numerous inconveniences brought about by gin abuse.[35] The general tax revision of 1896 installed a new system, based on the presumed production capacity. In April, a tax of 64 francs per hectolitre was proposed, but in July of the same year this was raised to 100 francs 'dans le cadre de la lutte contre l'alcoolisme'. In the motivation, budgetary needs had shifted to the background. The 1903 tax increase (to 150 francs per hectolitre) was motivated only in saying that raising the price of alcohol is the best means of limiting the ravages of alcoholism.

According to the officially registered statistics (see Appendix), these subsequent tax increases forced the alcohol consumption to diminish. This was particularly so with the 1903 tax rise: there was a reduction from about 9 litres per head and per year in 1900–02 to 5.5 litres in 1903–05. The government showed great satisfaction with this result. At first hesitatingly, but after a special inquiry into drinking habits in 1904, very self-confidently, it proclaimed the 'véritable triomphe remporté sur l'alcoolisme', thus announcing the end of the battle against alcoholism: 'le progrès est réel et définitivement acquis'![36] Hence, no further tax increases were applied. Only in 1913 was the consumption tax increased by another 30 per cent. However, this was solely motivated by the need to augment state income to pay for military expenditure; no mention whatsoever was made of alcoholism.[37]

The declining alcohol consumption and the official proclamation of the 'end of the battle' did not stop the ardour of the anti-alcohol movement. In the 1900s, per capita consumption data were increasingly seen as meaningless, and the focus was directed towards drunkards who could consume up to 90 litres of gin per year.[38] This view on statistics implied that efforts of the temperance movement should persist. A meek defeat of the *Enemy* would not suffice.

Vandervelde's severe 1918 and 1919 regulation may come as a surprise in reference to the halving of gin consumption, and to the perception of the alcohol problem by the government after 1903. This radical legislation may be explained by various elements, including the enduring propaganda of the anti-alcohol movement, the intense medicalisation with the benefit for the social status of doctors, the gigantic moralisation with the ensuing social and self-control, and, last but not least, Vandervelde's view in which total abstinence was part of his eugenic project.[39]

CONCLUSION

From about 1880 doctors tried hard to become the leaders of the anti-alcohol movement by picturing the drunkard as an *ill* person. In so doing, they adapted a chief element of *la question sociale* – ie the bourgeois designation of class relations – to their domain, thus adding to their influence and prestige. This medicalisation was welcomed for providing *scientific* evidence on heavy drinking, for it reinforced the moralising and incriminating discourse that had prevailed until then. Yet, the leading circles only hesitatingly accepted these medical allegations. It was the discord between tolerant doctors and doctors in favour of total abstinence that prevented the emergence of authoritative and concerted actions which would have given doctors the very lead in the movement.

Nonetheless, after 1890 the doctors' continuing efforts greatly contributed to the common sense about alcohol drinking, which in turn influenced anti-alcohol measures. The example of the absinthe prohibition shows that the medical profession had obtained an authoritative position by 1900: a construct (the imminent danger of absinthe with its ruinous image – though absinthe was hardly drunk in Belgium), led to regulation (total prohibition by law). *Mutatis mutandis*, a similar condition occurred after World War I: a construct (the imminent danger of massive drinking – though official statistics had registered a impressive fall since 1903, and principally during the war) led to regulation (Vandervelde's restrictive law). Thus, the anti-alcohol movement's discourse had such impact that subsequent measures could be applied not only during the *fléau* years, but also after 1903 and up to 1919, when gin consumption had actually decreased.

APPENDIX: CONSUMPTION OF ALCOHOL (OF 50°), ACCORDING TO TAX DATA, BELGIUM 1835-1913

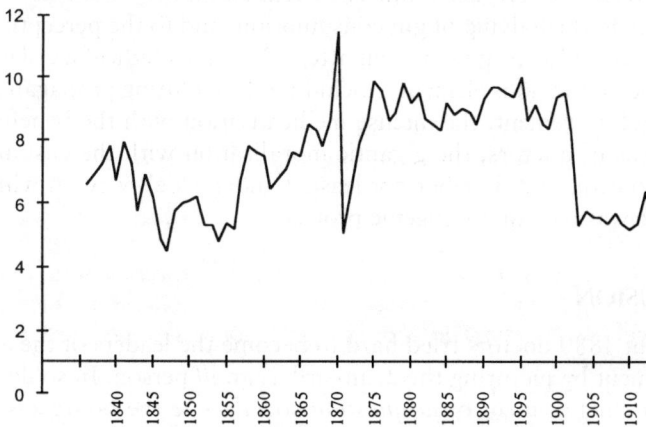

Based on Tableau général du commerce avec les pays étrangers *(Brussels, 1846); see van den Eeckhout & Scholliers (1981) 293–6.*

BIBLIOGRAPHY

L'action de l'état contre l'alcoolisme. Travaux des groupes d'études de la recon-struction nationale, Brussels, 1919.

Barella, Hippolyte. *De l'abus des spiritueux. Maladies des buveurs*, Brussels, 1878.

Bruylants, Dr. *L'influence de la composition des eaux-de-vie et alcools sur l'alcoolisme*, Brussels, 1895.

Bulletin de l'Association belge contre l'abus des boissons alcooliques, Brussels, 1882.

Bulletin de la société médicale belge de tempérance, Brussels, 1898–1914.

van Coillie, E. *Alcool et débauche*, Brussels, 1891.

Commission d'études relatives à la question de l'alcoolisme. Rapports généraux, 1895–7, Brussels, 1897.

Commission du travail, 4 vols, Brussels, 1887–8.

Documents. Chambre des représentants, Brussels, 1868, 1903–5, 1913.

Ducpétiaux, Edouard. *De l'intempérance et de l'ivrognerie dans la classe ouvrière*, Brussels, 1843.

van den Eeckhout, Patricia & Scholliers, Peter. De hoofdelijke voedselconsumptie in België, 1831-1939, *Tijdschrift voor Sociale Geschiedenis*, 9 (1983), 273–301.

Faure, Olivier. *Histoire sociale de la médecine XVIIIe–XIXe siècles*, Paris, 1994.

Gubin, Eliane. Les enquêtes sur le travail en Belgique et au Canada à la fin du 19e siècle. In Kurgan-van Hentenryck, Ginette ed, *La question sociale en Belgique et au Canada*, Brussels, 1988, 93–121.

van de Kerchove, Michel. L'organisation d'asiles spéciaux pour aliénés criminels et aliénés dangereux. In Tulkens, Françoise ed, *Généalogie de la défense sociale en Belgique 1880–1914*, Brussels 1988, 113–40.

Lockkamper, Nancy. 'Een situatieschets van de antialcoholische beweging in het laatste kwart van de 19e eeuw en het begin van de 20e eeuw', thesis, Brussels, 1994.

Mareska, J and Heyman, J. *Enquête sur le travail et la condition physique et morale des ouvriers employés dans les manufactures de coton, à Gand*, Ghent, 1845.

Moeller, Dr. Les alcoolisés en Belgique, *Mouvement Hygiénique*, August (1887), 285–97.

Moeller, Dr. *L'alcoolisme et ses remèdes*, Brussels, 1895.

Mommens, Thierry. *De Belgische voedingsnijverheid tijdens de 19e eeuw*, Leuven, 1993.

Le Mouvement Hygiénique Revue d'hygiène publique et privée, Brussels (1884–1914).

Parent, M. *Le rôle de la femme dans la lutte contre l'alcoolisme*, Brussels, 1890.

Petithan, Dr. *Répression de l'alcoolisme. Interdiction, collocation*, Liège, 1881.

Pirard, Joseph. *Le pouvoir central belge et ses comptes économiques, 1830–1913*, Brussels, 1985.

de Raes, Wouter. Eugenetika in de Belgische medische wereld tijdens het interbellum, *Revue belge d'Histoire Contemporaine*, 20 (1989), 399–464.

van Schoonenberghe, Eric. *Jenever in de Lage Landen*, Bruges, 1996.

Statistique comparative des octrois communaux de Belgique pendant les années 1828, 1829; 1835 et 1836, Brussels, 1839.

de Vaucleroy, Dr. *L'hérédité alcoolique*, Brussels, 1892.

Velle, Karel. *De nieuwe biechtvaders. De sociale geschiedenis van de arts in België*, Leuven, 1991.

NOTES

1 Pasinomie, 1919, 396, 'Exposé des motifs, Loi sur le régime de l'alcool'.
2 Annales Chambres, 1919, 1342–9, 1441–9, 1496. The law passed with 66 votes in favour, 51 against, and 4 abstentions.
3 Van Schoonenberghe, 1996, 94, 115–16.
4 Statistique comparative, 170. These figures are confirmed by Mommens 1993, table 6.
5 Ducpétiaux, 1843.
6 Mareska and Heyman, 1845, 109, 241.
7 *De l'abus des boissons enivrantes. Renseignements déposés par M le ministre des Finances*. Documents Chambre, 1868 no 136, 495–560.
8 Pirard, 1985, 997–1003. Tax augmented from 1 frs in 1842 to 5 frs in 1877 per production capacity of 100 hectolitres, but although this was a tangible increase, it was generally accepted that tax measures only slightly infuenced gin consumption.
9 Faure, 1994, chapters 5 to 8, and especially 98–106. A sign of the problems may be seen in the decline and stagnation of the ratio of doctors in Belgium from 1840 to 1880; Velle, 1991, 343.
10 *Bulletin de l'Association*, 1882, 64.
11 Petithan, 1881, 12. This demand had no consequence.
12 For this evaluation of the contest's impact, see Moeller, 1887, 287, who classified this contest as 'un fait qui exerça une grande influence sur l'opinion publique'.

13 *Mouvement Hygiénique*, 1885, 521–536.
14 Lockkamper, 1994, 65–7, 193. The number of members increased from 300 in 1883, to 700 in 1884.
15 *Mouvement Hygiénique*, 1885, 502–6.
16 Surprisingly, indeed, since doctors had played a prominent role in the inquiries of 1843, and 1869–70; see Gubin, 1988, 96.
17 Commission, 1887, I, 1092.
18 eg ibid, 1089.
19 Commission, 1887, III, 191–207.
20 Commission, 1888, IV, 99–107. These measures included a lowering of the beer tax, the limitation of the number of pubs, the fixing of the closing hour, the punishment of public drunkenness, and the promotion of temperance societies.
21 *Mouvement Hygiénique*, 1887, 289.
22 *Annales Sénat*, 1887, 518; *Annales Chambre*, 1887, 1645.
23 *Mouvement Hygiénique*, 1887, 246–51.
24 *Mouvement Hygiénique*, 1887, 293. Moeller mentioned that minister Beernaert met dr Petithan, the promoter of the collocation, who 'revint à la charge avec une nouvelle ardeur'.
25 eg Parent, 1890; van Coillie, 1891; de Vaucleroy, 1892.
26 Moeller, 1895, 4–5.
27 *Commission d'études*, 1897, 17–20.
28 van de Kerchove, 1988, 121. The law did not pass; the *loi de défense sociale* with regard to 'habitual delinquents' passed in 1930.
29 *Bulletin de la société*; 1898, 2.
30 *Bulletin de la société*, 1903, 433; 1905, 610.
31 *Documents Chambre*, 1905, 365–7; *Annales Chambre*, 1905, 1215. The vote in Senate was less clear : 50 yes, against 21 no and 2 abstentions.
32 *Bulletin de la société*, 1905, 657.
33 Lockkamper, 1994, 172–4, 203. In 1890 one society received 500 francs, in 1910, 15 societies obtained 68,450 francs.
34 eg the final report of the *Commission du travail*, III, 1887, 193, and the final recommendations of the *Commission d'études*, 1897, 52, that stressed that 'le prix du petit verre au détail soit au moins doublé' to show results.
35 Pirard, 1985, 1003.
36 'Budget des recettes et des dépenses. Exposé général', *Documents Chambre*, 1905, no 4, 25; *Documents Chambre*, 1906, no 4, 18.
37 Pasinomie, 1913, 531.
38 *Action de l'état*, 1919, 2.
39 De Raes, 1989, 441–3, in 1922 Vandervelde was elected honorary chairman of the Société belge d'Eugénique.

14   Food, fibres, and health

Jakob Tanner

Dietary fibres are a rather inconspicuous phenomenon whose historical analysis, however, reveals large-scale problems; for the discussion of how significant these indigestible elements of our diet is, and was – implicitly or explicitly – closely associated with the idea of physical health and social order.[1] Therefore, I would like to add some introductory remarks on the history of these metaphorical operations and symbolic analogies between food, body, and society, and explain the theoretical assumptions on which my paper is based.

THE SEMIOTICS OF FOOD

Health is an individual condition – and simultaneously a key term which helped crystallize the collective conception modern society acquired of itself in the course of the nineteenth century. Since the 1850s the 'protection of public health' had become the core of an entire agenda of 'biopolitical' measures,[2] with the help of which the social élites and middle-class strata of society strove to achieve a double objective: on the one hand, 'normal people' were to be defended against pathological menace and 'dangerous elements'; on the other, behavioural patterns and conditions of life were to be improved – above all, those sections of the population which were perceived as both endangered due to their underprivileged position and, at the same time, dangerous. Beside a broad range of hygienic reform measures, this included proposals on how to 'rationalize' the diet of the 'working classes'.[3]

The key slogan of a 'rational public diet' shows how very much the debates on public diet developed under the spell of different scientific disciplines. Food was endowed with a specific usefulness due to the diet-related knowledge acquired as to the composition of nutrients and an optimum functioning of human physiology. Around the turn of the century, the elaborate classification system of the chemically distinct components of food (carbohydrates, proteins, fats, water, and roughage) developed since the 1840s and empirically tested in laboratories, was enriched by more recently discovered groups of substances (vitamins, trace elements) and could now be linked to thermodynamic models.[4] It is essential to recognize that the newly acquired knowledge of the chemistry of nutrients and that of physiological functions were permanently and mutually dependent. A field of complementary as well as contrasting interpretations came into existence, and links between nutrients and properties conducive to health or causing diseases were established. Far from merely supplying nutrients or calories, foodstuffs now became the very symbols of the productivist order of industrial society and the physiological order of (working) man.[5]

Historical research on dietetics has long focused on an analysis of these semiotic processes and attempted to uncover the various strata of the semantics of edibles. This analysis again and again confirmed the insight that the attempt to put everything on a highly scientific basis, a process which can be detected all through the nineteenth century in the most varied areas of life, not only introduced new scales of evaluation but also affected the prevalent ideas in the society and the behaviour of man. Inverse influences, from everyday awareness to the scientific formation of hypotheses, can be detected as well. This interaction led to an overall dichotomization of thought. Science quite obviously based its findings on a clearly defined confrontation or comparison of right and wrong, mainly, however, on the binary opposites of 'healthy vs ill' or 'normal vs pathological'. A proper life-style implied healthy normality and thus always referred to its opposite and the possibility of its reversal into a social deviation. In this collective, imaginary scenario, pathologies up to collective degeneration represented the very opposite of what nutritional reformers were wont to designate as 'positive, unassailable, and glowing public health'.[6] By becoming the standard of expected behaviour, a scientifically legitimized 'correct diet', scientific research, and normative indoctrination were mutually supportive. Social progress, constituted by the idea that man could be perfected, was increasingly based on social disciplining. And because a 'perfect human being' was one who had internalized the 'correct' standard and adhered to it in a disciplined if voluntary way, these public, pedagogical reform campaigns were increasingly replaced by an 'inner voice', a so-called 'Zwang zum Selbstzwang' [compulsion to constrain oneself] (Norbert Elias).[7] And although the lament of experts about any wrong behaviour, in particular unsuitable dietary habits, did not stop in the twentieth century – it was, in particular in the last two decades, accompanied by new and intensive forms of self-control and a control of one's body in order to ameliorate its fitness, which was equally based on scientific findings.

THE SIGNIFICANCE OF FIBRES: TWO APPROACHES

This way of looking at the respective problems allows the logical linking of food, fibres, and health. Already in the nineteenth century, the industrialization of food was accused of destroying the simple harmony of natural food and replacing it with non-functional artificial foodstuffs. The more industrial societies mastered the centuries-old problems of hunger and poverty by an increase in productivity touching upon all sectors of the economy, the more this criticism increased. The traditional question of 'getting enough' was replaced by the modern problem of 'eating correctly'. The diagnosis that most of us did not nourish ourselves in a correct manner thus has long belonged among the *ceterum censeo* of dietary psychologists and the exponents of preventive medicine. In particular in the post-war period, critics began to focus on an abundance of food: we eat – and this dietary experts continue to tell us – too many calories, too much fat and cholesterol, too much sugar and salt. All the more interesting, therefore, to ask in which areas there is not so much an abundance but a latent (and sometimes even manifest) under-supply. If we restrict this question to nutrition, roughage or dietary fibres seem to have surpassed vitamins as the most important problem of nutritional deficiencies by now. The beginning of this problematic development can easily be dated. In his small standard paper published in 1979 on *Ernährung und Diätetik* [Nutrition and Dietetics], Karl Huth wrote that roughage had 'until a very few years ago' been considered 'a more or less incidental or even unwelcome food component'.[8] For somewhat more than a decade now, there has been a marked upwards trend of this topic.

From a historical perspective, it is interesting to distinguish between two approaches to the question: the first one is based on cultural history and links its 'significance' to categories of perception, patterns of interpretation, and symbolic ascription. The second asks for its 'significance' in a statistical-quantitative sense. According to this distinction, my paper is structured into two sections: the first and somewhat longer one will focus on the change of dietary patterns and their explanation; that is, on the significant semantic shift which turned those fibres once considered superfluous into something valuable. In the second chapter, I shall concentrate on some empirical findings which show how the roughage content of food changed over an extended period of time.

HEAVY INDUSTRIAL WORK AND 'EASILY DIGESTIBLE' FOOD

Modern dietetics developed in the nineteenth century and hardly focused on fibres at all. It considered the intake of food a remedying of its lack and was thus interested in the supply of calories and the three macro-nutrients: carbohydrates, proteins, and fats. As an example, we shall quote a paper on the 'rational feeding of our people, in particular the poor' of 1874. Conforming to the then prevalent opinion the author, Kallnach vicar Friedrich Küchler, wrote:

> The human body is subject to continual inner movement or chemical change, including the degradation of individual parts. The products of this process within the individual parts of the body are then excreted in various ways by the lungs, sweat, urine, etc. The breaks thus created have to be closed again, a matter which is handled by metabolism. The substances this is entrusted to are called food in the broadest sense of the word.[9]

Such a definition cannot properly focus on fibres; as substances which leave the body *per definitionem* in an unused state, they are simply superfluous.

This opinion was shared by the Glarus physician and Federal Inspector of Factories Fridolin Schuler who presented those chemical research methods in his paper *Über die Ernährung der Fabrikbevölkerung und ihre Mängel* [On the Diet of Factory Workers and Its Deficiencies] which, by way of animal experiments, could conceivably have allowed a precise determination of the 'food and drink requirements' of 'people of the most varied professions and life styles'. These 'exact studies' would have, according to the factory inspector, shown up 'a big mistake', 'made in evaluating foodstuffs earlier on'. This mistake he defined as follows: 'You should not calculate the worth of food according to certain chemical components if you wish to determine its nourishing value but by what the organism actually utilizes.' As an example he firstly mentioned black bread:

> If, due to theoretical reasons, hard-to-digest and coarse black bread was recommended, the fact that 30–40 per cent of it would be excreted undigested and that the presumed plus in nutritional value was thus changed into a minus was neglected.[10]

Here, roughage is considered a loss, and Schuler would probably have agreed with the rather negative designation of 'roughage'.

Given the accelerated process of economic growth and the expansion of factory-based industry, additional points of view appeared which helped add minus points to the indigestible parts of our diet. The mechanized, heteronomous work process within closed and more often than not badly ventilated and overheated spaces was considered a matter pertaining to the 'nervous' system. Thus, Fridolin Schuler wrote:

> However, the conditions necessary to assure the good digestion of a factory worker are by far less favourable than those of someone working in the great outdoors. (. . .) All of us (. . .) have already experienced a loss of appetite in sultry weather when the heat opened all our pores and we sweated abundantly. The skin is increasingly supplied with blood, its vessels expand – and the energy of our digestive organs diminishes at the same rate, as does the excretion of digestive liquids.[11]

The stomach was considered the centre of human metabolism and subject to malfunctions; it had to be fed light and easily digested meals. Roughage was exactly the contrary of this and thus a burden which, in the long run, might well ruin the stomach. 'Therefore, factory workers require more easily digestible food than most other workers, the food of farmers is not suitable for them', thus Schuler concluded. The more physically demanding the industrial work, the more the 'needle of the scale is pointing to the (. . .) side of the finer varieties of bread'.[12] With such statements, Factory Inspector Schuler, profiled 'factory workers' as pioneers of a lighter and in some ways 'more modern' dietary style. This should – in the commonly held opinion – triumph over food rich in fibres and carbohydrates when the income

of broad strata of society increases sufficiently. For once, this proved to be
a valid prognosis. In 1979, Karl Huth rather ironically stated: 'The rough-
age-free, so-called astronauts' diet seemed to represent the perfection of a
modern diet.'[13]

Therefore, it is hardly astonishing that leading social-political exponents
such as Schuler considered the application of the principle of industrialized
food production as a solution promising success. And because – such as
with relatively cheap but difficult-to-digest legumes – 'wrapping their nutritional substances in wood fibres (. . .)' impedes 'digestion', and because the
stomach may thus 'only partially use what is present', 'the food industry
(. . .) may substantially increase their nutritional value by a careful grind-
ing of the seeds.'[14] In the same year (1882) and on the basis of such considerations, Fridolin Schuler, along with mill owner Julius Maggi, decided
to launch a soup cube, which was not only considered a culinary panacea
against the prevalent drinking of alcohol but was also thought to eliminate
the bothersome presence of superfluous fibres by the use of modern technology.[15] Given this background, it is hardly astonishing that industrial society
considered fibre-poor meat something of a 'super food'. Meat conformed to
a dietary ideology which constantly feared the danger of a lack of proteins –
and was, moreover, suitable to protect the stomach against strain. Logically
enough, Schuler wrote in another, famous study on 'the dietary habits of
the working classes in Switzerland' in 1884, 'that people got more and more
accustomed to consider the amount of meat consumed as the best scale to
measure nutritional value by', and that it was 'not contested that for people
working within enclosed spaces and under conditions negatively affecting
digestion, meat was by far the best food.'[16]

THE RETURN OF 'NATURAL FOOD' IN THE
TWENTIETH CENTURY

When the term 'vitamins' was coined in 1911, there were already some coun-
ter-movements to the prevalent doctrine; reform-food and raw-food enthusiasts drew attention to invisible micronutrients which were acknowledged
to be infinitely small but indispensable biocatalysators of the digestive processes.[17] By proposing a vitamin-rich vegetable food, dietary reformers simultaneously propagated a type of food which was also increasing the supply of
roughage; this aspect was, however, rather a side effect and not a dominant
part of their awareness of the problem. This showed something which has
once again become important today: the supply of roughage depends less
on which value is accorded to (individual) parts of our food but rather on
which 'dietary models' are able to triumph at a given time. If 'healthy and
natural food' is *in*, the supply with fibres creates no problems. This is the
case whenever carbohydrates are in favour and play an important role in
nutrition. From this point of view, the period between the wars, which was
so intent on vitamins that some spoke of an actual *vitamania*, was rather

ambivalent. Once dietary reformers began to subject meat-rich food to a fundamental criticism, the attempt to judge meat as an indicator of wealth and a symbol of prestige on a scale of social evaluation became shaky. The intensive theoretical valuation of vegetable food was applied to culinary practices in a rather limited way, though.

During World War II, this was to change. After 1939, when supply bottle-necks forced an increased direct consumption of vegetable calories, this engendered a discussion of whether the 'war diet' striven for by a system of graded rationing was not – with some individual exceptions – healthier than normal food consumed in times of peace. There were various – above all younger – dietary experts who considered the improved supply of the population with vitamins and the declining consumption of sugar a bless-ing in disguise. But, as to fibres, whose share also increased along with the equally increasing amount of vegetables in people's food, scepticism still dominated. Here, it soon became clear just how strong the dietary tradition created by the industrialization and scientific approach of the nineteenth century was, which considered fibres to be a digestive problem mainly. The President of the Swiss Committee for War Diet, the Lausanne physiologist Alfred Fleisch, thus assumed in his extensive study on *Dietary Problems in Times of Want* (1947), a rather defensive attitude when he talked of the 'cellulose content of war-time food': 'If food such as our war-time meals contains a daily amount of 500g of potatoes and 400g of vegetables, and bread is made at a comminution rate of 90 per cent, the share of roughage is high and for many digestive tracts too high', he wrote and added, address-ing vegetarians and those eating only raw fruit and vegetables, that at least 'the criticism of some physicians concerning the lack of cellulose in pre-war food has stopped'.[18] A 'sensitive, irritable digestive tract reacts' – thus Fleisch quoted his colleague M Demole – 'with increased peristalsis and spasms to a high cellulose content.'[19] Alfred Fleisch, however, questioned the diagnosis that the increasing consumption of fibres was the direct cause of the increase of stomach and digestive-tract ailments. The fact that diges-tive problems and fermentative dyspepsia did not occur all that frequently in spite of the substantial increase in fibre content, he thought to be the result of a gradual adaptation of food consumption and a 'gradual habitua-tion' over a period of two to three years – which conforms to today's knowl-edge.[20]

All in all, Alfred Fleisch positively reacted to the development that had begun in 1939. Among other things, as President of the most important sci-entific committee in his field, he stressed the advantages and at the same time the unavoidability of the approach chosen. 'Swiss war-time food was frequently criticized for its high content of roughage – however also praised by others. However, it was not the special ideas of EKKE members which led to this high content of roughage but simply a necessity of war-time econ-omy.' Fleisch thereupon reminded the opponents of a food rich in roughage of 'some physiological facts' based on experiments executed on rabbits.[21]

The author again quotes E Demole to support his opinion. Demole determined on the basis of experiments with animal fodder 'that a certain proportion of indigestible ballast is absolutely necessary; for along with certain purified, totally assimilatable food mixtures, a conveying medium has to be added, for otherwise animals would soon die of autointoxication.'[22]

THE PROSPERITY OF LEAN BODIES SINCE THE 1960s

In 1950, when the so-called 'Korea boom' characterized the transitional phase leading to the long post-war period of prosperity, most Swiss households still had to scrimp and save. But once the 'American way of life' was assimilated in a typically Helvetian manner, a new image of the body became relevant for people's behaviour, characterized by sovereign slimness, glowing health, and a modern life-style. The economic upwards trend thus promoted 'high-energy' food: for the daily confrontation with the increasing demands of a high-performance society, only the very best seemed to be good enough. This implied a replacement of substances with low energy density by high-grade animal proteins and fats.

In particular the image of the till then most important provider of fibres, carbohydrates, was rather drastically tarnished: for two decades they were associated with being 'obese' and 'weak' – at a time in which everyone was continually able to afford something more, they recalled the long times of poverty and cut-backs. Since the end of the 1960s, physicians and dietary researchers began propagating breadless and reduced-carbohydrate food. Austrian physician Wolfgang Lutz, for example published his book *Life Without Bread* in 1967, depicting carbohydrates as villains who caused endless metabolic derailings and were responsible for the most important diseases of modern civilization such as obesity, diabetes, and arteriosclerosis.[23] At the end of the 1960s, Erna Carise followed in his steps with her book *Hurra – die Punktdiät ist da!* [Hurra – Here's the Point-by-Point Diet], which apostrophized carbohydrates as the 'arch enemy of gluttons'.[24] A reliable calculation of carbohydrate-based calories seemed to promise the key to success in life. The American physician Robert C Atkins went even further in his book *A Diet Revolution* published at the beginning of the 1970s and called carbohydrates 'pure poison' which played a 'deadly role' in the body.[25] To be just, we have to add that this rhetoric campaign against carbohydrates attacked a pattern of food consumption within which sugar and therefore 'empty energy providers' became more and more dominant. All in all, it seems logical that this combination of a cult of leanness, a quality-conscious approach and the modern 'steak religion' endangered the supply of the body with fibres.

In order to actually turn into a 'problem', people had to be made aware of this process, however, and it had to be interpreted. The cognitive categories to do so were provided by the science of dietetics, which developed in the same period a new biochemical-molecular understanding of the human metabolism. Even in spacecraft research, where only the internal environment of the space capsules and the flatus-producing effects of individual foodstuffs was studied, fibres now seemed to solve the problem in specific situations: 'It seems that the answer to excessive gas output is a two-day diet of water. If that does not appeal, a high-fibre diet makes it odourless.'[26]

Far beyond such special therapies, the definitely vital significance of fibres became clear.[27] And as always when experts diagnose new problems, the food industry started praising new solutions semantically linked with success. Thus, just as revitaminization became a profitable business in all industrial nations in the last half of the century, the enriching of snacks with roughage promises to become equally as profitable for some decades. The actual rehabilitation of fibres, however, goes far beyond such matters. Without exaggerating, we may say that a new concept of life was taking shape. This philosophy integrated old postulates of dietary reform into a Californian dream of life which abandoned the blue-eyed retrospect that former apostles of natural healing insisted on, and now presented itself as the *non plus ultra* of an active and modern way of life. Since the early 1980s, actress Jane Fonda became as an attractive icon of this attitude when she put her *Workout Studios* at the service of a relentless striving for physical fitness. The slogan of her enterprise, 'discipline is liberation', tries to provide the utilitarian behavioural model of the consumer society with new strategies 'to take control of one's own body'. The proposed 'high-fiber, complex-carbohydrate, low animal-protein, low-fat diet' characterized a new trend. In his study *Never Satisfied* (the source of this information), Hillel Schwartz emphasized that this 'new-found admiration for fiber (is) not just bran but moral fiber, resilience, resolve'.[28] These 'fibre' values are concomitant with 'structure', 'character trait', 'fitness' and represent a new approach to life. The term has jettisoned its historical ballast and become a metonym for a person acting according to the maxim of 'disciplined liberation'. This is good news not only for the 'roughage snack' available at delis and kiosks today but also for the breakfast industry which fills entire shelves in modern food stores with its many variants of breakfast cereals. These food companies advertise with the help of people such as Jane Fonda, and have discovered a new munition in fibres – for example in fighting the Mediterranean type of breakfast which consists of so little that any successful business would have to be conducted at an espresso bar.[29]

FROM AN ABUNDANCE OF ROUGHAGE TO A POVERTY OF FIBRES: THE CASE OF SWITZERLAND

In the following sections largely based on quantitative data, I shall confront the development just described with empirical findings of the supply of the Swiss population with food fibres. The transition to an industrial society brought – based on a roughage-rich food with a relatively low energy density such as had been prevalent in the centuries prior to this due to the vagaries of a chronic lack of food – a secular if not entirely linear shift of consumer preferences towards animal calories. This slow progress of animals in the food on offer was once again interrupted by World Wars I and II. As shown, war-time food was rich in roughage. In the decades of prosperity following 1950, there was a definitive renunciation of the economy of want of the 1940s. Since the 1960s, increasing real income and new body styles tended towards fewer carbohydrates and more animal nutrients. The downwards trend in roughage already tangible from the 1950s continued. Demand and the food on offer went in the same direction: the now accelerating industrialization of food resulted in an increasing share of foodstuffs being processed and converted by chemical, mechanical, and technical processes. As a rule, prefabricated 'convenience food' has no longer the same composition as the natural products it is based on, with dietary fibres once again losing out.

THE DOWNWARDS TREND OF THE POST-WAR PERIOD

Such trend statements are based on quantitative analyses of diet polls taken at different times are put into relation. According to the Second and Third Swiss Report on Nutrition, dietary-fibre consumption between 1956/57 and 1980 decreased from 27g to 22.4g (per day and person). For 1985–7, an average consumption of 20.3g was calculated.[30] This equals a decrease by a quarter over a 30-year period. However, the largest decrease took place in the period before 1956/57. Between 1943 and 1945, when food was distributed according to a graded rationing key, the respective 500g potatoes and 400g vegetables plus somewhat more than 200g bread per person per day amounted to about 50g in roughage.[31] There were added – I base my findings on the daily food rations on Ration Card A for the period mentioned – between 14.6g and 35.1g of cereals, 8.1g and 16.5g of pasta, about 10g of legumes, and so on. It is hardly astonishing that this overabundant supply of indigestibles we already mentioned engendered a discussion of stomach and digestive-tract ailments. Given the then existing level, a reduction of average dietary fibre consumption by about two thirds took place within a period of 40 years. How disparately this situation developed in spite of levelling tendencies even in post-war times, is shown by a study Fritz Verzár and Daniela Gsell published in 1962 under the title of *Ernährung und Gesundheitszustand der Bergbevölkerung der Schweiz* [The Nutrition and Health of the Swiss Mountain Population]. An approximate calculation showed that the contents of dietary fibre of the food in these mountain regions at the end of the 1950s was substantially higher than in the urban, industrial agglomerations of Central Switzerland. For the Lugnez (Grisons: 6 villages) and the Muggio Valley (Ticino: 6 communities), areas that were largely self-sufficient, values reached an identical 35g.[32] This was 30 per cent above the mean values for Switzerland at the time.

EMPIRICAL EVIDENCE FOR THE PERIOD BEFORE 1914

If we once again consider the time between World Wars I and II, we can see that the amount of roughage actually consumed was substantially below the peak values of the correspnding war years. Due to the increased consumption of complex carbohydrates, it was however also substantially higher than since the 1960s. An evaluation for the development before to World War I is based on the results of dietary studies executed at the time with a sample of wage-earners, all of them men. For 1914, there are two publications which can be evaluated: studies by Alfred Gigon and Moischa Linetzky on the so-called 'freely selected workers' food'.[33] Gigon, one of the important dietary physiologists of Switzerland, for the first time directly analysed 'the ready-to-serve meals selected by experimental subjects'. A table provided the amounts eaten by the eight workers and employees included in the study (building locksmith, boilermakers, gardeners, tram conductors, postmen, ribbon dyers, dyers, office secretaries) divided into 27 foodstuffs. The four with the highest roughage content – bread, potatoes, vegetables, and fruit – showed a combined roughage content of 38g; the overall amount was slightly higher than 40g.[34] Even considering food which was already strongly commercialized though freely 'chosen', this is double today's values. The findings calculated on the basis of Gigon's data are supported by (partial) calculations on the basis of Moischa Linetzky's thesis on the composition of ready-to-serve vegetable meals of the freely selected working man's diet.

If we go back even further and consider the situation prevalent in the nineteenth century, findings become more ambiguous and disparate. More recent calculations have shown that the real wages in Switzerland between 1890 and 1914 increased by a third, and that this increase in purchasing power on the one hand allowed for an improved provision of food, and on the other also accelerated the decrease of self-sufficiency. There are, therefore, good reasons to assume that vegetable, carbohydrate-rich foodstuffs played an important dietary role before this increase, that is, before 1890, and that, compared with today, meals were mainly based on vegetable substances. This statement conforms to the fear that the high amount of roughage might burden the stomach of workers, the way I quoted Fridolin Schuler for the beginning 1880s. Looking back at the 1840s, the Nuova Statistica della Svizzera published by Ticino statistician and later Federal Councillor

Stefano Franscini may provide some facts to allow for a rough estimate.[35] Starting with the daily per person consumption of wheat, potatoes, and fruit, these three items alone would account for about 50g of roughage a day. However, part of these foodstuffs probably served as animal fodder, an assumption which is supported by the already then comparatively high level of development of the Swiss livestock and dairy industry. But, for that point in time, all mean values are by far more erroneous than they are today. Regional differences were strongly emphasized, and earlier domestic statistics – for instance the work of Armand Chatelanat submitted in 1873 – also show to what great extent access to animal foodstuffs depended on social classes and privileges.[36] Large parts of the population only rarely had meat on their table, and here the above estimation of 50g of roughage may not be too low.

SUMMARY

To sum up, we may therefore state that the industrialization of the food industry and the modernization of dietary culture was linked to a marked shift in the composition of foodstuffs. From today's point of view, this negatively affected the supply of roughage in the long run. Modern consumer society has eliminated the old problem of want. The danger of a notorious lack of food and, in particular, the lack of proteins which characterized earlier ages and even the nineteenth century, was removed by a secular process of economic growth and a substantial increase of industrial and agrarian labour productivity. The same process, however, created a new and much more subtle lack which was less directly realized. Vitamins and – as a more recent problem – roughage were substances which showed a tendency to be scarce in spite of the increased overall supply with food. This shift also resulted in a change of diseases; there are epidemiological studies which clearly prove that those diseases whose aetiology may be linked to a lack of roughage were comparatively rare until the beginning of the post-war economic growth.[37]

In conclusion, I wish to put the two different analytical perspectives on which my explanations were based in relation to one another. It has become apparent that the term of 'significance' was characterized by certain contradictory movements. To the extent in which dietary fibres becamse scarce due to technical production methods and 'more refined' consumer preferences, their value for the medical prevention and evaluation of dietary behaviour increased – even though with a certain time lag. Today, the lack of dietary fibres has so-to-say conquered the last few fibres of the debate on our food culture. This is a situation which seems to recall the 'cognitive dissonance':[38] we know perfectly well we ought to eat more roughage to assure an optimum diet. Any dietetics with practical objectives is thus confronted with the age-old question of how enlightened discussions on food may be translated into equally as enlightened eating habits. Unfortunately, there never was an easy answer to the wealth of habits, desires, and seductions such as eating and drinking have ever been.

NOTES

1 For the connection of eating and order, cf Wirz, Albert. *Die Moral auf dem Teller, Zürich*, 1993.

2 Foucault, Michel. *Dispositive der Macht*, Berlin, 1978; ibid. *Resumé des cours 1970–1982*, Paris, 1989.

3 Tanner, Jakob. *Fabrikmahlzeit. Ernährungswissenschaft, Industriearbeit und Volksernährung in der Schweiz, 1890–1950*, Zurich, 1999.

4 Rabinbach, Anson. *The Human Motor. Energy, fatigue, and the origins of modernity*, Berkely/Los Angeles, 1992.

5 Sarasin, Philipp and Tanner, Jakob, eds. *Physiologie und industrielle Gesellschaft. Studien zur Verwissenschaftlichung des Körpers im 19. und 20. Jahrhundert*, Frankfurt a M, 1998.

6 Bircher, Ralph. *Hunsa. Das Volk, das keine Krankheit kennt*, Erlenbach-Zürich 1980, 5.

7 Elias, Norbert. *Über den Prozess der Zivilisation. Soziogenetische und psychogenetische Untersuchungen*, Frankfurt a M, 1976.

8 Huth, Karl. *Ernährung und Diätetik*, Heidelberg, 1997, 50. The term 'roughage' includes all not enzymatically digestible and non-reabsorbable food components. Essentially these are: cellulose, hemicellulose, lignin, pectin, mucilage, and gum. Note that these various plant-fibre substances show quite different dietetic and metabolic effects due to their chemical and physical properties; therefore, the term 'roughage' has to be differentiated. Frequently, filling and swelling substances are distinguished. Cf Hüdepohl, Mattias. *Stoffwechsel-Erkrankungen in der Praxis*, Stuttgart, 1987, 39.

9 Küchler, Friedrich. *Die rationelle Ernährung unseres Volkes, insbesondere der Armen. Ein volkswirtschaftlich-sozialer Versuch*, Bern, 1874, 3 f.

10 Schuler, Fridolin. *Über die Ernährung der Fabrikbevölkerung und ihre Mängel*, Zurich, 1882, 6 f.

11 ibid, 11

12 ibid, 43.

13 Huth, 1979, 50.

14 Schuler, 1882, 44.

15 Cf Schuler, Fridolin. *Die Leguminose als Volksnahrung. Gutachten abgegeben im Auftrag der SGG*, Zurich, 1885.

16 Schuler, Fridolin. *Die Ernährungsweise der arbeitenden Klassen in der Schweiz und ihr Einfluss auf die Ausbreitung des Alkoholismus*, Bern, 1884, 21.

17 Wirz, 1993.

18 Fleisch, Alfred. *Ernährungsprobleme in Mangelzeiten. Die schweizerische Kriegsernährung 1939–1946*, Basel, 1947, 358.

19 ibid, 467.

20 ibid, 358.

21 ibid, 359 f.

22 ibid, 467.

23 Lutz, Wolfgang. *Leben ohne Brot*, Munich, 1981, (1st edition 1967).

24 Carise, Erna. *Hurra – die Punktediät ist da. Die gastronomische Wunder-diät in Punkten,* Vienna, 1966.
25 Atkins, Robert C. *Diätrevolution,* Frankfurt a M, 1981, 35 and 12: a synop-tic view of this type of diet may be found in: Thomas, Berthold and Koerber, Karl W. *Ernährung ohne Brot? Risiken kohlenhydratarmen Ernährung-srichtungen,* Heidelberg, 1983.
26 Tannahill, Reay. *Food in History,* London, 1988, 195.
27 Cf for instance Burkitt, D P. Epidemiology of cancer of the colon and rectum, *Cancer,* 28, no 3 (1971); Trowell, H. Ischemic heart disease and dietary fiber, *American Journal of Clinical Nutrition,* 25 (1972); ibid, Food and dietary fibre, *Nutrition reviews,* 35, no 6 (1977): for a summary of the results, see Huth, 1979, 51.
28 Schwartz, Hillel. *Never Satisfied: a cultural history of diets, fantasies and fat,* New York/London, 1986, 335 f.
29 Schlettwein-Gsell, Daniela. Impact of Socio-Cultural Food Patterns, *Medi-terranean Diet. A Symposium of the Swiss Society for Nutritional Research,* Lugano, September 30/October 1, 1994: Extended Summaries of Oral Pres entations, 73 f.
30 Schweizer, T F and Amadò, R. Nahrungsfaser. In Stähelin, Hannes B et al, ed, *Dritter Schweizerischer Ernährungsbericht,* Bern, 1991, 79–84.
31 I calculate this on the basis of the calculation factors listed by Alfred Fleisch in his book. Recent studies list a lower roughage content e.g. for fruit and vegetables – with good reason because they thus meet the 'more refined' qual-ity of these foodstuffs. See *Die Zusammensetzung der Lebensmittel. Nähr-werttabellen 1989/90, gegründet durch Siegfried W. Souci et al,* revised by Scherz, Heimo and Senser, Friedrich, ed, Deutsche Forschungsanstalt für Lebensmittelchemie, Garching-Munich/Stuttgart, 1989.
32 Versár, Fritz and Gsell, Daniela. *Ernährung und Gesundheitszustand der Bergbevölkerung der Schweiz,* Bern, 1962; calculated according to the tables on pp 105 ff and 179.
33 Gigon, Alfred. *Die Arbeiterkost nach Untersuchungen über die Ernährung Basler Arbeiter bei freigewählter Kost,* Berlin, 1914; Linetzky, Moischa, *Die* Zusammensetzung vegetablischer tischfertiger Speisen der freigewählten *Arbeiterkost,* Basel, 1914.
34 Gigon, 1914, 9.
35 Franscini, Stefano. *Nuova Statistica della Svizzera,* 2 vol, Lugano, 1847; for a summary of the results cf Ziegler, E. *Betrachtungen über den säkularen Wandel der Ernährung in der Schweiz,* Bern, 1975 (series of papers of the Swiss Society for Nutritional Research, 12), 5 f.
36 A synopsis of these papers may be found in: Strahlmann Berend, Erhe-bungen über den Lebensmittelverbrauch der schweizerischen Bevölkerung in historischer Sicht, in Brubacher, Georg and Ritzel, Günther, eds. *Zur Ernährungssituation der schweizerischen Bevölkerung. Erster sch-weizerischer Ernährungsbericht,* Bern/Stuttgart/Vienna, 1975, 42–56.
37 Cf eg Kiple, Kenneth F, ed. *The Cambridge World History of Human Dis-ease,* Cambridge, 1993.
38 Festinger, Leon. *A Theory of Cognitive Dissonance,* Stanford, 1962.

15 The discovery of vitamins: laboratory research, reception, industrial production

Hans J Teuteberg

A representative poll in 1992 indicated that probably 76 per cent of Germans know that vitamins strengthen their defences against disease.[1] Although 20 per cent have never heard of vitamin C, the majority has a most positive attitude towards them in general. Vitamins are not only offered in foodstuffs, but also in the form of dragées and effervescent tablets, and are combined with drugs and shampoos. Vitamin admixtures are well-known for encouraging sales; people who buy a product with vitamins believe they are not doing anything wrong. So vitamin consumption has become a part of healthy nutrition and the modern lifestyle. But it is interesting to realise that only a few have a deeper knowledge of the physiological effects and the development history of vitamins. This paper tries to fill this gap by sketching the discovery of the most important vitamins and putting their results into practice. Of course, we have to restrict ourselves to some base-lines.

WHAT ARE VITAMINS?

The expression 'vitamins' can be traced back to the Polish chemist Casimir Funk. He regarded a new chemical substance, which he had in 1911 isolated from rice pollard, as the organic base Amin. Assuming correctly that this compound is essential for human life he combined in 1913 this expression Amin with the prefix 'Vit' (Latin, *vita*, life).[2] This general term continued till today, although it was realized later that there is a larger set of vitamins with quite different chemical ingredients. Several early efforts were made then to define these 'additional nutritive substances' or 'accessory food factors' more precisely.[3] The researchers recognized by these terms (which were used more than the word vitamin up till the 1920s) firstly all unknown nutritive substances which do not belong to protein, fats, and carbohydrates nor to water and 'salts' (ie minerals and trace elements) and are indispensable for growth and conservation of life, although only tiny quantities are necessary. There was in the beginning of vitamin research, of course, no agreement about the nature and their effects on the human being. In 1920 a well-known German encyclopedia of dietetics showed that medicine recognized under these 'additional food factors' all chemical compounds which are essential for life, but which the body cannot produce by itself; and at that time the ingredients were still not clear.[4]

In the meantime we have learnt that vitamins produce no energy, but that they are indispensable for the catalytic functions of metabolism. A deficiency of vitamins always emerges during periods of incorrect or insufficient nutrition which have become, of course, rare in modern prosperous societies. Vitamins are the first line compounds of enzymes, ie albuminous bio-catalysts which are necessary for metabolism and the decomposition of protein, fats and carbohydrates; especially vitamins of the B-group can be classed here. Another group of vitamins do not belong to the enzymes, the most important vitamins A, C and D rank among them. Moreover vitamins can be divided into fat soluble (A, D) and water soluble (B-group and C). We can give the following general view:[5]

A GENERAL VIEW OF VITAMINS

Name of vitamin or vitamin group	Synthesis and main functions in the body	Typical vitamin deficiencies and diseases
Vitamin A (Retinol)	Originates mainly in the body from pro-vitamin ß-carotine or in carotionids originating from plants	Important for the seeing process, the mucous membrane and perichondrium
Vitamin D (Ergocalciferol, Cholecalciferol)	Vitamin D_2 (Ergocalciferol) originates from ergosterine in plants which is synthesized in the body through ultraviolet light. Vitamin D_3 (Cholecalciferol) is formed through photogenetic reaction of the skin, caused by dehydrocholesterin which is created in the liver from cholesterin. The D-vitamins assist the absorption of calcium and phosporous which are stored in the bones. Butter, milk, fish, egg yolk, and mushrooms, for instance, contain D-vitamins	Rickets
Vitamin E (Tocopherole)	This vitamin group covers most different activities, for instance, the protection of fatty acids. It protects the cells against oxygen-radicals and therefore influences the process of growing old	Deficiencies of muscular metabolism, membranes and neurotic disturbances
Vitamin K	Originates especially in the intestine and plays a part in the synthesis of coagulation substances	Diseases of intestinal bacteria or bile obstruction
Vitamin B_1 (Thiamin)	This vitamin is richly available, especially in corn. It plays a role	Loss of appetite and weight, muscular atrophy, weariness,

Name of vitamin or vitamin group	Synthesis and main functions in the body	Typical vitamin deficiencies and diseases
	as co-enzyme in the metabolism of carbohydrates	depression. Often nervous disturbances which cause a loss of memory and paralysis, heart insufficiency and oedema
Vitamin B_2 (Riboflavin)	This vitamin is a part of co-enzymes which are relevant for the supply of body tissue with oxygen and therefore for respiratory exchange	Reddening, formation of scale at mouth, nose, and eyes, atrophy of the mucous membrane of the tongue, change of nails and horny skin, dislike of light, lachrymose conditions
Niacin	General term for nicotinic acid and nicotinic acidamid. Part of two co-enzymes which assists the metabolism of hydrogen. Niacin contributes to the synthesis and decomposition of carbohydrate, fats and amino-acids. The body can partly change the amino-acid Thryptophan into nicotinic acids	Pellagra, especially in former times in those regions where people were living primarily on millet or maize. Inspissation and deposition of pigments in the skin, digestive troubles with diarrhoea, nervous inflammations, paralysis and depression
Vitamin B_6 (Pyrodoxin)	To this vitamin group counts pyridoxol, pyrodoxal and pyridoxamid which can be blended. Their active agent is pyridoxal$_5$-phosphate. As co-enzyme of a larger group of enzymes it takes part in the metabolism of protein	Disturbances of growth and reproduction, skin changes, anaemia and spasms
Vitamin B_{12} (Cyanobalamin)	This complex of vitamin factors with cobalt comprises several chemical compounds. They are formed by micro-bacteria only in animal bodies. The absorption takes place in the stomach. The colabalamine which are formed in the great gut of the human body are alone not sufficient. As a co-enzyme vitamin B_{12} takes part in the formation of blood and the cell substance, it is therefore indispensable for growth processes.	Anaemia, too large blood corpuscles (erythrocytes), degeneration of spinal cord and nervous complaints
Vitamin C (Ascorbic acid)	This vitamin which is part of fruit and especially of lemons and oranges, is very sensitive to oxydation and shows a loss of concentration after longer storage, preservation and cooking. Unlike most animals the human body cannot produce ascorbic acid by itself. This vitamin assists the transport of electrons, the reception of iron and the bio-synthesis of hormones, blocks the	Classical disease is scurvy with gum bleeding, wrist and ankle inflammations, effusion of blood in the skin, muscles and gut, disturbances of the bone growth

Name of vitamin or vitamin group	Synthesis and main functions in the body	Typical vitamin deficienies and diseases
	nitrasamines causing cancer and protects other vitamins as well as in the resistance against infectious diseases	
Biotin	This vitamin is primarily in food-stuffs with protein. The co-enzyme takes part in the synthesis and decomposition of certain fat and amino acids as well at the formation of cholestrine; biotin is formed by intestinal bacteria	Pathological changes of the skin after extreme unbalanced nutrition
Folic-acid	This vitamin which originates in the liver and green plants, is formed by intestinal bacteria and takes part in the division and regeneration of cells	Pathological changes of the skin and mucous membranes, disturbances of the digestive tract, decrease of resistance against infections and changes in the bones.
Patothen acid	A composition of co-enzymes which is a key factor in the process of metabolism. Patothen acid is wide-spread and therefore is not lacking in normal foodstuffs	Deficiency of growth, loss of weight, changes of skin, nervous disturbances and of the intestinal tract, loss of hormones in experiments with animals

SCURVY AND THE FIRST TREATMENTS

Probably from very early times it was noticed that an enforced unbalanced diet, after a while, causes certain health defects. Such problems arose regularly when a large group of persons had to be provisioned in a relatively small room or area. Within besieged towns or ships' crews, in hospitals, poor houses and prisons, especially during famines, pathological symptoms appeared similar to scurvy. In Greek and Roman literature and in the legends of the Vikings we find some first vague hints in this direction.[6] As far as we can tell this insidious sickness began to spread from the start of the European overseas discovery voyages in the fifteenth and sixteenth centuries. Portuguese, Spanish and Dutch, and then French and English seafarers lost so many sailors because of diseases on their expeditions that always only a small number of them returned. The reports of Vasco da Gama, Fernando de Magellan and Jacques Cartier show that 'lemon water', the juice of certain leaves and roots, the blood of seals and whales, also water-cress, 'scurvy grass' and sauerkraut were seen as remedies against this 'plague of the sea', but the causes remained unknown.[7] The first more detailed but still imperfect descriptions by the British Admiral James Lancaster after his voyages to Brazil and East-India in 1591 and 1603 (who learnt from the experiences of the famous filibuster Richard Hawkins), and of the Austrian military physician J G H Kramer who had seen thousands of soldiers dying through scurvy epidemics in the wars against the Turks in the late seventeenth century, were not taken notice of by medical science and there was no change in ships' provisions.[8]

A turning-point in scurvy research came with the Scottish ship's doctor James Lind (1716–94). In 1748, he started systematic experiments which he presented in a 400 page volume in 1753.[9] When the sailors in his ship showed the first symptoms of scurvy, he divided them in groups and one of them received the juice of two oranges and a lemon per day. Lind was in this way very successful and defined citrus fruit as the best medicine. His investigations, written unusually not in Latin but in English, placed accidental experiences on a controlled basis; now it was certain that there was a remedy against the 'plague of the sea'. But it was still impossible to explain why this tropical fruit had this healing effect and what it had in common with pickled cabbage, seals' blood or the extracts of certain plants.

Lind's results were of great benefit to James Cook when he sailed as an officer with the British ship 'Endeavour' between 1768 and 1772 to Tahiti. He made more experiments and included sauerkraut, being much cheaper than tropical fruit, in the ship's provisions. Although from his crew of 94 seamen only 34 returned after three years, nobody had died of scurvy.[10] This experiment had the effect that in English harbours 'sauerkraut manufactories' were erected and from 1782 every sailor of the Royal Navy was provided with a certain amount of pickled cabbage per week. Cook was made an admiral and charged to undertake a second voyage to the South Seas between 1772 and 1776. This time he carried with him 60 barrels of sauerkraut as well as citrus fruit. On his way Cook in addition tried always to get fresh vegetables and fruit for his crew. This was a revolution in ship's provisioning and the first break-through in healing scurvy, and for these reasons he was made a member of the Royal Society.[11]

But the nature of scurvy remained a riddle. In 1874/5 the Medical Society of Paris expressed the opinion that the symptoms were caused by bacterial infection. So throughout the nineteenth century severe scurvy epidemics recurred, for instance, in the American Civil War 1861–5 and the German-French War 1870–1, and also later in prison camps during World War I. As a list of sources indicates there were 114 large scurvy epidemics between 1556 and 1857 (40 in besieged towns and 33 in hospitals and poor houses), and between 1872 and 1952 in Europe as a whole 91,241 cases of scurvy.[12]

THE DEVELOPMENT OF VITAMIN RESEARCH IN THE LATE NINETEENTH AND EARLY TWENTIETH CENTURIES

The discovery of the B-vitamins

The first experimental research with vitamins in a laboratory concerned beriberi disease which appeared in world regions where rice was the staple food, especially in East Asia. Reports of the symptoms can be traced far

back in ancient China, and a Dutch ship's physician gave the first description of them in the seventeenth century. Disastrous beriberi epidemics
occurred after 1860 when steam rice-mills removed the husks with the help
of a newly invented machine while another one polished the rice, so that
the rice gained a white colour. This very old food became through these
processes more palatable and more digestible, but lost its vitamins. More
and more plantation hands, mining workers, soldiers, sailors and inmates
of hospitals showed beriberi symptoms: stiff limbs, fever, spasm, muscular
atrophy, later on disturbances of respiration and sight, loss of hair (alo-
pecia), weariness, apathy and loss of weight, and eventually abscesses, intes-
tinal infections and depression were observed.

The Japanese military physician Kanehiro Takaki (1849–1937), in 1882,
observed *c* 1000 sailors and fed half of them, besides the usual rice portion,
with meat, bread fruit, and vegetables.[13] His carefully written measures
show that the beriberi cases decreased drastically, but he could not explain
his success and assumed this had to do with the extra meat. Another
beriberi epidemic in 1885 in a prison at Batavia on the Dutch colonial
island of Java, which spread out quickly to the native population, led to
a special Commission being set up by the Dutch governor. Christiaan Eijkman (1858–1930), a former student of the famous bacteriologist Robert
Koch (1845–1910) from Berlin, with some beriberi experiences in Java, was
able to prove that this had nothing to do with bacterial infections as other
members of the Commission had assumed. Looking for the real causes a
lucky chance helped him: when feeding fowls in his laboratory at the Royal
Dutch-Indian Research Institute of Bacteriology and Anatomy in Batavia,
he noticed one day that they suddenly showed all the symptoms of beriberi
which then disappeared some days later. These test animals had for a short
time been fed polished rice without husks from a military kitchen. He supposed that the disease 'polyneuritis gallinarum' was connected with this different feeding. More experiments with pigeons showed that beriberi could
be initiated through withdrawal of certain food substances, as for instance,
the husks. This success encouraged him and his assistant Gerrit Grijns to
start further experiments with human beings. Then came a second lucky
chance: the Inspector of Sanitary Conditions in Java told him that the
280,000 inmates of prisons were provisioned partly with unpolished and
partly with polished rice. Eijkman estimated that in prisons with polished
rice the beriberi cases were 300 times higher than in those with unpolished
rice.[14] At first there was much criticism of his methods, but when new
experiments after 1900 by other scholars confirmed his findings, the Far
East Association of Tropical Medicine gave him their overdue approval. In
1929, together with Frederick Gowland Hopkins (1861–1945), he received
the Nobel Prize for medicine.

Hopkins, a British chemist from Cambridge, introduced another important scientific finding. Justus Liebig, who had a dominating influence on the
emerging science of nutrition in the late nineteenth century, had detected

since 1842 that the triad – protein, fats, and carbohydrates, together with water and 'salts' – are the constituents of all animal and human nutrition.[15] But new vitamin research indicated more and more after 1900 that no life is possible without certain additional substances which were rather mysterious. Hopkins defined them as 'accessory food factors'.[16] After experiments with test-rats he concluded that:

> no animal can live upon a mixture of pure protein, fat and carbohydrate, and even when the necessary inorganic material is carefully supplied, the animal cannot flourish. The animal body is adjusted to live either upon plant tissues or other animals and these contain countless substances other than proteins, carbohydrates and fats . . . The field is almost unexplored, it is only certain that there are many minor factors in all diets, of which the body takes account. In diseases, such as rickets and particularly in scurvy, we do not have many years' knowledge of dietetic factors, but though we know how to benefit these conditions empirically, the real errors in diet are to this day obscure. They do, however, certainly comprise those animal qualitative factors that I am considering. Scurvy and rickets are conditions so severe that they force themselves upon our attention, but many other nutritive errors affect the health of individuals to a most important degree and some of them depend on unsuspected dietary factors.[17]

With this chain of reasoning Hopkins became the real 'spiritual father of vitamin theory'.[18]

There were some other scholars like the Dutch bacteriologist Cornelius Pekelharing from Utrecht who at the same time came very close to his conclusions, but unlike Hopkins they gave up their vitamin research in the belief that they could not get more results. Hopkins, using Eijkman's findings, explained definitely that there are certain diseases solely caused by faults of food composition. Like Liebig in the middle of the nineteenth century, he summarized the whole knowledge of his time so brilliantly that the scientific world was convinced. His theory of 'accessory foodstuffs' was introduced to all nutrition science handbooks. Now it was quite clear that the lack of certain substances in foodstuffs, which the German chemical physiologist Emil Abderhalden called by the general term 'nutritive dystrophy', was responsible for many diseases.[19] But it was true that scholars up to World War I did not know very much about the chemical compounds in this connection. On the other hand the first laboratory experiments created a base for numerous subsequent investigations. In 1911 Casimir Funk (1884–1967) extracted in the course of four months 170 g of an unknown mixture of crystalline substances. He could demonstrate that only centigrams of this was enough to cure the paralysis of polyneuritic pigeons. Eijkman's analysis was thus shown by biochemistry to be absolutely correct.

The Polish chemist, Funk, also contributed to the progress of vitamin theory.[20] He called all diseases caused by vitamin shortages by the general term 'avitaminosis' and made the expression 'vitamin' synonymous for a new miraculous weapon of medicine, with revolutionary expectations.

There was much criticism of his word-creation. He was attacked because the term vitamin was not very precise and clearly not enough to cover all the necessary effects on nutrition. Others said that the 'amines' had nothing to do with all vitamins. But all proposals for another expression failed against Funk's inspired catchword[21] as being too complicated or leading to the belief that the new substances were not really essential. In 1931 an international conference in London organized by the League of Nations agreed finally to the term vitamin and set out the different segments alphabetically. A US commission, headed by the nutritionist Elmar Verner McCollum from Baltimore, had earlier settled disagreements with the nomenclature and made a general difference between fat soluble and water soluble vitamins. Also in 1931, a special journal for vitamin research (*Zeitschrift für Vitaminforschung*) was started in Germany.

THE DISCOVERY OF VITAMIN A

The first reliable observations about deficiency symptoms connected with vitamin A did not appear until the end of the nineteenth century. In 1890 the Japanese physician Inoyue observed especially in children an epidemic eye-disease which he named Xerophtalamy (Greek *xeros*, dry; and *ophtalamos*, eye). The organ of sight became dim because the lachrymal gland and connective tissue were dry and therefore germs penetrated the eyeball, destroying it by inflammation.[22] This sickness, which had in former times different names, was traditionally cured with fish-oil and liver of fowls. The Japanese doctor noticed moreover that this eye-complaint appeared more in the interior parts of the islands where fish was not, as in coastal regions, the main foodstuff. His casual observations were forgotten till his professional colleague Mori, already informed about the vitamin discussion, directed public attention again towards these findings. But all this remained without an experimental background and therefore without academic or public response.

The first pioneering tests in a laboratory were started by the German chemist Wilhelm Stepp. In 1909 he noticed, like Eijkman and Hopkins, that Liebig's three nutritive substances, protein, fats and carbohydrates, are indeed not sufficient to maintain health. He fed white mice with wheat bread baked in milk and an extract of alcohol and ether. During his experiments he found proof that within the last named additions there must be an another unknown soluble substance which is indispensable for all beings. Stepp called these new agents 'lipoids' (Greek *lipos*, fat; and *eides*, similar).[23] His results had little influence at first, perhaps because communication between chemists was hindered by language barriers. In 1927 Hopkins made the same discovery as Stepp, without knowing of those earlier experiments. His rats fed with milk indicated that the missing substance in the food was, in contrast to the known B-vitamins, fat-soluble. Stepp called the fat-soluble vitamin 'factor A' and the water-soluble vitamin 'factor B'. In the

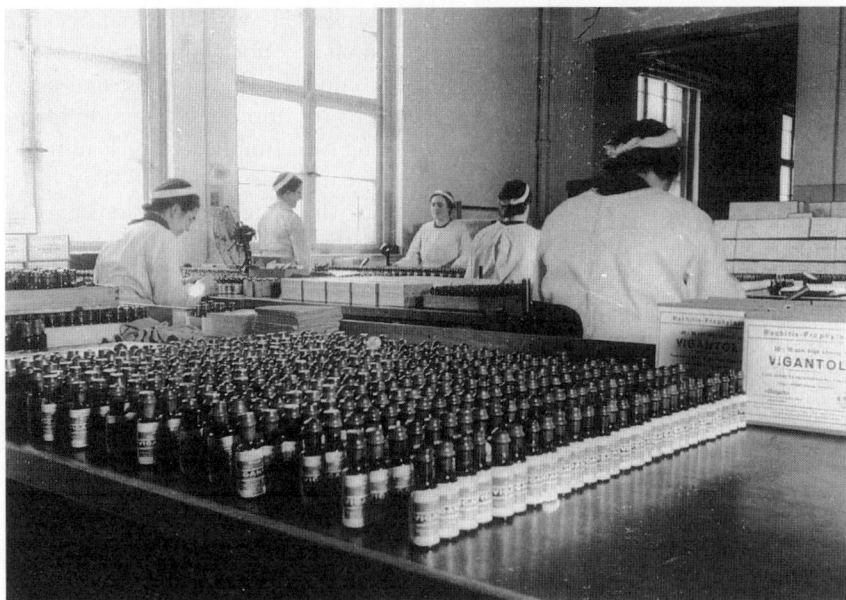

Fig.1. *Vitamin products of the Merck Company, Darmstadt, around 1930*

course of his laboratory tests he was able to show that vitamin A in animals had its origin in plants. This meant that the content of vitamin A in animal foodstuffs could be manipulated by feeding. The importance of the milk fat was then confirmed by an involuntary large test. When during World War I the neutral country Denmark raised its butter exports by a large amount for bargaining reasons, there were after a short time, beside other deficiency diseases, hundreds of Danish people with xerophtalamy. This health problem ceased at once one year later, when Denmark stopped its fat exports.[24] The discovery of carotine as a first-step (pro-vitamin) for forming vitamin A, by the Zürich chemist Karrer in 1932, paved the way for more research into the chemical structure of this vitamin and its application.

THE DISCOVERY OF VITAMIN C

The experiments of Eijkman inspired the Norwegian researchers Axel Holst and Theodor Frölich in 1907 to begin similar investigations on beriberi in Oslo.[25] They supposed that polished rice was not the only reason for this disease and detected that green vegetables were also suitable for test animals. They were able to demonstrate that citrus juice, sauerkraut and onions were not only suitable for prophylaxis but also for curing beriberi. Since the new additive factor dominates in citrus fruit and the letter 'B' was already being used, the British nutritionist Jack Drummond and Casimir Funk chose the expression 'vitamin C' for the new substance.

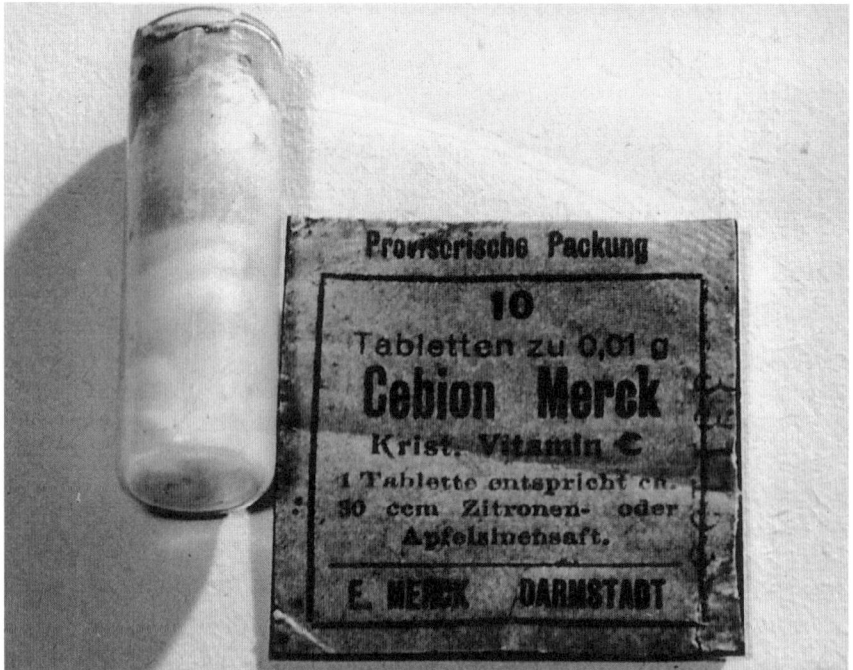

Fig. 2. *The first Vitamin C- preparation of the Merck Company, Cebion, in 1933*

Twenty years after, in 1928, the Hungarian chemist Albert Szent-Györgi was a leader in this field of research. Working at Hopkins' biochemistry laboratory in Cambridge he extracted from the cortex of the suprarenal gland a new white powder which was soluble in water and alcohol. Together with his American colleague J L Sviberley, he succeeded in 1932 to show that this new substance, first named by him 'hexuron acid', was identical to vitamin C. Szent-Györgi, then nominated as a professor in Budapest, was crowned with more success: he managed to give evidence that paprika (red pepper), which is very common in Hungary, has more vitamin C than the suprarenal gland, so that the extraction process could be made easier and much cheaper. In January 1933 he had extracted 430 g of pure vitamin C-powder and therefore the research could be pushed ahead much quicker. Nearly at the same time the nutritionist J Tillmans from Frankfurt-upon-Main had demonstrated independently that hexuron acid is identical to vitamin C. In co-ordination with Szent-Györgi the new vitamin-powder was called 'ascorbic acid' because of its marked healing effects on scurvy.[26] The following work in this field can be characterized as an international collaboration of several research-groups which do not need further detailed description here. Only noteworthy is that in 1934 the Swiss chemist Reichstein succeeded in detecting grape sugar (D-glucose) as a first stage for vitamin C- production.

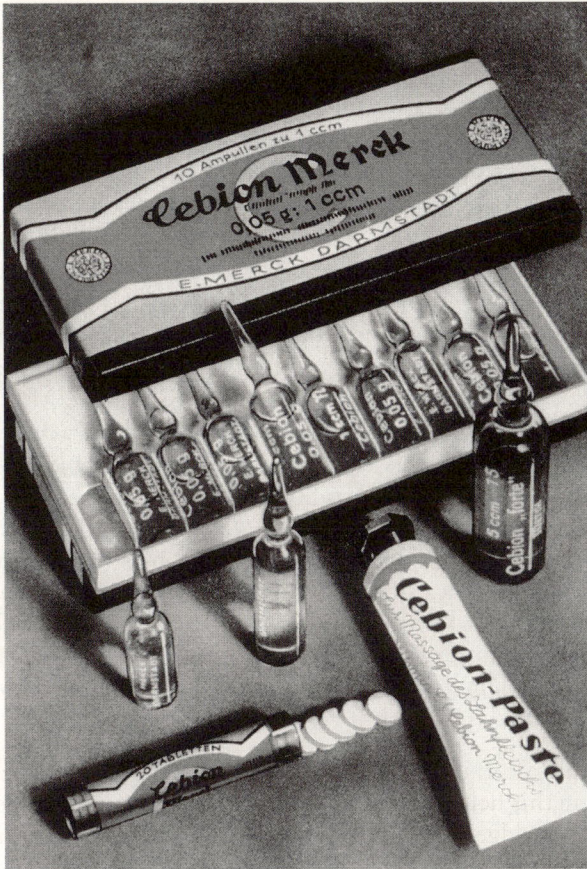

Fig. 3. *Some of the Merck Company's Cebion products*

THE DISCOVERY OF THE VITAMIN D

In the middle of the seventeenth century a physician had already described a widespread illness, especially in England, called rickets which we know today as rachitis: large deformities of the bones, anaemia, relaxation of the muscles and pale skin. Much later it was recognised that this had to do with phosphate and calcium metabolism caused by lack of sunlight and insufficiency of vitamin D.[27] The Saxon pathologist Schurl from Dresden in 1909 first hinted at insolation as a medicine for curing this disease, in close connection with this naturally occurring medicine, recommending walking societies, sports movements and nudism, but the majority of the researchers regarded nutrition and bad housing conditions as the main causes of this sickness. Rickets was seen as a result of the 'labour question' because urban worker families mostly suffered from this sickness.

Edward Mellanby, an English physician, was the first to unmask this dangerous disease as a shortage of vitamins in 1919.[28] He showed with his experiments that animal fat contains an anti-rachitic factor. Since the new substance was fat-soluble he had first mistakenly thought it might be identical to the newly discovered vitamin A. At the same time the paediatrician Kurt Huldschinsky from Berlin was able to demonstrate with other tests that radiation with ultra-violet light also had absolutely curative effects. This was confirmed by the new method of X-ray examination which had been introduced from the United States shortly before. Of course, this meant a wide division between Mellanby and Huldschinsky regarding what was the best therapy for curing rachitis. But further explorations, by the American chemists Hess and Steenbock in 1923, ended this controversy. They showed that a combination of both methods was also successful. Foodstuff radiated with ultra-violet light had the same anti-rachitic effects as direct radiation of the body.

Elmar Verner McCollum then produced startling evidence in a book about the anti-rachitic effects of cod-liver oil, and that there was an additive vitamin essential for the metabolism of the bones. The anti-rachitic substance was named on his suggestion vitamin D.[29] The chemist Adolf Windaus, carrying out optical experiments at Göttingen, discovered finally that very small quantities of mushrooms and yeast contain an attendant substance of cholestrine which is a pro-vitamin or, in other words, the first stage for the formation of the vitamin D-group.[30] New control tests confirmed that the tiny amount of 0.15 million of a gram of this newly invented Ergosterine, irradiated with ultra-violet light, is sufficient to give protection against rachitis. Since 1927 the chemical nature of the anti-rachitic vitamin D had been definitely unmasked and now a base has been laid for its industrial production. In 1935 Windaus received the Nobel prize in chemistry for his discovery.

THE RECEPTION OF VITAMIN RESEARCH IN SCIENCE AND PRACTICE

Academic controversies

The investigations into vitamins remained till the end of the nineteenth century a controversial field of activities with casual and dispersed individual analysis. Not before 1900 can we speak of systematic research presenting results in scientific journals of chemistry, pharmacy, biology and medicine. Two lines can be distinguished. On the one hand there were short reports about experimental results, without evaluations. For instance, in a German journal of biochemistry and biophysics, founded in 1898 in Leipzig, there were year after year several very short research notes. The volumes between 1913 and 1921 show that the editors adhered to the older term 'accessory nutrition substances' and often had a sceptical opinion of them, but all aspects of this new field of research were observed carefully.[31] On the other hand we see also a first and modest forum for discussion and exchange of ideas. Worthy of remark are the rejections of the 'vitamin hurly-burly' by leading German nutritionists. The field of vitamins was in their eyes not qualified enough to become a new discipline within the nutrition sciences, because a varied and good mixture of food had enough 'additional food factors'.[32] This broad rejection of vitamin research is easy to explain: Germany had been in the late nineteenth century a stronghold of the emerging nutrition sciences, and the theories of Liebig, Pettenkofer, Voit, and Rubner ranked as dogmas. The new ideas of 'accessory nutritive substances' flooding in from abroad were seen as unpleasant rivalry in a conquered area, and therefore they tried to ignore or demean the whole area of vitamin research. In this disagreement the Hamburg physician Friedrich von Hahn stood out especially. In numerous articles he spoke against the vitamin nuisance, and criticised especially the new industrially produced artificial vitamin compounds which claimed to replace vitamins in natural foodstuffs. Hahn called the vitamin researchers a 'danger to the people's common food', and 'guilty of careless bodily injury'.[33] When he attacked the products 'Eviunis' and 'Vitiphos' of the Swiss firm Castello from Thusis, a court procedure was launched. The German High Court (Reichsgericht) exonerated him in 1932 because he had argued only in a scientific connection. But the judges focused the public attention on a legislative gap: the sale of industrial vitamin products which could be dangerous to health could not be stopped by law. This problem was recognized at the same time in other European states. In 1932 the Netherlands made a first bill against vitamin swindling. This was an occasion for the German government to issue a 'Decree on the Trade of Foodstuff containing Vitamins'. The sale of these products now needed a licence from the National Board of Health.[34] These waves of criticism caused the small group of vitamin researchers in Germany to publish some easily understandable summary outlines on vitamins and to organise public lectures in 1925, using the new broadcasting system.[35]

But it should not be overlooked that vitamin researchers were often in a state of feud with each other when they stepped into this *terra incognita*. Obviously this was a fertile field for such rivalry. So Casimir Funk published in 1924 a first historical overview of the development of vitamin research during the previous twelve years. After praising Hopkins he reproached his British colleague for going public rather late in 1912, probably because he was not quite sure about his results. Funk considered himself therefore as the first and real discoverer of the vitamin B complex, since he had announced his research one year earlier. Hopkins answered that in 1906 he had already begun his experiments but according to Funk's own notes not before 1911. The British scholar had given a report to a Biochemical Club during this period and Funk admitted in a footnote that he got information about this lecture by 'private communication'. The merit of Funk was, in Hopkin's view, that his Polish colleague had given a good summary of the whole arc of vitamin research and a significant hypothesis, but nothing more.[36] He gave Funk due praise, but was not willing to give up his place as discoverer of vitamin B. Why Hopkins kept back his important results for so many years and why he made his publication after Funk remains unclear.

VITAMINS IN COOKERY AND HOUSEKEEPING BOOKS

As usual the transformation of new scientific findings into practice happened with a certain delay. All authors of cookery and housekeeping books till 1930 held fast to Liebig's triad of protein, fats and carbohydrates.[37] Vegetables and fruit were still considered luxury foodstuffs – certainly healthy, but not nutritious and with few exceptions not absolutely necessary. Not before 1927 is the expression 'additional substances' mentioned in this literature. From that time green and fresh vegetables are understood to be not only a supplement for alternative purposes but also a vehicle for substances essential for life. Although the functions of the vitamins were for the time being almost unknown, the women readers were now becoming familiar with the terms vitamin A, B, and C. Their importance was described as follows:

> Modern nutritional science recognises two words which were totally unknown to our mothers and which the housewife nowadays has to work with: vitamins and calories. Everyday health depends for a large part on correct nutrition. Therefore, German housewife, read this short transaction! What do we know about vitamins? These are primarily elements, additional substances which we cannot explain totally, but it is clear that they have the greatest importance for the human body.

Before World War I the speakers of the popular health-reform movement and especially the small sect of orthodox vegetarians had already discussed the 'protein superstition' and praised the consumption of green raw vegetables together with allotment gardening for urban dwellers, but this had been more a matter of a quasi-religious confession. Now the consumption of vegetables received for the first time a scientific legitimation. There was now quite new information for the housewife: cooking for too long destroyed the vitamins, the 'good butter' contained, unlike the 'bad margarine', vitamin A; preference had to be given to traditional unpolished rice; and fresh vegetables, potatoes, and fruit were important bearers of the essential vitamin C. A special vegetarian cookery book promised a fare which included many vitamins and therefore vigour as well as power to resist diseases. Vegetables and fruit could help, moreover, in keeping slim.[38] All authors were against factory-made vitamin-products. In 1929 a handbook for housekeeping offered for the first time recipes which not only show the already known three nutritive elements and calories but also the tabulated vitamin content.[39] Knowledge of vitamins in cookery and housekeeping books was growing in the 1930s. Of course, it was inevitable that sometimes dubious or wrong information was given. It was insisted in one cookery book, for instance, that the more fat there is in cheese or fish the more vitamins there are in these victuals. The transfer of complicated biochemical and medical knowledge into cookery books was extremely difficult, because special teaching was lacking. The chemists and physicians were used to producing their ideas only for a small élite circle of colleagues and had no contact with the sporadic and private consumer advisory groups.

THE INDUSTRIAL PRODUCTION OF VITAMINS AND THEIR MARKETING

At the end of the nineteenth century the pharmaceutical industry began to blossom in the wake of the quick progress of biochemical science. Looking for new profitable markets these entrepreneurs ventured during the 1920s to turn to the field of vitamins. The firm Merck in Darmstadt started in 1927 to produce the cod-liver oil 'Vigantol', containing vitamin D, which had been developed earlier by Bayer enterprise and Nobel prize-winner

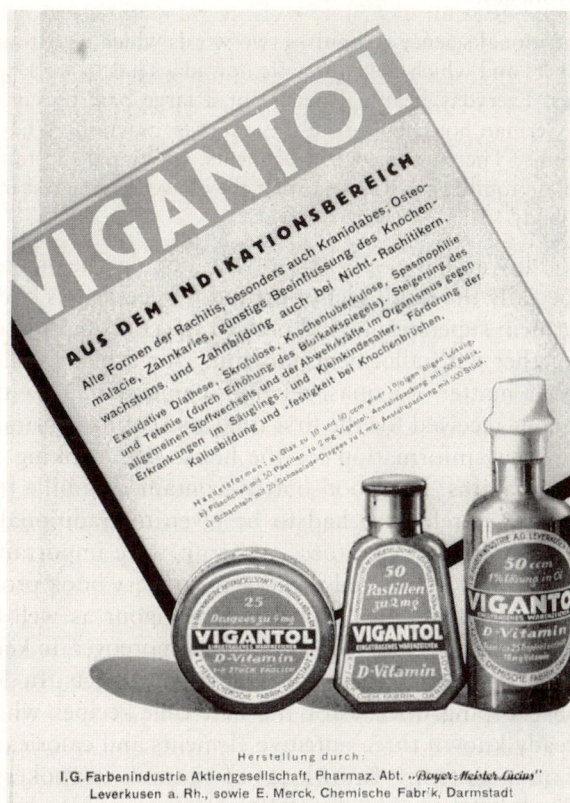

Fig. 4. *The Vigantol cod-liver oil products of the Merck Company*

Adolf Windaus. The new preparation against the 'English disease', rickets, replaced cod liver-oil, and was an immediate success and the prelude for other factory-made vitamin products.[40] In 1932 Merck began laboratory experiments to isolate pure vitamin C from different sorts of cabbage, Swedish turnips, currants, oranges, and rosehips. The vitamins in cabbages and oranges had to be extracted very quickly, as the vitamin concentration decreased through storage. Paprika proved to be much more profitable with its very high content of vitamin C. Therefore during the early 1930s there began an increasing import of this red pepper from Hungary and Italy. After several further tests scientists succeeded in producing raw crystals which could be changed into ascorbinic acid. In subsequent research into vitamin C Hungarian, Swiss and British scholars worked closely together. In 1933 the Swiss chemists Reichstein and Güssner succeeded in making a synthesis of ascorbinic acid which greatly reduced the expense. Industrial production independent of weather and harvests was now possible. After this synthesis Merck, on 8 July 1933, registered its first vitamin C-preparation 'Cebion' for protection as a trademark. At that time 12 kg of pure vitamin C had been produced – the breakthrough had arrived. The demand for this artificial vitamin C was now rising very quickly globally. The production capacity which amounted in 1964 to 5,000 t per year increased to 50,000 t in 1991. Two thirds of this output were delivered directly to the food industry for improving the quality of their products. From 1935 the number of industrial vitamin preparations could be extended and for the first time combinations of several vitamins were offered. The multi-vitamin product 'Opticon', a combination of liver extract, iron, manganese, caffeine, glycerophosphate, and amara, 'Scottin' with vitamins A and D and 'Sanastol' with the vitamin mixture A, B, C, and D can be named here.[41] Up to 1939 Merck had competition from the other big pharmaceutical-combines Hoffmann La Roche and Bayer who offered their ampoules and tablets with similar combinations and prices.[42]

It is remarkable that from the end of the 1920s in some countries a similar public awareness for vitamins began to rise. In the United States, for example, there were now frequent recommendations for a higher consumption of fresh milk and green vegetables to overcome the lack of the vitamins A and C. The big food company Standard Brands boasted from the early 1930s that its yeast cakes, rich in vitamin B₁, were good for many complaints. Three 'slimy cakes' a day would clear up pimples, spots, and acne, increase energy and cure 'poor digestion', 'unfed blood', and constipation.[43] The leading 'nutrition apostle' Henry C Sherman, perceived in vitamins a real 'fountain of youth'. Milk, eggs, fresh fruit and vegetables not only protect against diseases but would also lengthen life. In 1934 the Californian fruit growers declared, quoting a physician from Chicago, that orange and lemon juice can stop all tooth decay in children. Therefore the American Dental Association debated in the same year whether this vitamin C would be more effective than the toothbrush. Vitamin D was praised for saving

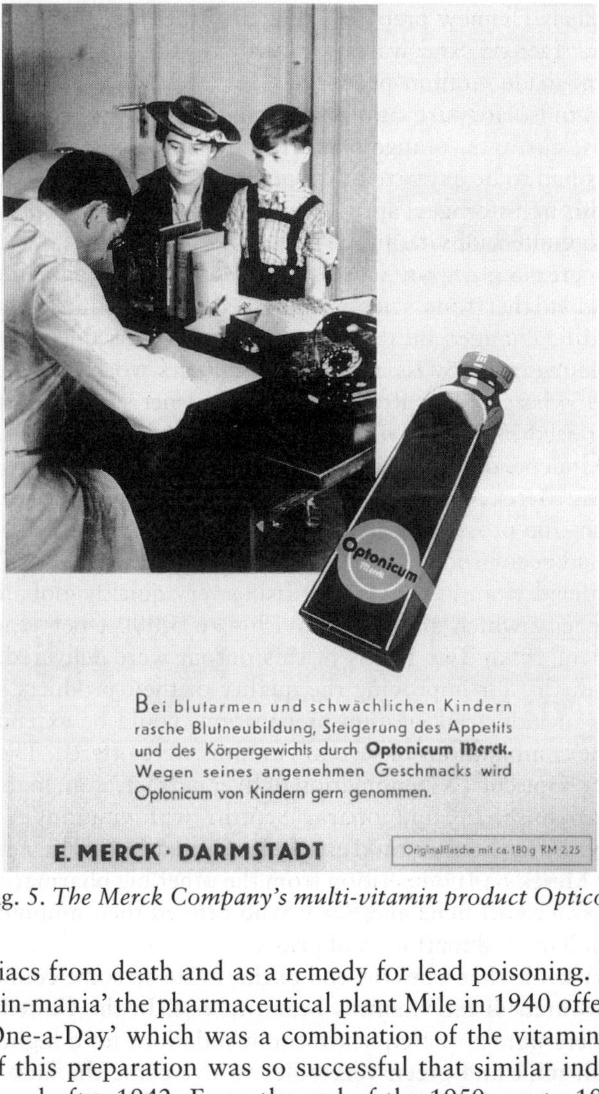

Bei blutarmen und schwächlichen Kindern rasche Blutneubildung, Steigerung des Appetits und des Körpergewichts durch **Optonicum Merck.** Wegen seines angenehmen Geschmacks wird Optonicum von Kindern gern genommen.

E. MERCK · DARMSTADT Originalflasche mit ca. 180 g RM 2.25

Fig. 5. *The Merck Company's multi-vitamin product Opticon*

haemophiliacs from death and as a remedy for lead poisoning. Induced by this 'vitamin-mania' the pharmaceutical plant Mile in 1940 offered its new product 'One-a-Day' which was a combination of the vitamins A and D. The sale of this preparation was so successful that similar industrial products followed after 1942. From the end of the 1950s up to 1983 this US enterprise, since 1979 part of the Bayer combine, increased its turnover from $350m to $16b.[44]

From the end of the 1920s, vitamins became an object of advertizing. Because in the beginning so little was known about their functions and how much was needed for health purposes, there was immense scope for exaggerated claims. Because there were no standardized methods to measure these factors, false promises were made. The German firm Vitam GmbH announced in 1930 a newly invented product with the name 'VITAM-R'. This preparation, 'similar to butter', was praised as 'a highly active driving power', especially for the cold winter time, with a good taste, refreshing not

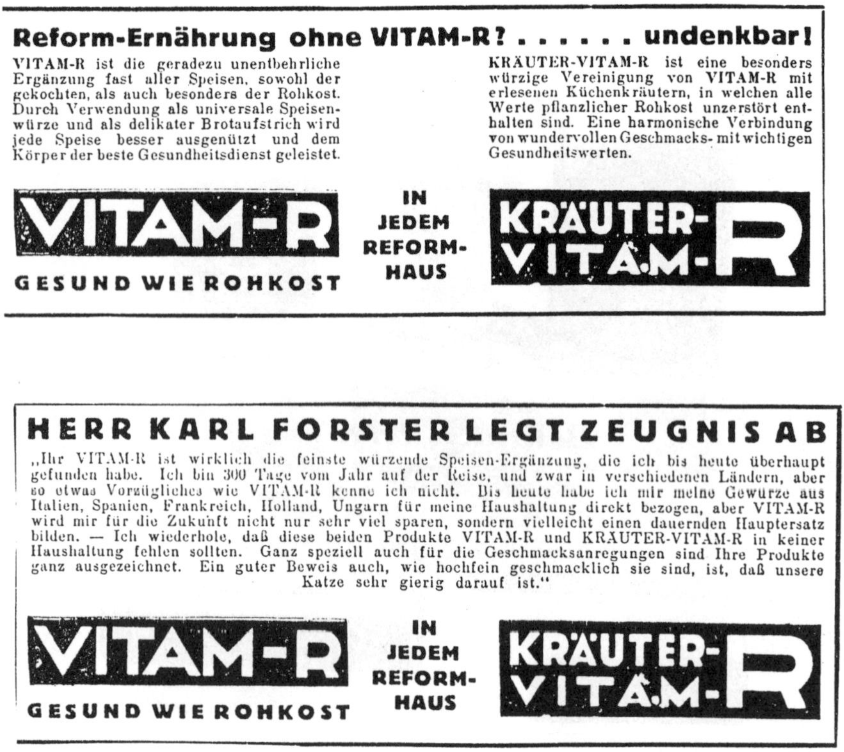

Reform-Ernährung ohne VITAM-R? . . . . . . undenkbar!

VITAM-R ist die geradezu unentbehrliche Ergänzung fast aller Speisen, sowohl der gekochten, als auch besonders der Rohkost. Durch Verwendung als universale Speisenwürze und als delikater Brotaufstrich wird jede Speise besser ausgenützt und dem Körper der beste Gesundheitsdienst geleistet.

KRÄUTER-VITAM-R ist eine besonders würzige Vereinigung von VITAM-R mit erlesenen Küchenkräutern, in welchen alle Werte pflanzlicher Rohkost unzerstört enthalten sind. Eine harmonische Verbindung von wundervollen Geschmacks- mit wichtigen Gesundheitswerten.

VITAM-R

GESUND WIE ROHKOST

IN JEDEM REFORM-HAUS

KRÄUTER-VITAM-R

HERR KARL FORSTER LEGT ZEUGNIS AB

„Ihr VITAM-R ist wirklich die feinste würzende Speisen-Ergänzung, die ich bis heute überhaupt gefunden habe. Ich bin 300 Tage vom Jahr auf der Reise, und zwar in verschiedenen Ländern, aber so etwas Vorzügliches wie VITAM-R kenne ich nicht. Bis heute habe ich mir meine Gewürze aus Italien, Spanien, Frankreich, Holland, Ungarn für meine Haushaltung direkt bezogen, aber VITAM-R wird mir für die Zukunft nicht nur sehr viel sparen, sondern vielleicht einen dauernden Hauptersatz bilden. — Ich wiederhole, daß diese beiden Produkte VITAM-R und KRÄUTER-VITAM-R in keiner Haushaltung fehlen sollten. Ganz speziell auch für die Geschmacksanregungen sind Ihre Produkte ganz ausgezeichnet. Ein guter Beweis auch, wie hochfein geschmacklich sie sind, ist, daß unsere Katze sehr gierig darauf ist.“

VITAM-R

GESUND WIE ROHKOST

IN JEDEM REFORM-HAUS

KRÄUTER-VITAM-R

Fig. 6. *The Vitam-R reform diet (1932)*

only the whole body but also the spirit'. One advertisement had the headline: 'Reform diet without VITAM-R? – Unthinkable!' Obviously these products had enormous success, although no further information about the content and method of consumption was given. Sometime later this enterprise offered a 'Herbal VITAM beef cube'.[45] These and other newly induced vitamin preparations were aimed at the supporters of the popular health-reform movement in Germany focusing on the educated urban middle classes with higher household budgets. Advertisements in the leading *Zeitschrift für Volksernährung* in 1938 show that nearly all industrial vitamin products still used the pre-fix 'vit' in order to reflect the expression vitamin. The vitamins were seen more and more as a medium for a healthy diet and modern lifestyle.

From the early 1930s there were also some vitamin products outside the 'reform diet'. So we find a special 'Heart Vitamin-Bread', a 'Vitamin Plant Margarine', a vitaminized powder of cocoa-malt mix with the curious name 'Düs-co-lade' (which is reminiscent in German of chocolate) and a 'Herbal Vitamin Tablet' which promised 'to free the body from waste matter and especially the gut from poisoned putrefactions'. With the production of vitamin tablets a completely new market with large consumer

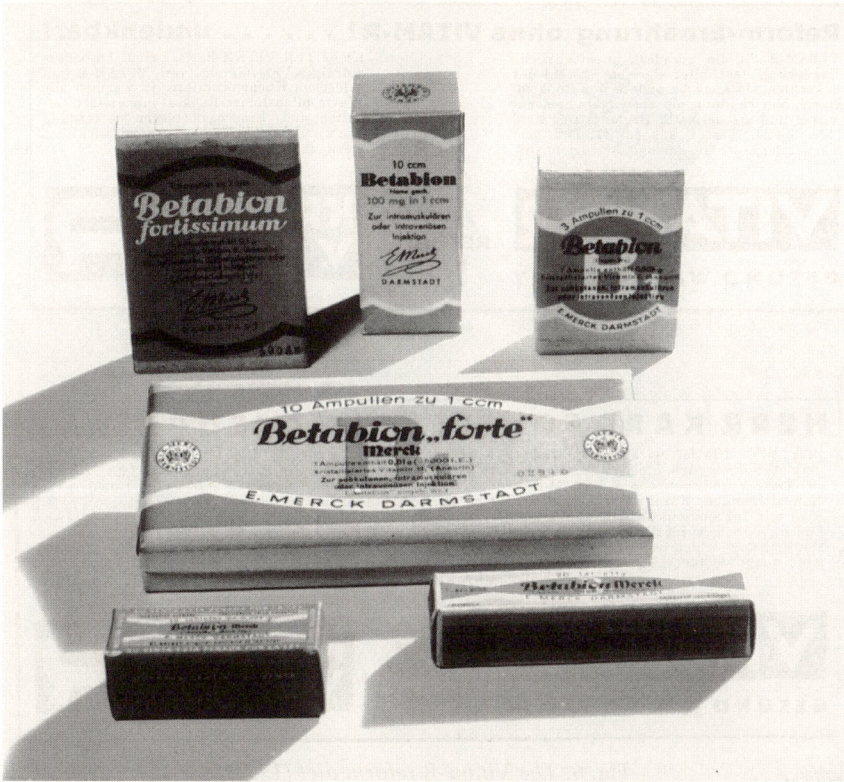

Fig. 7. *The Merck Company's product Betabion, 1937*

potential was created. But only the international pharmaceutical combines prevailed in the vitamin market. Only they had enough financial and intellectual resources for the fast growing and expensive research and marketing. As the advertisements for the products 'BETABION' (1937) and 'DIBIONTA' (1939) from Merck demonstrate, there was now always a detailed chemical analysis and other necessary information about the contents for the consumers.

RÉSUMÉ

The results of this contribution can be summarised as follows:

- The question of who was the discoverer of each individual vitamin or vitamin-group cannot be answered exactly. The Nobel prize given to three vitamin researchers does not mean that the rise of this new discipline is due only to some ingenious scholars. For centuries there was empirical knowledge about remedies against some epidemic diseases. This had only to do with vitamin deficiencies, but the bio-

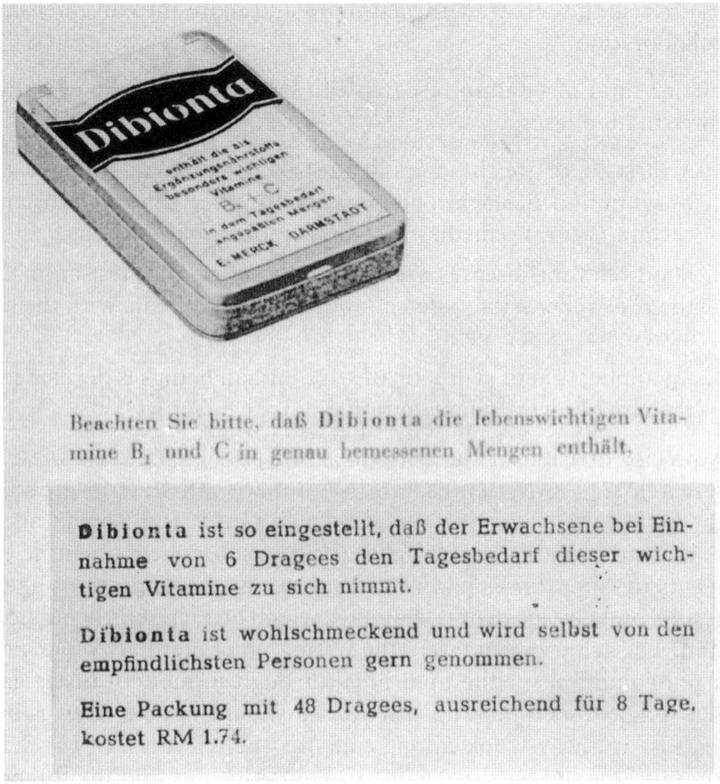

Beachten Sie bitte, daß Dibionta die lebenswichtigen Vitamine B, und C in genau bemessenen Mengen enthält.

Dibionta ist so eingestellt, daß der Erwachsene bei Ein-
nahme von 6 Dragees den Tagesbedarf dieser wichtigen Vitamine zu sich nimmt.

Dibionta ist wohlschmeckend und wird selbst von den
empfindlichsten Personen gern genommen.

Eine Packung mit 48 Dragees, ausreichend für 8 Tage,
kostet RM 1.74.

Fig. 8. *The Merck Company's product Dibontia, 1939*

chemical proceedings and their connection as well as the general
meaning of these 'accessory food substances', being tasteless and invisible, remained obscured. The dispersed experiences and speculations
could not be ascertained and were becoming lost again in part, for
lack of a systematic methodology of natural sciences.

- After 1900 the first reliable results from laboratory experiments on
  vitamin diseases were presented. But the dominance of the then most
  successful bacteriology and especially the insistence on Justus Liebig's
  triad of protein, fats, and carbohydrates plus water and 'salts' as sole
  elements of all human nutrition, as well as the rigid maintenance
  of quantitative measurements, turned out to be serious obstacles for
  this new research. Since nearly all leading German nutritionists at
  first ignored or underestimated the role of the 'accessory nutritive substances' and criticised the 'vitamin hurly-burly', they lost their international leading position in nutritional science[46]. So, vitamin researchers
  of several other nations were the ones to make progress during the
  first two decades of the twentieth century. It is remarkable that vita-

min research thereafter turned more and more into an international collaboration.

- The method of vitamin research can be divided chronologically into three main phases:

  1. At first there are therapies against some epidemic diseases caused by vitamin deficiencies; people see only external symptoms and use certain natural remedies based on empirical knowledge.

  2. Food relevant diseases are artificially induced in test-animals and the researcher tries to detect optimal medicaments with the help of systematic experiments.

  3. An application of synthetic diet for human beings is developed with the aim of identifying additional nutritive factors.

- A precise division of the periods is not possible because these three research stages overlap each other. But we can state in general that the first phase in Europe stretches from Greek and Roman antiquity to the end of the nineteenth century. The subsequent scientific experiments in laboratories had in the beginning no connections and their results only an accidental character which attracted little public attention. The achievements were the setting-up of methods which became a pre-condition for the final breakthrough to modern investigations. The single epoch-making discoveries should not be over estimated, because it always took a long time for the relevance of the detected vitamin, for the nutritive value to human beings and the life process to be discerned. The vehement academic controversies on the recognition of this new discipline of nutritional science did not end until 1930.

- The detection of the vitamins took place in laboratories, but the results had then to be put into practice. In the handbooks of nutritional science this important transfer process has been overlooked till today. As cookery and housekeeping books show, the acceptance of vitamin knowledge began after much delay at the end of the 1920s. From this turning point we can speak of the first influences of vitamin research on normal households and their meals. The lack of public nutrition advisory boards probably hindered the uptake of new recommendations to improve food quality in this way.

- The increasing lack of knowledge of the correct vitamin balance created for a short time a sort of 'gold-rush atmosphere'. A number of small quack-doctors tried to make profits with quick self-manufactured 'vitamin preparations' which were not scrutinized by the authorities. Advertisements from the early 1930s demonstrate that they tried to follow in the wake of the popular health reform movement. But these rather ridiculous products with their boasting promises to solve many health complaints disappeared as soon as the first legal norms for vitamin production were issued and international pharmaceutical enterprises conquered this market with their highly effective and safe vitamin preparations. These products with detailed information about the content and prescriptions for their use by the consumer became a sort of symbol for improving health and a modern lifestyle. These 'artificial' vitamins made people independent from natural barriers and harvest variations, and the food processing plants acquired, besides modern preservation methods, a new prop for their efforts to raise the quality of food.

• The expansion of nutritional science through vitamin research can be interpreted as a change of paradigm, if we follow the theory about the structure of scientific revolutions of the American physicist and natural philosopher Thomas S Kuhn[47]. As we have seen here the theoretical base of a valid dogma reached a point of rising scientific uncertainty and consciousness of new expectations which could not be served by the old system. Liebig's theory of the triad protein, fats and carbohydrates as a unique base for all life was definitely called into question at the beginning of the twentieth century; his quantitative aspects were supplemented by qualitative ones and a totally new paradigm was gained. The traditional doctrine therefore had to be changed in a revolutionary manner.

BIBLIOGRAPHY

Abderhalden, Emil and Schaumann, H. Beitrag zur Kenntnis von organischen Nahrungsstoffen mit spezifischer Wirkung, *Pflügers Archiv*, 172 (1918), 11.

Aberhalden, Emil and Mourriquand, G. *Vitamine und Vitamintheorie*, Bern, 1948.

Ackerknecht, Emil H. *Kurze Geschichte der Medizin*, 3rd edn, Stuttgart, 1975, new ed, 1997.

Ankenbrand, Lisbeth. *Die Rohkostküche. Gesundheit durch vitaminreiche Nahrung*, Stuttgart, 1928.

Aron, Hans. Referat über Casimir Funk, Die Vitamine, ihre Bedeutung für die Physiologie und Pathologie mit besonderer Berücksichtigung der Avitaminosen, *Zentralblatt für Biochemie und Biophysik*, 16 (1913/14); Ueber akzessorische Nährstoffe und ihre Bedeutung für die Ernährung des Kindes, *Berliner Klinische Wochenschrift*, 55 (1918), 546–50.

Aron, Hans and Gralka, K. Vitamine und akzessorische Nährstoffe, *Oppenheims Handbuch der Biochemie*, 6, 2nd edn, Leipzig, 1924.

Backstrom, J F. *Observationes circa Scorbutum*, Leyden, 1734.

Bässler, Karl-Heinz and Lang, Konrad. *Die Vitamine*, Darmstadt, 1975.

Bätz, E. *Mitteilungen der Deutschen Gesellschaft für Natur; und Völkerkunde Ostasiens*, vol 1882, no 21

Bayer, Wolfgang and Schmidt, Karlheinz. *Vitamine in Prävention und Therapie*, Stuttgart, 1991.

Beaglehole, J C. *The Journals of Captain Cook I: The Voyage of the Endeavour*, Cambridge, 1955.

Berg, Ragnar. *Die Vitamine. Kritische Übersicht über die Lehre von den Ergänzungsstoffen*, Leipzig, 1922.

Bickel, Adolf. *Vitamine, Fermente, Salze in der Nahrung*, Berlin, 1927.

Biggar, H P. *Early Trading Companies of New France*, Toronto, 1901; *The Voyages of Jacques Cartier*, Ottawa, 1924.

Bömer et al, eds. Allgemeine Bestandteile der Lebensmittel. In *Handbuch der Lebensmittelchemie*, Vol 1, Berlin, 1933.

Bomskov, Christian. *Methodik der Vitaminforschung*, Leipzig, 1935.

Böttcher, Helmuth M. *Das Vitaminbuch*, Köln and Berlin, 1965.

Brauchle, Alfred. *Geschichte der Naturheilkunde in Lebensbildern*, Stuttgart, 1951.

Budd, G. *Tweedie's System of Practical Medicine*, Philadelphia, 1840.

Castro, J de. *La géographie du faim*, Paris, 1953.

Carpenter, Kenneth J. *The History of Scurvy and Vitamin C*, Cambridge, 1986.

Cray, William C. *A Centennial History*, S l, New Jersey, 1984.

Drummond, Jack C and Wilbraham, Anne. *The Englishman's Food. A History of five centuries of English diet*. A rev edn with a new chapter by Dorothy Hollingworth, London, 1957.

Duin, Nancy and Sutcliffe, Jenny. *Die Entdeckung der Vitamine*, A d Engl, Köln, 1993.

Eddy, W H and Dalldorf, G. *The Avitaminosis*, Baltimore, 1944.

Eijkman, Christiaan. Das antineuritische Vitamin und die Beriberi, Nobel-Stiftung, Stockholm edn, *Autorisierte Ausgabe aller Texte und Dokumente zum Nobelpreis für Medizin in deutscher Sprache*, Zürich, s.a.

Fähndrich, Wilhelm. Klinik und Therapie der Vitamin-C-Mangelkrankheiten, Lang, Konrad and Schoen, Rudolf eds, *Die Ernährung. Physiologie, Pathologie, Therapie*, Berlin, 1952.

Foster, W. *The Voyage of Sir James Lancaster to Brasil and the East Indies, 1591–1603*, London, 1940.

Fragner, Jiri. *Vitamine*, Jena, 1964.

Friedrich, Wilhelm. *Handbuch der Vitamine*, München/ Wien /Baltimore, 1987.

Fulton, John F. *Selected Readings in the History of Physiology*, 2nd edn, Yale, Conn, 1966.

Funk, Casimir. On the chemical structure of the substance which cures Polyneuritis in birds, induced from a diet of polished rice, *Journal of Physiology*, 43 (1911), 395; Über die physiologische Bedeutung gewisser bisher unbekannter Nahrungsbestandteile, der Vitamine, *Ergebnisse der Physiologie* 13 (1913), 125-205; Die Vitaminlehre, ihre wissenschaftliche und praktische Bedeutung, *Die Naturwissenschaften*, 2 (1914), 121–5.

Funk, Casimir. *Die Vitamine. Ihre Bedeutung für die Physiologie und Pathologie*, 3rd edn, München, 1924.

Funk, Casimir and Macallum, Archibald. Die chemischen Determinanten des Wachstums, *Zeitschrift für physiologische Chemie*, 92 (1914), no 1, 13–20.

Grmek, Mirko D. *Geschichte des medizinischen Denkens*, München, 1997.

Grünewald, Max. Die Bedeutung der Vitamine der Nahrung, *Metallarbeiterzeitung*, 46 (1927), 313.

Gubler, J C. *Handbook of Vitamins*, New York, 1984.

Hahn, F V von. Vitaminhaltig?, *Die Volksernährung*, 4, (1929), 299–300; Von der Vitaminbedeutung für unsere Ernährung und vom Vitaminunfug in modernen Kochbüchern, *Die Volksernährung*, 4 (1929), 41–3; Ist die Bekämpfung des Vitaminschwindels möglich? *Zeitschrift für Volkserährung und Vitaminkost*, 8 (1933), 83–6.

Harris, L J. *Vitamins in Theory and Practice*, Cambridge, 1955.

Haushaltungsschule Mönchengladbach eds. *Die Haushaltungsschule. Ein Lehrbüchlein für die Schülerinnen der Haushaltungsschule, herausgegeben unter Mitwirkung von führenden Fachlehrkräften*, Mönchengladbach, 1929.

Hawkins, Richard. *Voyage into the South Sea in the Year 1593*, London, 1622.

Hess, Alfred F. *Scurvy: past and present*, Philadelphia/London, 1920.

Hirsch, A. *Handbuch der historisch; geographischen Pathologie*, 1, Erlangen, 1860.

Hoffmann La Roche, ed. *Vitamin Basics*, Basel, 1994.

Hofmeister, Franz. Die Vitamine, *Blätter für Volksgesundheitspflege*, 21 (1921), 74–6.

Hopkins, Frederick Gowland, Die Anfangsgeschichte der Vitaminforschung, Nobelstiftung Stockholm. In Hopkins, F G, ed, *Autorisierte Ausgabe aller Texte und Dokumente zum Nobelpreis für Medizin in deutscher Sprache*, Zürich, 1929.

Huhle-Kreutzer, Gabriele. *Die Entwicklung von arzneilichen Produktionsstätten aus Apothekerlaboratorien*, Stuttgart, 1989.

Huisgen, Rolf. Liebigs unvergängliches chemisches Werk, Zeitschrift für Landwirtschaftliche Forschung, Sonderheft 3: *J v Liebig im Lichte der Forschung des 20. Jahrhunderts*, Frankfurt a M/Darmstadt, 1953.

Huldschinsky, Kurt. Rachitis, Klemperer, Georg and Klemperer, Felix, eds. *Handwörterbuch der Medizin*, Berlin, 1932, 367–8.

IFAK; Studie (Westdeutschland). Bekannheitsgrad von Vitaminen wächst, *EVIAKTUELL Hrsg Arbeitskreis Ernährungs- und Vitamin – Information e V*, no 1, Frankfurt a/M, 1992.

Ihde, Aaron and Becker, Stanley. Conflict concepts in early vitamin studies, *Journal of History of Biology* (1971), 1–33.

de Knecht-van Eekelen, Annemarie. Uit de bibliotheek van het Nederlands Tijdschrift voor Geneeskunde: Speculum Scorbuticum; opvattingen over ontstaan, behandeling en preventie van scheurbuik, *Nederlands Tijdschrift voor Geneeskunde*, 139 (1995), no 39, 1156–1553.

Koch- und Haushaltungsbuch für Schule und Haus. Bearbeitet und herausgegeben von Hauswirtschaftslehrerinnen in Barmen, 6th edn, Barmen, 1921.

Koelliker, Oscar. *Die erste Umsegelung der Erde durch Fernando de Magellanes und Juhan del Cano 1515-1522*, Leipzig, 1908.

Kramer, J G H. *Medicina Castrensis*, Nürnberg, 1735, new edn, 1983; *Disputatio epistolica de Scorbuto*, Nürnberg, 1737.

Lang, Konrad and Schoen, Rudolf, eds. *Die Ernährung. Physiologie, Pathologie, Therapie*, Berlin, 1952.

Leicester, Henry M. *Development of Biochemical Concepts from Ancient to Modern Times*, Cambridge, Mass, 1974.

Levenstein, Harvey. *Paradox of Plenty. A Social History of Eating in Modern America*, New York/Oxford, 1993.

Lieben, Fritz. *Geschichte der physiologischen Chemie*, Leipzig/Wien, 1935.

Liebig, Justus. *Die Thier-Chemie oder die organische Chemie in ihrer Anwendung auf Physiologie und Pathologie*, 3rd edn, Braunschweig, 1846.

Liljestrand G. Laudation. Christiaan Eijkman für die Entdeckung des antineuritischen Vitamins und Sir Frederick Gowland Hopkins für die Entdeckung des wachstumsfördenden Vitamins 1929, in Nobelstiftung Stockholm, ed, *Autorisierte Ausgabe aller Texte und Dokumente zum Nobelpreis für Medizin in deutscher Sprache*, Zürich, 1929.

Lind, James. *A Treatise of the Scurvy*, Edinburgh, 1753. Deutsch: *Abhandlung vom Scharbock. Nach der zweiten Ausgabe aus dem Englischen übersetzt von Johann Nathaniel Pezold*, Riga/Leipzig, 1775.

McCollum, Elmer Verner. *A History of Nutrition. The sequence of ideas in nutrition investigations*, Boston, Mass, 1957.

Mani, Nikolaus. Die wissenschaftliche Ernährungslehre im 19 Jahrhundert, Heischkel-Artelt, Edith, ed, *Ernährung und Ernährungslehre im 19. Jahrhundert*, Göttingen, 1976, 22-75.

Noorden, Carl von and Salomon, Hugo. *Allgemeine Diätetik*, Berlin, 1920.

Nowell, C E. *Magellan's Voyage Round the World*, Evanston, 1962.

Platen, Moritz. *Die neue Heilmethode. Lehrbuch der naturgemäßen Lebensweise, der Gesundheitspflege und naturgemäßen Heilweise. Neu bearbeitet von Ärzten, Hygienikern und Pädagogen*, vol 1, Berlin, 1913.

Possehl, Ingunn. *Modern aus Tradition. Geschichte der chemisch-pharmazeutischen Fabrik E Merck Darmstadt*, 2nd edn, Darmstadt, 1994.

Pschyrembel. *Klinisches Wörterbuch*, 255th edn, Berlin/New York, 1986.

Quenzer, Emma. *Das süddeutsche Koch; und Haushaltungsbuch*, 4th edn, München, 1930.

Ravenstein, E G. *A Journal of the first Voyage of Vasco da Gama, 1477–1499*, London, 1898.

Regin, Cornelia. *Selbsthilfe und Gesundheitspolitik. Die Naturheilkundebewegung im Kaiserreich, 1889 bis 1914*, Stuttgart, 1996.

Reyher, P. Der gegenwärtige Stand der Vitaminforschung, *Die Volksernährung*, 4 (1929), 67 ff.

Röhmann, F. Über die Ernährung mit Mäusen mit einer aus einfachen Nahrungsstoffen zusammengesetzten Nahrung, *Biochemische Zeitschrift*, 64 (1914).

Rote Liste. Preisverzeichnis deutscher pharmazeutischer Spezialpräparate. Hrsg von der Fachgruppe Pharmazeutische Erzeugnisse der Wirtschaftsgruppe Chemische Industrie, 3rd edn, Berlin, 1939.

Royal Society, ed. *Philosophical Transactions*, vol LXV, abridged vol XIX, London, 1809, 58–60.

Schadewaldt, Hans. Die Ernährung der Seeleute, Heischkel-Artelt, Edith, ed, *Ernährung und Ernährungslehre im 19. Jahrhundert*, Göttingen, 1976, 318–49.

Scheibler, Sophie Wilhelmine. *Allgemeines Deutsches Kochbuch*, 47th edn, Leipzig, 1927.

Scheunert, Arthur. Vitamine, in Böhmer et al, eds, *Handbuch der Lebensmittelchemie. Ernährung und allgemeine Lebensmittelgesetzgebung*, Berlin, 1933.

Schneck, Peter. *Geschichte der Medizin-systematisch*, Bremen, 1997.

Stepp, Wilhelm. Die Bedeutung der akzessorischen Nährstoffe. Referat, erstattet in der gemeinschaftlichen Sitzung der Abteilungen für Physiologie, Pathologie, Innere Medizin und Kinderheilkunde der 86. Versammlung deutscher Naturforscher und Ärzte in Bad Nauheim 1920, *Zeitschrift für ärzliche Fortbildung*, 18 (1921), 95–9, 124–8.

Stepp, Wihelm and Görgy, Wilhelm, eds. *Avitaminosen und verwandte Krankheits-zustände*, Berlin, 1927.

Stepp, Wilhelm and Kühnau, Joachim. Übersicht über die Ergebnisse der Vitamin-forschung in den Jahren 1926–1931, Bethge et al, eds, *Handbuch der normalen und pathologischen Physiologie*, 18 (1932), Berlin.

Sukup, Sophie. *Iß dich schlank! Eine Auswahl kalorienarmer Rezepte*, Stuttgart, 1921.

Venzmer, Gerhard. *Lebensstoffe unserer Nahrung. Was jeder von Vitaminen wissen muß*, Stuttgart, 1935;

Die Wirkstoffe des Lebendigen. Von Hormonen, Vitaminen und anderen Lebens-reglen, Stuttgart, 1948.

Verein für wirtschaftliche Frauenschulen auf dem Lande Bayerischer Verein, ed, *Kochbuch*, 9th rev edn, München, 1927.

Virchow, C. Die Bedeutung der Nährsalze, *Die Gesundheit in Wort und Bild* (1908), 246–9.

Vogel, Martin. Kapitän Cook als Ernährungsreformer. Ein Beitrag zur Geschichte des Skorbuts, *Zeitschrift für Ernährung*, 3 (1933), no 8, 240–3.

Wintermeyer, Ursula. *Vitamin C. Entdeckung, Identifizierung und Synthese*, Stutt-gart, 1981.

NOTES

1 IFAK-Studie, 1992.
2 Funk, 1913, 125–205; see Scheunert, 1933, 769, 773 ff; Funk, 1914, 121;125; Funk, 1924.
3 Röhmann, 1914, 30; Hofmeister, 1921, 74–6; Stepp, 1921, 95; Scheunert, 1933, 775.
4 Noorden and Salomon, 1920, 6.
5 Venzmer, 1948, 161 ff; Pschyrembel, 1986, 161 ff; See Bässler, 1975; Gubler, 1984; Bayer, 1991.
6 Hirsch, 1860, 522; Hess, 1920, 1–6; Lieben, 1935, 166; Venzmer, 1935, 38 f; Lang and Schoen, 1952, 418 ff, 53, 557f ; McCollum, 1957; Böttcher, 1965, 56, 85.
7 Carpenter, 1986. Here are early notes of scurvy symptoms and their remedies; see also Böttcher 1965, 58; Biggar, 1901, 18–62; Biggar, 1924; Koelliker, 1908; Nowell, 1962; Fragner, 1964, 17; Abderhalden and Mourriquand, 1948; Castro, 1953; probably the older German expression *scharbock* – scurvy (Dutch *scheurbuik*) stems from the famous physician, humanist and friend of Luther Enricius Cordus (August Heinrich Simtshausen, 1486–1534); See Fragner, 1964, 17; de Knecht–van Eekelen, 1995, 1553–6.
8 Kramer, 1737; See Backstrom, 1737; Foster, 1940; Hawkins, 1622; Schade-waldt, 1976, 318–49; Carpenter, 1986, 17–19.
9 Lind, 1753; See Drummond et al, 1957, 133–46.
10 Beaglehole, 1955; Vogel, 1933, 240–3; Schadewaldt, 1976, 339; Carpenter, 1986, 79–80.
11 Royal Society, 1809, 58–60; Wintermeyer, 1981, 15.
12 Hirsch, 1860, 537–51; Fähndrich, 1952, 537 f; see also Budd, 1840.
13 McCollum, 1957, 154; Böttcher, 1965, 30; Funk, 1924, 13 ff; Friedrich, 1987, 220.

14 Detailed descriptions of Eijkman's experiments in Böttcher, 1965, 42 ff; see
    Funk, 1924, 14; Funk, 1913; Duin and Sutcliffe, 1993, 122; Bickel, 1927, 76;
    Fulton, 1966, 454; the first German report about beriberi in East Asia by
    Bätz, 1882, no 21; see Eddy and Dalldorf, 1944; Harris, 1955.
15 Liebig, 1846.
16 Lieben, 1935, 181 f; Scheunert, 1933, 774; before Hopkin's epoch-making
    transaction in the *Journal of Physiology*, 44 (1912), 425, Dumas, 1871,
    Lunin, 1881, Soci (1891), Hall, 1896, Häußermann, 1897, Falta and Noeg-
    gerath, 1905, Henriques and Hansen, 1905, Pekelharing, 1905, Jacob, 1906
    and Stepp, 1909 had given hints of an unknown additional food substance
    which had an important influence on human life, although the quantities are
    tiny. Hopkins reached the climax of this debate and culminated the results.
17 Funk, 1924, 9–10; Böttcher, 1965, 73 ff; Fulton, 1969, 457.
18 Hoffmann La Roche, 1994, II.
19 Funk, 1924, 146.
20 Abderhalden and Schaumann, 1918, 1; see Funk, 1911, 395.
21 An overview of the debate on the nomenclature in Scheunert, 1933, 769, 773
    ff; See Stepp and Györgi, 1927, 8–9; Virchow, 1908, 246–9; Berg, 1922, 6;
    Funk and Macallum, 1914, 13–20; Stepp and Kühnau, 1932.
22 See Venzmer, 1948, 200 ff; McCollum, 1957, 229 ff.
23 Stepp and Györgi, 1927, 5 ff; Böttcher, 1965, 75 ff.
24 Venzmer, 1948, 200.
25 Wintermeyer, 1981, 16–36.
26 Böttcher, 1965, 212 ff; Venzmer, 1948, 195; Wintermeyer, 1981.
27 A good overview on the rachitis disease in Huldschinsky, 1932, 367 ff.
28 Scheunert, 1933, 820 ff.
29 Friedrich, 1987, 93.
30 Venzmer, 1935, 209 ff; Friedrich, 1987, 93.
31 *Zentralblatt für Biochemie und Biophysik*, 1913/14–1921. For the adher-
    ence to the term 'accessory nutritive substances' and the critics on Funk's new
    expression 'vitamin' see Stepp, 1921, 95; Aron, 1913/14, 758–60.
32 Aron, 1918, 546-50; Reyher, 1929, 67; Aron, 1924.
33 See F V von Hahn's articles against vitamins in *Zeitschrift für Volk-
    sernährung*, 4 (1929), 41–3, 299–300, and 5 (1933), 83–6. About similar
    controversies in the United States reports Ihde, 1972, 1–33.
34 Hahn, 1933, 83–6.
35 *Zeitschrift für Volksernährung*, (1925/26), 153 ff; (1928), 103 ff; (1936),
    165 ff; (1937), 312 ff.
36 Hopkins, 1929, 460 ff; the birthright of Hopkins confirms also Röhmann,
    1916; see Funk, 1924, 9-10.
37 See *Koch- und Haushaltungsbuch*, (1921), 577; *Verein für wirtschaftliche
    Frauenschulen*, (1927), 6.
38 Scheibler, 1927, 577; *Verein für wirtschaftliche Frauenschulen*, (1927), 6;
    Ankenbrand, 1928; Sukup, 1921, 17; for first recommendations for fresh veg-
    etables and attacks against the 'protein legend' before World War I see Regin,
    1996, 187–8; Platen, 1913, 352 ff; Brauchle, 1951.
39 *Die Haushaltungsschule*, (1929), 18 ff.
40 Huhle-Kreutzer, 1989, 145.
41 Rote Liste, 1939.

42 Rote Liste, 1939, 80–2, 118, 127, 732.
43 See for the following Levenstein, 1993, 13 ff.
44 Cray, 1984, 55; 66.
45 *Die Lebensreform*, 9 (1932), no 8, 502; ibid no 7, 387; ibid no 11 last cover page.
46 Lieben, 1935, 15ff; Ackerknecht, 1997, 193 ff; Mani, 1976, 22–-75.
47 Kuhn, 1976.

16 Between medical ideals and financial restraints: standards of German hospital food in the nineteenth and early twentieth centuries

Ulrike Thoms

In the year 1842 the diet scheme of Berlin's famous Charité was discussed. One comment stated the usefulness of the so-called small portion, and of rolls instead of a normal bread portion, and explained that:

> on the one hand in strong and full fleshy individuals ... scabies is stubborn, so that often laxatives and small portions are necessary in support of the cure; on the other hand, a great number of the sick are homeless and work-shy subjects, for whom the Charité means a welcome asylum, and care for their health, and therefore – despite all controls – they avoid following medical instructions so as to slow down the healing of their illness for as long as possible. For these people hunger is the single means of making their stay in the hospital unpleasant for them and forcing them to follow the instructions more thoroughly. Yes, in the last years, I have found myself compelled to deprive the sick, who retarded the cure on purpose, of the roll as well.[1]

Contrary to what one might expect, the author of this letter was not the treasurer of the Charité, but the medical director of the gynaecological clinic Karl Alexander Kluge. Especially striking is his intermingling of such different aspects as the institution's economy, medical treatment, social differentiation and discipline. In Kluge's view, very small portions for those showing scabies served several purposes: it was part of the medical treatment, it educated the sick and poor to follow medical advice, it saved the hospital a lot of money by not giving the sick much expensive food and it prevented the sick from coming back soon, which created places for others.

What took place here was an essential part of the process of social disciplining in the seventeenth and eighteenth centuries, as analyzed and described by Michel Foucault.[2] This process resulted in making the patient a suggestible and therefore controllable individual and was developed in institutions such as prisons and hospitals, where the knowledge necessary for disciplining people could be gathered. As controls are already in place here, a further disciplining process is not required: not only are they obedient and reliable, but efficient and can act independently as well.

This paper shows how hospital diet was involved in this process. It will describe the way in which an order of diet, a system of norms within the institutions, was developed and how it worked. It concentrates on the question of the influence of medicine and the developing nutritional physiology on nutrition, which appear to have been overestimated in former works.[3] But the interesting questions of social differentiation, which occur within the institutions themselves, are not treated here.

Thus it goes beyond the recently prevailing attempts to use data on institutional diet instead of the scarce data for the diet of the underclasses. This approach generates insights into the general development of consumption, but diet in institutions shows many differences from ordinary diet. Most important is the fact that inmates of an institution cannot freely choose their diet, but are stuck with what is thought to be appropiate in terms of health, economy, social class and so forth.

One has to remember that the German hospital of the eighteenth and early nineteenth centuries served a number of functions: it was not a clinic in the strict sense of Foucault, which he described as a place of formation of medical knowledge, but a place to care for the poor in different ways. So the Berlin Charité was at the same time hospital, academy for military medicine, lunatic asylum and workhouse up to the beginning of the nineteenth century.[4]

Though it is clear that the development of the clinic had consequences for the hospital as far as medical treatment and its innovations through scientific research were concerned, there was only a little medical treatment within the eighteenth-century hospital. Several factors, which cannot be fully described here, led to nursing instead of treating the ill, and thus an overall approach of economical housekeeping dominated.[5] This did not necessarily harm the patients. As Johann Theodor Eller stated in 1730: 'where good nutriment is missing, medicaments can help only a little':[6] good nutrition could achieve much more than medicine, especially in the case of the poor, often undernourished patients.

With the beginning of the nineteenth century, the situation changed dramatically for a great number of hospitals and their own financial situation became worse and worse. At the same time the number of poor grew dramatically. Most hospitals suffered from a lack of funds, and had to endure scarcity. Another point was the professional training of the medical staff, taking place within the process of medicalisation.[7] Though the hospital's finances were not all that interesting to them, it remained an important place for them.

Above all, the clinic was important for gathering and organising information on the process of nutrition in health and disease and on nutritional needs. In this respect, the general acceptance of Descartes' view on nutrition as a circuit model of eating and digesting, dominated by the question of nutritive values and the economy of nutrition, was most important.[8]

Secondly, the hospital was the ideal place to test the new power and professional authority of the medical practitioners. The inmates were dependent, as they were poor and would get no treatment elsewhere. They had neither the money, the knowledge, nor the social position, to defend themselves against the different medical and disciplinatory procedures to which they were subjected.

There can be no doubt that by the early nineteenth century physicians were always asked for their opinion on feeding the inmates. But it was the administration's view on financial economy, and not the medical view on economy of the body's functions, that was decisive. In fact, most of the hospital physicians were neither interested in what the inmates were served, nor were they able to say positively what would be good for them. At least, they could and would say, what should be omitted from the diet to preserve the sick from serious harm. It is important to note that medicine and dietetics on the whole had reached a deadlock in the 1830s.[9] Whereas the old dietetic practice, heavily impressed by Hippocratic and Galenic opinions, slowly disappeared with the new laboratory science of nutrition, nothing new or useful was set up. What was missing was a system capable of integrating the numerous and partly diverging results of the basic research of chemistry and biology. A number of basic problems had to be solved first and then to be put together for a conclusive picture to be reached and made applicable in the end.[10] Despite the fact that the importance of a healthy diet was stressed by the physicians, the dietetic rules imposed on the institution's inmates were only rough formulae. But around the middle of the nineteenth century, important changes took place. In his famous work, *Organic Chemistry in its Application to Physiology and Pathology*, (1840), Justus Liebig interpreted the countless, seemingly diverging results of researchers like Magendie, Prout, Dulong, Despretz, Mulder and Boussingault.[11] His *Animal Chemistry*, published two years later, traced the development of the whole nutritional and dietetic science over the following decades.[12] It was based on the belief that it was possible to list the patients' precise need for the various nutrients. Hence this concept was deeply indebted to Descartes' view of the human body as a machine. Liebig's work pointed in two directions: firstly, the role of the different nutrients, especially the qualitative role of protein; and secondly, the energy side of the nutritive process. It was the latter direction that led to a kind of quantitative euphoria and consequently laid the foundation for the formulation of dietetic norms. Most important for institutional diet was Liebig's concentration on the question of how much protein man needs, as protein metabolism basically summed up metabolism to him. The general problem was that proteins were the most expensive nutrients of all, and therefore were traditionally scarce in the institutional diet.

In Germany, norms for institutional diets including formulae of that kind, were set up since the late 1840s. At first, they were published within general works on nutrition.[13] From 1850 there were publications dealing particularly with the diet of institutions; from then on the amount of medical expertise upon institutional diets increased, and about 1870 nutritional physiology was decisive for reforms of the dietary schemes of different institutions. This is mainly due to the work of Carl Voit. He declared that he wanted to make use of the existing results of science to improve the diet of institutions' inmates.[14]

But it took a long time to spread the new knowledge. Tradition was very strong and of great influence. An impressive example of this is the diet prescribed in fever. In the medicine of the eighteenth century, fevers were the most common diagnosis: between 1731 and 1742 nearly 10 per cent of all persons received at the Charité, in Berlin, had fevers. Only infections and injuries had higher percentages. Between 1754 and 1772 fevers still stood top of the list: 19 per cent of male and 12.7 per cent of female patients were received at the Charité because they were suffering from fever.[15]

In Hippocratic and Galenic medicine fevers had played an important role, being not only a symptom as now, but the illness itself. Additionally, most diseases were accompanied by fevers, which were said to have a purifying effect. This doctrine was passed on almost unchanged throughout medieval and early modern times. But as Hippocrates had postulated a moderate diet, his later followers tended to exaggeration and practised a so-called emptying diet. Feeding the sick only small portions dominated up to the second half of the nineteenth century, now based on diverse medical theories, but ending in the same treatment. The Iatrophysicists such as Friedrich Hoffmann (1660–1742) interpreted illness as a disturbance within the mechanical processes of the body, as obstruction of the smallest vessels. To remove this obstruction, one had to follow a modest diet, if not an abstinent one. Vitalistic concepts such as the most discussed one of John Brown (1735–1788) with its irritability theory tended to assert the same, but put the old practice into a new theoretical frame. To Brown, life depended on the effect of nervous irritation, caused by outer and inner stimuli, being warmth, air and food, and the movement of muscles, muscle tissues or emotions, respectively. The lack as well as excess of stimuli was supposed to lead to illness. Brown called these conditions 'asthenie' and 'sthenie', the latter of which was indicated by fever. The main purpose of nutrition was to reduce or to improve the irritation, to bring the body back to its natural balance. Either irritation was avoided, for example by doing without hot spices or fried meat, or irritation was aimed at by administering substances like alcohol, opium and camphor. It is important to note Brown's conviction that most people fall ill because of sthenie, so that nutrition has to be reduced. This mostly resulted in a diet consisting simply of water soups. And it culminated in a sort of nutrition, paradoxically called 'absolute diet', in which the patient did not get any food at all.[16]

This theory spread especially through the importance exerted by the General Hospital (Allgemeines Krankenhaus) at Bamberg, which has been characterised as a model institution.[17] Here Röschlaub and Marcus, the famous German protagonists of the irritation theory, held their clinical lectures. Many doctors of influence, for example Johann Christian Reil and Christian Wilhelm Hufeland, travelled to Bamberg in order to acquaint themselves with the organisation of the hospital as well as with Andreas Röschlaub's and Adalbert Marcus's doctrines.[18] In fact, the experts asked for their opinion about the best diet scheme for the Charité, and referred to the medical authorities of John Brown and Albrecht Haller and the example of the hospital at Bamberg.[19]

And indeed, in the nineteenth century the diet in a great number of hospitals was divided into full, half, quarter and eighth forms, as was usual there. In the Charité there was a number of followers of Brown's theory. Here the said division of diet was introduced in 1811 and practised until the 1840s, though revised several times in between.[20] It is worth noting that taking over a certain scheme from another institution was furthered by the existence of a kind of information tourism on the one hand and a vivid information exchange between the different institutions on the other. The famous philanthropist John Howard was the most famous to undertake such journeys and found a number of followers.[21] Institutions were ready to serve the interest in information not only by answering questions by letter, as happened very often, but even by receiving visiting guests, who sometimes even had to pay an entrance fee.[22] The passing on of information was formalised later on, for example through handbooks on hospital management and by associations of hospital administrators with their periodicals and annual meetings. All this had the effect that the organisational structures or a certain number of their organisational traits were copied in others.[23]

But let us get back to the question of fever diet. Around the turn of the nineteenth century, the French physician François Broussais (1772–1838) changed to a physiological view of illness. In his theory, so-called inflammations were most important. All of them were caused or at least accompanied by a gastroenteritis, which therefore had to be the most important tackling point of therapy. For him, the giving of plenty of food to sick persons meant to nourish and to breed the fever itself.[24]

Though a change took place in the proofs of practices, the norms for feeding the ill did not change during the first half of the nineteenth century, but remained the same as in the eighteenth century. The quantity of food was still kept low though, because they were afraid of doing harm by giving too much food and of 'overthrowing the convalescent', as an eighteenth century source stated.[25] Another spoke of the 'severe conducting of diet', which clearly points to its disciplinary aspects.[26] In fact, the consequences for the patients were harsh. On the occasion of an epidemic of putrid fever in the workhouse at Münster in 1787, its physician P M Roer stated: 'The convalescents hurry away from the room for the sick, because they are so hungry, therefore more food must be admitted to them, when they, urged by hunger, promise to work the full number, so I cannot hold them back.'[27]

As one follows the calculation according to the requirements of the different diet schemes as of 1824, it becomes clear that these did not mean qualitative as much as quantitative differences. The whole diet contained about 85 kg of meat a year, 301 kg of bread, 9.1 kg of butter, 58 kg of different cereals and 13 kg of dried peas, different vegetables and potatoes, whereas the quarter diet contained no vegetables, only 30 kg of meat, 20 kg of cereals, 3 kg of butter and 5 kg of bread, and the eighth only included broth made of 130 kg of meat and nothing else. Naturally, this resulted in expenditures which differed considerably between the various diet forms. The whole diet required expenditures nearly three times as high as that for the quarter diet.[28]

This dietary scheme resulted from a reform conducted in 1822. Its discussion makes clear the importance of the monetary factor that was still prevalent then. The administrative director stated: 'By the way, the physicians are of my opinion, that the prescription of the first and the three-quarter diet should not be handled too generously.'[29] In fact, the budgets always calculated that most of the sick would fall into one of the inferior diet schemes, whereas the whole diet was only scheduled for a small proportion of them. Following the budget for 1819, only a third of all patients were to receive the full, but nearly 60 per cent the half and 14 per cent the quarter diet.[30] The one of 1830/31 had further reduced the number of the full diet's recipients, but introduced a three-quarter diet, planned for roughly 21 per cent of all inmates. A third of the patients should get the half diet. So about 50 per cent of the sick were assigned the quarter form![31]

As has been shown above, the physician's efforts for professional training had had some success around the turn of the century. From now on they were accepted as specialists in questions of diet. But this does not mean that the arrangement of diet really did change. First, there was the role of the doctrine of economy, which remained strong. The discussion of the needs for certain diet schemes shows that these were initially thought to render the costs of feeding calculable. In the beginning of the nineteenth century they were mostly discussed within the general parameters of the budget and of financial reorganisation of the institution. So controllability played an important role, whereas medical aspects had to play second fiddle. In a report on the grievances within the hospital from 1819, the medical and administrative director of the Charité, stated that, in general, the physicians should be subject to regulations as little in the matter of diet as of nursing. On the other hand, a freely handled prescription would and did not only provoke mistakes in the distribution of diet, but especially could lead to cases of fraud. To the administrator, the doctor's task consisted only in bringing the different diet forms into an appropiate relationship, for in this way, medical and economical purposes were served all in one.[32] This proves once again that the view of medical knowledge on nutrition was deeply indebted to economical thinking. Doctors and physiologists themselves thought this would be their most important task. So Carl Voit clearly declared in 1877 that, to him, the task of the modern physiologist in relation to institutional diet was to satisfy man's needs in the cheapest way.[33]

Relating to the diverging interests of scientists, doctors and administration, this opinion could be shared by all, as it promised the acceptance of professionality as well as the acceptance of financial restraints. And we must not forget the fact that the doctors accommodated to the pressures of economy so as not to endanger their new, but still weak professional and power position. In consequence, the dietary schemes were further minimised with the help of the calculations about physical needs.

So it can be stated that the creation of uniformity and minimilisation were the most important traits in the development of hospital diet at the beginning of the nineteenth century. They met general medical beliefs, as the explanations on the theory and therapy of fevers have shown, as well as the standpoint of physiology, which was dominated by the search for the subsistence level.

There can be no doubt that the hospital doctors at that point had finally succeeded in the general acceptance of their professional autonomy as regards the question of food. This was mainly due to the acceptance of the importance of their formal knowledge of nutrition. It is striking that complaints about the quantity of food arose after the dietary schemes had been reformed according to the modern physiological knowledge of those days. In fact, reforms mainly resulted in the reduction of fibrous foodstuffs, such as pulses and brown bread and in increasing albuminous and easily digestible foodstuffs. As the latter were the more expensive, the difficult to digest but filling, fibrous foodstuffs had to be reduced as much as possible to avoid the increase in expenses. In consequence, some of the patients might have been constantly hungry. In 1894, in a general discussion about the grievances within the Charité, even diet was criticised as being too low. In a report to the minister, medical arguments were used by the administration to support their view that the portions served were largely sufficient.

> But it does happen, that the sick in their opinion are always hungry during their stay in the hospital, because they are used to the mostly greater amounts of vegetables outside and deceive themselves about the nutritional value of the less voluminous food they get within the hospital. They judge a diet by the filling of their stomach and the deceptive feeling of satiation, and feel a kind [sic] of hunger, as soon as their stomach is not filled that much [. . .] – therefore it has happened, that the sick spread the opinion that they had been starving for food while in hospital.[34]

According to this view, the professional autonomy of medicine had developed so far that it alone was believed to have the defining power in questions of physical needs. Neither the administration nor the patients themselves were seen as deciding instances, even if the sick were the only ones feeling the hunger.

As this had not been the case before, even the doctors were clever at finding a way of encompassing professional autonomy, holding their ground in struggles with administration as well as with patients. Using their professional knowledge, the physicians answered the administration's efforts to reduce the prescription of extra items with the argument that some patients needed certain extra dishes or foods for medical reasons or simply for the fact that the normal diet was too bad.[35] As a matter of fact, they succeeded in using the so-called 'extraordinary prescriptions' to balance out a seemingly insufficient diet in relation to both quality and quantity. Initially, extra food was restricted to a very small number of patients, as it was expensive. But in course of time the variance and number of prescriptions rose. Whereas the diet scheme for 1798 allowed only 13 different articles, eg white bread, broth, wine, eggs, dried fruit and milk, in 1817 this number had already risen to 21, in 1830 to 23, in 1894 to 25 and in 1910 to 48 different standard articles. At first, extra prescriptions had been an exception, so that in the year 1833 only about every second patient got one extra portion per day, if at all. Though the administration sharply controlled the extra prescriptions and asked the doctors to reduce them according to the diet scheme, as early as 1876 this number had risen to three and a half extra portions per day, but it kept rising further up to nearly five extra portions. From 1894 a certain number of extra food articles, introduced as maximum allowances, in fact were given as standard allowances for every diet scheme.[36]

So one can conclude, that a liberalisation within the prescription of extra food for the sick had taken place. But a certain deviation from the diet scheme was only accepted if ordered by a doctor from the hospital. The administration, in fact being unable to judge whether or not there was a medical need for extra food, had imposed a formal procedure for this. Every single prescription had to be permitted and was registered. If the order, once set up, seemed to be endangered, this danger was fought against. First, the staff was punished severely if they abused the order. The working contracts contained appropriate paragraphs and threatened severe punishment, to avoid, for example, embezzlement. A deviation from these instructions was punished with the workhouse or dismissal.[37] Second, the physicians were often admonished to reduce the numbers of extra prescriptions, if they seemed to be too high to the administration. Third, the patients were more and more forbidden to eat anything else than the prescribed food, as the order of diet was considered good and sufficient. This latter practice was extended during the nineteenth century. In a number of hospitals, there was a shop where the sick could buy whatever was sold and they wanted. The list of foodstuffs of, for example, the Charité shop contained coffee, tea, tobacco, sugar, syrup, milk, rolls, butter, beer, lemons, bitter beer, and spirit.[38] Again, it was the doctors who took the initiative in stopping this custom in the first decade of the nineteenth century, because with these shops, the diet of the inmates was out of their disciplinary reach. Without regard to the fact that most of the inmates were simply too poor to pay for extra food, they argued that the sick did harm to themselves by eating the wrong food at the wrong time and relapsed into the illness from which they just had recovered. In other words, they claimed regulating power, founded on their professional knowledge. The shop was closed in 1816.[39] Some years later, the same arguments were used for justifying the prohibition of the bringing in of food by visitors. The doctors stressed that every sick person received the diet suitable for him without suffering from a lack of food. Again it was argued that the additional food was not under medical control and therefore could do serious harm to the sick.[40] So visitors were forbidden to bring in food if they did not have a doctor's permit, which was controlled at the entrance.[41] In the Charité, it was not handled severely in times of poor diet resulting from the hospital's financial problems. As the economic situation had improved, the prohibition was renewed again in the 1820s and was still in operation at the beginning of the twentieth century.

In fact, the arguments used against selling food within the hospital, or against gifts of food, resemble the arguments used in the discussion of fever diet. It has already been explained that this diet was not only prescribed for medical, but also for economic reasons. On the whole, the general opinion concerning food necessities did change around the middle of the century, due to the research done by Liebig. So did the theory on fever-diet, in which revolutionary changes took place. The Englishman Robert James Graves (1796–1853) was of the opinion that 'the starving system has, in many instances, been carried to a dangerous excess, and that many persons have fallen victim to prolonged abstinences in fever.'[42] Inanition, a weakness following from a general loss of strength, was the most dangerous consequence of fever to him, which was at least re-inforced, if not provoked, by low diet.[43] Therefore he required a plentiful diet during fever to prevent this. His investigations were confirmed by Charles Chossat (1796–1875).[44] The experiments Chossat had undertaken over several years had shown that certain symptoms of fevers were identical with those of inanition, so that a strongly withdrawing diet only increased the dangers of fever instead of lowering them. A great number of doctors concluded that it was necessary to rather give a fattening diet to the fever patients. In their view, alcohol was ideal for this purpose, because it had only little volume, but a high energy value.

And indeed there was a rising consumption of alcoholic beverages within the hospitals. Nevertheless, this could be interpreted as a consequence of the irritability theory, as alcohol was seen as a means to irritate the nerves of the sick. However, the overwhelming number of sick were to suffer from an excess of irritation. But neither the dietary system itself nor the practice of prescription really changed until the very end of the nineteenth century. Despite a general improvement of quality and quantity, the basic structures remained the same, as once again the example of the Charité shows. The full or first diet still consisted of what was believed to be the food of healthy working men at home, ie coffee and bread in the morning, vegetables and a portion of meat for lunch and soup with bread in the evening. The other

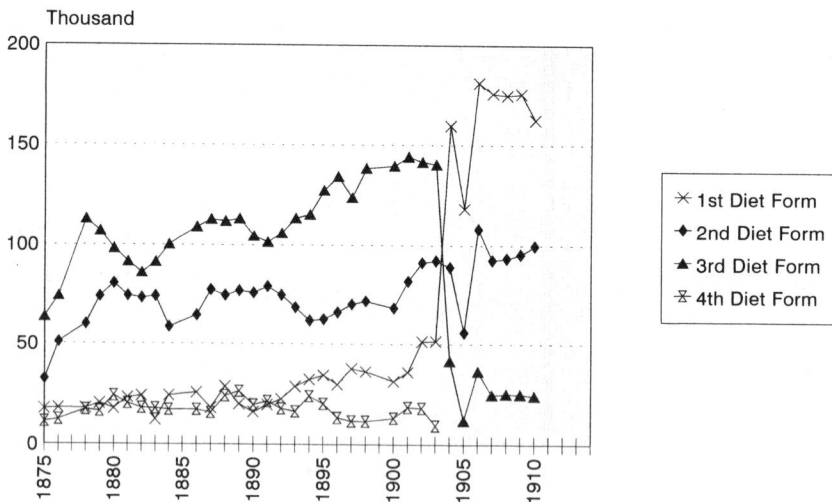

Fig. 1. *Distribution of the different Diet Schemes in the Hospital in the Friedrich-shain, Berlin, 1875–1910 (number of catered days a year). Source: Verwaltungs-Bericht (1876)ff.*

forms varied mainly in what was given for lunch. The second form contained a portion of meat as well, but with rice cooked in milk or mashed
potatoes. In the third form broth, some weak vegetables and meat were
given, whereas lunch for the fourth form still simply consisted of broth.[45]
It has already been mentioned that the hospital budgets calculated for a
high number of inmates ranked in the inferior diet forms. This was not only
wishful thinking on the part of the administration, but was indeed put into
practice. As a report from 1891/92 proudly stated, 53 per cent of all sick
were fed in the cheap dietary schemes, which were held to be valid for most
of the severely ill and equally for fevers.[46] Some hospitals, as for example
the Clemens Hospital at Münster, did have a full diet form, but not a single
patient got the full diet between 1877 and 1900. Here, about 90 per cent of
the ill were regularly fed the half diet.[47] There was clearly no general change
until the beginning of the twentieth century, as the following graph for the
Hospital in the Friedrichshain, Berlin, demonstrates.

Again, the vast majority got the third diet up to the year 1903, when
a new diet scheme was introduced and the fourth diet was entirely omitted. The increase in the number of the first diet form and the decrease in
those of the third diet, does not indicate a general change in the prescription practice. It results from the nature of the reform itself, as this simply
replaced the first with the third and the third with the first diet form, as far
as concerned the quality and quantity of the food.[48] Even the fact that the
cost of the first diet fell about 30 per cent during these years had no significant influence. As stated above, there can be no doubt that financial reasons

Thousand Marks

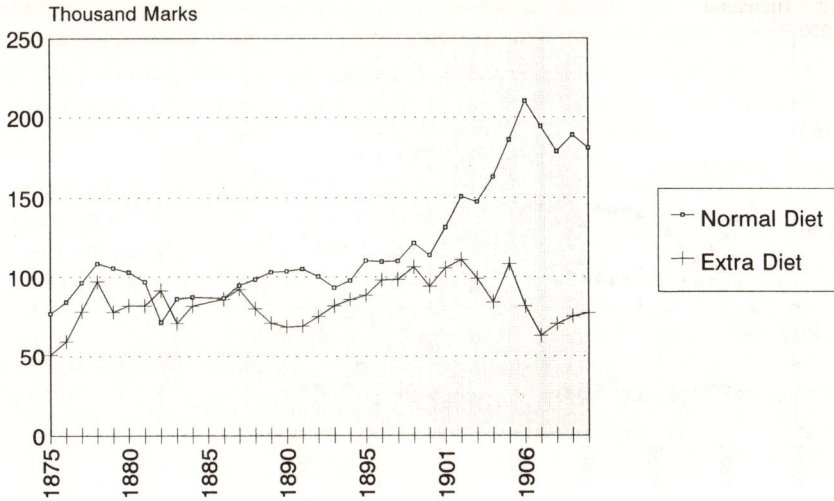

Fig. 2. *Expenses for extra diet in the Hospital in the Friedrichshain, Berlin, 1876–1910. Source: Verwaltungs-Bericht (1876)ff.*

dominated this practice. In 1875 the hospital had to pay 91 Pfennigs for a patient's daily diet in its first form, but only 63 Pfennigs in its second, 58 in its third and 33 Pfennigs in its fourth.[49] Still, the doctors switched to the extra diet to be sure that their patients got enough. This is shown by the figures for the food expenses (see Fig 2).

In 1875 the expenses for extra food were about 66 per cent of those for the normal diet and were still increasing during the following years. It was not until the improved diet reform of 1903 that these percentages fell again.

To the modern reader it is obvious that the complicated combination of normal diets and extra portions caused the administrative as well as the medical personnel a lot of work and increased the waste of food and therefore unnecessary expenditures. Nevertheless, it took until the beginning of the twentieth century for the administration to understand how efficiency depended on individualisation. One can see that the diet schemes from the beginning of the twentieth century onwards give only rough guidelines and in many points resemble cookery books, especially in the great variation of food and dishes. From 1904 the inmates of the Charité got as much bread as they wanted, and no longer as regulations prescribed. As the administration proudly stated, this procedure was much more economical as it reduced waste and thus saved much money.[50] Another symptom is marked by the changes in the diet schemes of the military hospitals. From 1912 there was no longer any strict diet scheme. From then on, hospitals had only a limited budget, within which they could organise the diet as they liked according to medical purposes and specific preferences. This meant the victory of individualisation. The question of the monetary, physiological and medical economics of nutrition had been generalised and standardised to such an extent that exact and dictatorial regulations of hospital diet were no longer needed within the hospital, whether on economic grounds, or for medical purposes.

ARCHIVES

UAHU (Universitäts-Archiv der Humboldt-Universität Berlin), Charité-Direktion, Nr. 60–3; 1361; 1368; 1584–87; 1588; 1594; 1606.
Stadtarchiv Münster, Stadtregistratur, Fach 203, Nr. 10.
STAMS (Staatsarchiv Münster), Fürstentum Münster, Kabinettsregistratur, Nr. 2833.
GStA (Geheimes Staatsarchiv Merseburg),Rep 76, VIIIA, Nr. 3644, 224.

BIBLIOGRAPHY

Artelt, Walter. *Medizinische Wissenschaft und ärztliche Praxis im alten Berlin in Selbstzeugnissen*, Berlin, 1948.
Bemerkungen eines Reisenden durch die königlich preussischen Staaten in Briefen, 2. Theil. Altenburg, 1779.
Berliner Krankenhäuser, Berliner Rettungswesen, Berlin, 1909.
Chossat, Charles Jacques Etienne. *Recherches expérimentales sur l'inanition. Mémoire auquel l'Academie de Sciences a décerné en 1841 le prix de physiologie expérimental*, Paris, 1843.
Zur Einführung, *Zeitschrift für Krankenanstalten*, 1 (1905), H. 1, Sp. 1.
Eller, Johann Theodor. *Nützliche und auserlesene Medicinische und Chirurgische Anmerckungen*, Berlin, 1730.
Engstrom, Eric J and Volker, Hess, eds. Zwischen Wissens- und Verwaltungsökonomie. Zur Geschichte des Berliner Charité-Krankenhauses im 19. Jahrhundert, *Jahrbuch für Universitätsgeschichte*, 2 (2000).
Foucault, Michel. *Die Geburt der Klinik. Eine Ärchaologie des ärztlichen Blicks*, Frankfurt a M, 1988.
Foucault, Michel. *Überwachen und Strafen. Die Geburt des Gefängnisses*, 8th edn, Frankfurt a M, 1989.
Frevert, Ute. *Krankheit als Politisches Problem 1770–1880. Soziale unterschichten in Preussen zwischen medizinischer Polizei und staatlicher Sozialversicherung*, Göttingen, 1984.
Goerke, Heinz. Anstaltsernährung im 19 Jahrhundert. In Edith Heischkel-Artelt, ed, *Ernährung und Ernährungslehre im 19. Jahrhundert*, Göttingen, 1976, 303–317.
Graves, Robert J. *Clinical Lectures on the Practice of Medicine*, 1841, 2 vols, 2nd edn, Dublin/London, 1848.
Guttstadt, Albert. *Die naturwissenschaftlichen und medicinischen Staatsanstalten Berlins. Festschrift für die 59. Versammlung deutscher Naturforscher und Ärzte*, Berlin, 1886.
Hildesheim, W. *Die Normaldiät*, Berlin, 1856.
Horn, Ernst. *Öffentliche Rechenschaft über meine zwölfjährige Dienstführung als zweiter Arzt des Königl. Charité-Krankenhauses zu Berlin nebst Erfahrungen über Krankenhäuser und Irrenanstalten*, Berlin, 1818.

Howard, John. *The State of the Prisons in England and Wales with Preliminary Observations and an Account of some Foreign Prisons and Hospitals*, 2nd edn, Warrington, 1780.

Howard, William. *An Account of the Principal Lazarettos in Europe, with Various Papers Relative to the Plague. Together with further observations on some foreign prisons and hospitals and additional remarks on the present state of those in Great Britain and Ireland*, Warrington, 1789.

Huerkamp, Claudia. *Der Aufstieg der Ärzte im 19 Jahrhundert. Vom gelehrten Stand zum professionellen Experten: Das Beispiel Preussen*, Göttingen, 1983.

Hufeland, Christoph Wilhelm. *Hufeland. Leibarzt und Volkserzieher. Selbstbiographie*, new edn and introduction by Walter von Brunn, Stuttgart, 1937.

Jahresbericht über den Stand der Gemeinde-Angelegenheiten der Stadt Münster, für das Jahr 1885ff, Münster, 1886ff.

Kessler, Georg Wilhelm, ed. *Der alte Heim. Leben und Wirken Ernst Ludwig Heim's aus hinterlassenen Briefen und Tagebüchern*, 2nd edn, 1846.

Kleinspehn, Thomas. *Warum sind wir so unersättlich? Über den Bedeutungswandel des Essens*, Frankfurt a M, 1987.

Leyden, Ernst von. Allgemeine Therapie der Ernährung. In Ernst von Leyden, ed, *Handbuch der Ernährungstherapie und Diätetik*, vol 1, Leipzig, 1898, 217-281.

Lichtenthaeler, Charles. *Geschichte der Medizin*, vol 2, 3 edn, Köln, 1982.

Liebig, Justus. *Die organische Chemie in ihrer Anwendung auf Agricultur und Physiologie*, Braunschweig, 1840.

Liebig, Justus. *Die Thier-Chemie oder die organische Chemie in ihrer Anwendung auf Physiologie und Pathologie*, 2nd edn, Braunschweig, 1843.

Mani, Nikolaus. Die wissenschaftliche Ernährungslehre im 19 Jahrhundert. In Edith Heischkel-Artelt, ed, *Ernährung und Ernährungslehre im 19 Jahrhundert*, Göttingen, 1976, 22–75.

Moleschott, Jacob. *Physiologie der Nahrungsmittel. Ein Handbuch der Diätetik*, 2nd edn, Giessen, 1859.

Murken, Axel Hinrich. *Vom Armenhospital zum Grossklinikum. Die Geschichte des Krankenhauses vom 18. Jahrhundert bis zur Gegenwart*, 2nd edn, Köln, 1991.

Petersen, Julius. Zur Geschichte der Ernährungstherapie. In Ernst von Leyden, ed, *Handbuch der Ernährungstherapie und Diätetik*, vol 1, Leipzig, 1898, 1–15.

Rothschuh, Karl E. *Geschichte der Physiologie*, Berlin/Göttingen/Heidelberg, 1953.

Rothschuh, Karl E. Krankenkost in alten Tagen, *Deutsches Medizinisches Journal*, 12 (1961), 117–23.

Scheibe, O. Zweihundert Jahre des Charité-Krankenhauses zu Berlin, *Charité-Annalen*, 34 (1910), 1–178.

Seidler, Eduard. *Geschichte der Pflege des kranken Menschen*, 4th edn, Stuttgart et al, 1977.

Tsouyopoulos, Nelly. Reformen am Bamberger Krankenhaus. Theorie und Praxis der Medizin um 1800, *Historia Hospitalium*, 11 (1987), 103–22.

Verwaltungs-Bericht des Magistrats zu Berlin pro 1875ff No X: *Bericht über die Verwaltung des städtischen allgemeinen Krankenhauses im Friedrichshain*, Berlin, 1876ff; since 1894 published as No 14: *Bericht der Deputation für die städtischen Krankenanstalten, I: Krankenhaus im Friedrichshain*, Berlin, 1895ff.

Voit, Carl von, ed. *Untersuchung der Kost in einigen öffentlichen Anstalten. Für Ärzte und Verwaltungsbeamte zusammengestellt*, München, 1877.

Winau, Rolf. *Medizin in Berlin*, Berlin/New York, 1987.

NOTES

1 Rust to the administration of the Charité on 9 Dec 1842, UAHU, Charité-Direktion, nr 1585, 170.
2 Foucault, 1989; Foucault, 1988.
3 Goerke, 1972.
4 For the history of the Charité see: Scheibe, 1910; Winau, 1987, 76ff; Engström/Hess, 2000.
5 See the description in Artelt, 1948, 69.
6 Eller, 1730, 24.
7 Cf Huerkamp, 1985; Frevert, 1984.
8 Kleinspehn, 1987, 301f.
9 Seidler, 1977, 137; cf Lichtenthaeler, 1982, 472.
10 Rothschuh, 1953; Rothschuh, 1961, 122; Mani, 1976, 28.
11 Liebig, 1840.
12 Liebig, 1842.
13 Hildesheim, 1856; Moleschott, 1859.
14 Voit, 1877, Introduction, 3ff.
15 Winau, 1987, 94.
16 Leyden, 1898, 235; Petersen, 1898, 16.
17 Murken, 1991, 43ff.
18 See Tsouyopoulos, 1976, 110–14.
19 See the several statements by experts on the reform of the Charité's diet from 1799, in: UAHU, Charité-Direktion, Nr. 1584, 6–10.
20 Cf UAHU, Charité-Direktion, Nr. 1584, 109–12. The etat for 1840/42 mentioned a division into first, second and third diets, UAHU, Charité-Direktion, Nr. 1368, 46–52; Hufeland, 1937, 90f.
21 Howard, 1770; Howard, 1789.
22 See Heim's experiences with hospitals in London and Paris, Kessler, 1846, 158, 171. In the archive of the Humbolt University of Berlin there exist four big files, containing letters with questions on the most varied topics of daily life within the Charité, covering the nineteenth to the twentieth centuries, UHAU, Charité-Direktion, Nr. 60–3.
23 Zur Einführung, in *Zeitschrift für Krankenanstalten*, 1 (1905), H 1, 1, 222ff; Kessler, 1846, 158, 171; *Bemerkungen eines Reisenden*, (1779), 20.
24 Lichtenthaeler, vol 2, 1982, 488f; Petersen, 1898, 16; Foucault, 1991, 198ff.
25 *Bemerkungen eines Reisenden*, (1779), 20.
26 UAHU, Charité-Direktion, Nr. 1585, 10.
27 STAMS, Fürstentum Münster, Kabinettsregistratur, Nr. 2833, 11.
28 UAHU, Charité-Direktion, Nr. 1584, 103–6. With a calculated expenditure of about 49 Taler, the half diet was the most expensive, because white instead of brown bread was given.

29 ibid, Nr. 1585, 38.

30 ibid, Nr. 1361, 182.

31 ibid, Nr. 1368, 232.

32 ibid, Nr. 1585, 8–11; Horn, 1818, 98f. This becomes even clearer in the discussion of prison diet.

33 Voit, 1877, 11. There were a number of scientists working on the so-called 'Nährgeldwert', a theory of the best relation of nutrients to price; see the hints in Voit, 1877, 11.

34 GStA Merseberg, Rep 76 VIII A, Nr. 3544.

35 In this sense the explanations of Kluge, see UAHU, Charité-Direktion, Nr. 1586, 172 cf the discussions of the year 1861, UAHU, Charité-Direktion Nr. 1587, 225ff.

36 For the permitted numbers see: UAHU, Charité-Direktion, Nr. 1584, 26; Nr. 1585, 609, 634, Guttstadt, 1886, 54; Scheibe, 1910, 143; for the real figures UAHU, Charité-Direktion, Nr. 1586, 31; Nr. 1587, 144, Nr. 1588, 53; 133, 199; Scheibe, 1910, 143.

37 UAHU, Charité-Direktion, Nr. 264, 14.

38 ibid, Nr. 1606, 4.

39 Horn, 1818, 128f.

40 See the letter of the doctor Förster to the administration of the Charité from 24 July 1826, UAHU, Charité-Direktion, Nr. 1594, 1.

41 UAHU, Charité-Direktion, Nr. 1585, 474.

42 Graves, 1848, 117.

43 ibid.

44 Chossat, 1843.

45 See Scheibe, 1910, 142.

46 GStA Merseberg, Rep 76 VIII A; Nr. 3644, 224.

47 Stadtarchiv Münster, Stadtregistratur, Fach 203, Nr. 10; Jahres-Bericht 1886ff.

48 For a comparison see the Diet Scheme of 1875 in Verwaltungs-Bericht, 1875, 5 and that of 1903 in *Berliner Krankenhäuser,* (1909), 163–205.

49 Verwaltungs-Bericht, 1876, 6; ibid, 1903.

50 UAHU, Charité-Direktion, Nr. 1589, 41.

Part 3

Food products and health

17 From cordial waters to Coca-Cola: soft drinks and health in Britain

John Burnett

1. In 1970 soft drinks accounted for 6.4 per cent (by volume) of all drinks consumed in the United Kingdom except tap water: in 1995 they represented 20 per cent – greater than the share of alcohol (15 per cent) and the same as that of coffee. This ranks as the greatest change in British drinking habits in recent times, following a trend first established in the United States, though still lagging somewhat behind consumption levels in Germany, France and Italy.[1] Nevertheless, soft drinks are the fastest-growing sector of all food and drink sales in Britain with an annual value of £6.4 billion and an advertising expenditure of £89 million, replacing lager as the most heavily promoted drink. Mass-produced and -marketed soft drinks, led by American companies, have achieved world-wide penetration ('Coca-Cola' is the second most universally recognised word on earth[2]): this paper focuses on the growth of consumption in Britain during the last two centuries, but begins with a brief survey of the historical origins of soft drinks and the importance which from the first attached to their health claims.

2. Four principal origins of soft drinks may be identified. The first was the range of 'cordials' and 'elixirs', which were important components of folk medicine from medieval times until the nineteenth century. Influential works such as those by Nicholas Culpeper taught that herbs and their distilled essences stimulated the natural 'Life Force', enabling the body successfully to fight disease:[3] a wide variety of native plants, herbs, flowers, berries, fruits and nuts, supplemented by imported spices, was employed in making 'cordial waters' or 'draughts', their concoction being a recognised part of the housewife's skill at all social levels. Some cordials were primarily medicinal, others simply pleasantly-flavoured drinks, but many had a dual function as therapeutic and enjoyable: almost all were sweetened with sugar or honey and many were considered particularly appropriate for ladies as aids to digestion or restoratives for any mild affliction. Spices such as nutmeg, cinnamon, mace and ginger were often added, while some cordials such as Rosa Solis and Aqua Vitae contained distilled spirits of wine and were similar to liqueurs. But herbs remained the principal constituent, which as well as having curative powers were believed to influence the emotions. 'Every appetite, mood, fear, aberration and abnormality had its

own appropriate restraining herbs':[4] they could assuage grief, subdue passions, strengthen the nerves, stimulate the appetite, aid digestion, and act as rejuvenators and aphrodisiacs. The most widely-read receipt book of the first half of the eighteenth century, Eliza Smith's *The Compleat Housewife*, included the Great Palsey Water ('of excellent use in all swoonings, weakness of heart and decay of spirits'), Lady Allen's Water, Aqua Mirabilis, King Charles II's Surfeit Water and The Golden Cordial (containing gold leaf) as well as Clary and Orange and Lemon Waters, described as 'fine entertaining waters'.[5] Treats and treatments were sometimes distinct, sometimes indistinguishable, while Eau Divine and Eau d'Amour could be respectable subterfuges for intoxicating draughts.

By the later eighteenth century the growing urbanisation of Britain offered fewer opportunities for home-made cordials but more for commercially manufactured products. The two attributes of cordials – the therapeutic and the pleasurable – now tended to separate, some becoming patent medicines or quack nostrums (Olbion Cordial, Duffy's Elixir, Godfrey's Cordial, etc.[6]) while others concentrated on providing a refreshing drink which may or may not have had incidental 'health' benefits. Nineteenth-century recipe books continued to give directions for home-made cordials, often using ready-prepared extracts of herbs and fruits which were now widely available,[7] but many people preferred to buy the proprietary sweetened cordials like those made by Stones, distillers and vintners since 1740, whose well-known Ginger Ale sold 240,000 gallons in 1848: some of this firm's traditional cordials such as Lovage, Clary and Peppermint continued to be marketed until the 1960s.[8]

The line between cordials and simple fruit juices – the second source of modern soft drinks – was a thin one. Tudor and Stuart herbals recommended spring medicines for 'purifying the blood' at a time when many people were in a pre-scorbutic condition after the restricted winter diet: apples, gooseberries, rhubarb and blackcurrants were the principal constituents at this time. The development of citrus fruit drinks, which were to become a mainstay of the soft drinks industry, depended on the expansion of imports of oranges and lemons from Mediterranean countries, the availability of greater and cheaper supplies of sugar from the Caribbean, and the emergence of a demand for non-alcoholic drinks which fitted into new patterns of fashionable consumption. Lemonade and orangeade were known at the time of the Restoration and sold in the proliferating coffee houses, though there was no equivalent in England of the French 'limonadiers' who sold lemonade in the streets and were granted the rights of a 'Companie' in 1676. In some wealthy households citrus drinks came to be incorporated into the reformed menus of people of taste in the eighteenth century, a change which began in Italy and France and involved the rejection of heavy, Baroque meals in favour of lightness and moderation. Strong flavours and smells were now unfashionable; chicken was preferred to coarse meat, heavy wines were diluted or replaced by iced fruit drinks, a guide to 'haute cuisine' in 1807 listing 72 varieties.[9] In England, where the cooler climate encouraged a preference for the new, hot beverages tea, coffee and chocolate, the adoption of citrus drinks was more limited, though they were popular in summer in the numerous Tea Gardens and at domestic entertaining occasions.

By the eighteenth century it was also becoming recognised that citrus fruits, especially lemons, possessed preventive and curative properties for the dreaded disease of scurvy, which caused distressing symptoms of swollen limbs and ulcerated mouths, often resulting in death: it was a major cause of casualties in European navies and armies deprived of ascorbic acid from fresh fruit and vegetables. Its diagnosis was long hindered by the belief that the disease took two distinct forms – 'land scurvy' and 'sea scurvy' – which required different remedies: land scurvy was treated with infusions of plants, especially scurvy-grass, cresses, sorrel and brooklime,[10] but on his voyage to the South Seas in the 1590s Sir Richard Hawkins carried oranges and lemons as a 'certain remedy' for sea (muriatic) scurvy with good results. Yet it was only in 1795 that the Royal Navy required a daily dose of lemon juice after six weeks at sea – the 'grog' consisting of 1 gill of rum to 3 of lemon juice and water, the rum acting as a preservative as well as encouraging take-up.[11]

The long debate over scurvy and its treatment ultimately had important consequences for the domestic consumer. The fact that of an adult male population in 1801 of two million, 120,000 served in the Navy during the Napoleonic Wars disseminated knowledge and appreciation of citrus drinks. Further, a direct link can be established between the therapeutic uses of fruit juices at sea and their commercial development as refreshing soft drinks for the home market. From 1854 Merchant Shipping Acts required vessels likely to be away from port for ten days or more to carry lemon or lime juice. A firm of ships chandlers in Leith, Rose's, began supplying ships with West Indian lime juice: Lachlan Rose patented a method of preserving the juice without the use of spirits, so establishing Rose's Lime Juice, the first commercially-made concentrated fruit juice in Britain, 'delicious, cooling and refreshing ... eminently suitable for family use'.[12]

A third source of soft drinks was 'small beers', drinks which bore some resemblance to the product of malt and hops but were usually home-made from native herbs and plants.[13] Of many regional varieties the commonest were dandelion and burdock, horehound, spruce beer, sarsaparilla and root beer (sassafras): in Lancashire nettle beer was popular and in Yorkshire sweet gale (or bog myrtle) beer.[14] By the nineteenth century some of these had passed from the domestic to the commercial stage, with ginger beer becoming the most widely-known in the north of England and Scotland where more than a thousand trade names have been identified.[15] Home-brewing of small beers also continued with the availability of ready-prepared extracts of herbs and flavours, among the most widely advertised Kemp's Compound Essences and Mason's Extracts, 6d bottles of which

would make eight gallons of liquid. They had particular appeal to Victorian teetotallers, as cheap, respectable alternatives to 'the demon drink':
Mason's, for example, advertised their products as giving 'herbaceous fla-
vour and a creamy head like bottled ale . . . always acceptable at Picnics or in
the home'.[16] The Church of England Temperance Society advocated 'Stokos'
(oatmeal and lemon), 'Cokos' (cocoa and oatmeal) and 'Hopkos' (hops and
ginger), the last particularly recommended for the harvest field in place of
the traditional liberal supplies of beer,[17] (it is not known to what effect.)

Since medieval times certain English springs and wells had been credited
with curative powers, and by the seventeenth century spas had developed
at some of these, providing facilities for 'taking the waters' as well as rec-
reational amenities. Wealthy visitors to Bath, Harrogate, Buxton and other
spas did so partly for their supposed cures of rheumatism, gout or excessive
indulgence, partly for amusement and social intercourse. The importance
of spas in the history of soft drinks lies in the fact that at an early date their
waters began to be marketed to a wider public who were thereby familiar-
ised with consuming a bottled, labelled drink in their own homes. By the
early eighteenth century 'the movement of people to the spas was matched
by the movement of spa waters to the people':[18] of 65 English spas at this
time 9 had their waters bottled and distributed to most parts of the country,
while London wholesalers also imported the famed waters of Spa, Pyrmont
and Seltzer.[19]

Natural mineral waters indirectly bridged the gap between the traditional drinks so far described and the modern, science-based soft drinks
industry. Through the seventeenth and eighteenth centuries chemists began
to analyse the solid constituents of spa waters,[20] but particular interest cen-
tred on attempts to imitate the effervescent Continental waters which were
popular but most expensive and difficult to transport. Here the crucial discovery of 'fixed air' (carbon dioxide gas) was made by Joseph Priestley in
1767: he could now carbonate ordinary water by pumping the gas into it
and produce what he believed to have superior medicinal properties to Pyrmont water. Production on a large scale was due to Jacob Schweppes, a
Genevan watchmaker, who in partnership with an engineer, Nicholas Paul,
established a factory in London in 1792: from 1798 what was now generally
known as 'soda water' was advertised as good for gout, complaints of the
bladder, stone and indigestion, and for 'invigorating the system and exalt-
ing the spirits'.[21]

Aeration was the key process which enabled effervescent waters to be
manufactured in quantity and to be charged with a range of fruit syrups
and herbs to produce flavoured drinks. Surprisingly, Schweppes did not
market an aerated lemonade until 1835 and their Quinine Tonic Water until
1858, though their position as Britain's leading manufacturer was established when they gained the concession to supply the Great Exhibition in
1851 and sold over a million bottles of soda water there.[22] The transition
from medicinal to purely pleasurable uses was, however, mostly the work

of smaller, local manufacturers who could set up business on little capital: inventions by Hamilton and Bramah made it possible easily to compress carbonic acid gas, and in 1813 Plinth patented a 'Portable Fountain' which could be mounted in shops or on a cart for street sale.[23] London in the 1840s had more than 50 soft drinks manufacturers, often now using proprietary essences in a sugar syrup rather than natural juices and flavours. Henry Mayhew believed that in 1850 there were some 1,500 street-sellers of soft drinks in London during the summer months, many of whom made their own drinks at home from lemon-acid, essence of cloves, ginger, yeast and sugar: they sold ½ pint bottles for 1d (up to half froth is 'considered very fair'). A somewhat superior product was sold from the street 'Fountains', handsome machines of mahogany and glass with pumps for the injection of gas, but Mayhew was told that some sellers added oil of vitriol (sulphuric acid) 'to bring out the sharpness'.[24]

By the last quarter of the nineteenth century a number of large-scale manufacturers had emerged in the soft drinks industry, either processing their own materials or buying from specialist firms like C W Field (established 1870) and Stevenson and Howell (established 1882) who employed trained chemists to produce concentrates, essences and essential oils. By then the industry was becoming sharply divided between large, science-based manufacturers who supplied hotels, restaurants and the better-class domestic market, and small, local producers who relied on artificial ingredients and sold their penny bottles at sweetshops rather than at respectable family grocers. The widespread location of manufacturers by the end of the century (for example 28 in Dorset, 24 in Norwich, 37 in Glasgow, 11 in Falkirk[25]) suggests the growth of a new mass market for soft drinks in late Victorian Britain which reflects important social changes. From the mid-1870s disposable income was rising, especially in the working-classes, as a result of major reductions in the prices of bread, meat, tea and sugar: shorter working hours and the growth of holidays encouraged more leisure expenditure. Furthermore, alcohol consumption reached a nineteenth-century peak in 1876 (beer 34 gallons/head/year; spirits 1.1 gallons/head/year) from which high point it began a slow, though irregular, secular decline. This was probably not so much directly due to the propaganda of the organised Temperance Movement as to the general development of 'respectability' among the working-classes, improved diet and housing standards and the growth of countervailing alternatives to the public house.

The expansion of the soft drinks industry also depended crucially on increased supplies and lower costs of raw materials, especially fruit and sugar. United Kingdom sugar consumption rose dramatically in the second half of the century, from 25 lbs/head/year in 1850 to 85 lbs in 1900:[26] previously heavily taxed, the duty of 14/- a hundredweight in 1854 was totally abolished in 1874, thereby halving the price of raw sugar.[27] At the same time the commercial development of tropical and sub-tropical regions of the world greatly expanded the availability and range of fruits, which could

now be transported in refrigerated holds: it is estimated that imports of
fruit increased tenfold between 1870 and 1908 to thirteen million hun-
dredweights, more than half of which were citrus fruits.[28] Statistics of production and consumption of soft drinks at the end of the century must
be uncertain in view of the large numbers of small manufacturers whose
output was probably under-recorded, but estimates suggest a rise in United
Kingdom consumption from 66.7 million gallons in 1870 to 87.9 million by
1900,[29] around sixteen pints per person per year.

3. Despite the continued existence of much small-scale production, by 1914
the British consumer was beginning to become familiar with a number of
branded soft drinks, widely advertised on a national or regional basis. The
precedent for this change came largely from the United States, where by
1870 there were already 387 manufacturing plants.[30] America in the late
nineteenth century was besieged by proprietary nostrums, appealing to a
nation experiencing the strains of transition from scattered, rural communities to an urban, competitive society: it was also strongly influenced by
the temperance movement, which had powerful support from organised
religion and women's groups. 'Hines Root Beer' was patented in 1876 as
'The Nation's Temperance Drink' and also claimed to purify the blood:
Dr A C Ayer's 'Sarsaparilla' promised to 'dislodge and expel any lurking
taint of Scrofula from the system', while Dr Pepper's cherry soda drink of
1885 'aids digestion and restores vim, vigor and vitality.'[31] The immediate
antecedent of Coca-Cola, however, was a French drink of 1863, 'Vin Mariani', a concoction of wine and coca leaves which was strongly advertised
in Europe and America with alleged testimonials from President McKinley,
Queen Victoria and three Popes. In 1885 Dr John S Pemberton of Atlanta,
Georgia, added an imitation of 'Vin Mariani' to his range of cough and
headache cures, but also included the West African kola nut, which possessed similar properties to coca.[32] The same year, Atlanta adopted Prohibition: Pemberton dropped the wine from his formula, experimented with
numerous fruits, herbs and essential oils, and in 1886 launched 'Coca-Cola'
as a temperance drink and 'brain tonic . . . a cure for all nervous affections'.
Asa Candler, who acquired Coca-Cola on Pemberton's early death, played
down the therapeutic claims, and when public concern over the contents
of patent medicines resulted in the Pure Food and Drugs Act, 1906, he
removed the traces of cocaine from the product and in future presented it
primarily as a leisure drink, refreshing and enjoyable but also associated
with health, youth and activity.
    This combination of health with pleasurable gratification in a cheap, mas-
sively advertised drink influenced the development and marketing of new
products in Britain. Schweppes produced a kola drink in 1885 though it
did not appear regularly in their price lists until 1916.[33] Much more successful were two new drinks which bore some resemblance to the constituents
and promotional methods of Coca-Cola – 'Iron Brew' produced by Robert

Barr, a mineral water manufacturer of Falkirk in 1901 and promoted as a stimulating tonic, restorative and hangover cure,[34] and 'Vimto' (originally 'Vimtonic') invented by a Manchester druggist, John Joel Nichols, in 1906 as a temperance drink and 'Health Tonic'. Containing 29 ingredients known only to two people (like Coca-Cola) and first intended to supply temperance bars and cafes, it established its reputation as a healthful leisure drink mainly in the north of England before 1914 but subsequently with an international market.[35] 'Iron Brew', 'Vimto' and 'Tizer' ('The Appetizer') were strongly-flavoured drinks which bore some resemblance to the earlier home-made herb beers, but the mass production of fruit juices also developed strongly at the turn of the century, with Stower's Lime Juice rivalling Rose's, and 'Idris' and 'Kia-Ora' (established 1911) setting new standards of quality for citrus juice.

This growth in the soft drinks industry was not maintained in the 1920s after wartime restrictions on output and sharp price rises: production fell to 44.8 million gallons in 1922, recovering to 75.9 million in 1932 and thereafter increasing rapidly to 110.2 million in 1938,[36] equivalent to around 20 pints/person/year. This suggests that disposable income for what was still regarded as a luxury in the 1920s was restricted by high prices (1920 average price of soft drinks 6.6d/pint) and economic instability, but increased in the more favourable climate after 1932, aided by a large fall in sugar prices: by 1938 average soft drinks prices had fallen to 3.6d per pint. As yet soft drinks were not regularly found in British homes with the exception of soda and tonic water used mainly as 'splashes' for spirits by some of the middle-classes; strongly associated with leisure, soft drinks were mainly consumed in cafes, Temperance Bars, herbalists' shops, cinemas and dance-halls. They were for special occasions, not for everyday use: consumption was encouraged by the spread of holidays with pay, mass attendance at sporting events, the growth of personal mobility by bicycles, cars and motor coaches and by the popularity of 'hiking' and exploration of the countryside. Some soft drinks continued to be advertised as temperance beverages as a guarantee of their suitability for family use, but more often stressed were broad health claims in the form of generalised 'tonic' values: 'Vimto', for example, stated that it 'eliminates that out-of-sorts feeling', and that 'You will feel the benefit from the very first glass'. Nor did it hesitate to adopt 'the new knowledge of nutrition', an advertisement at Christmas, 1929, stating that 'Vimto' was 'not only delicious, but good for you too because it is rich in the vitamins that you need so badly in wintry weather'.

World War II had both positive and negative effects on the soft drinks industry. Under the powers of the Ministry of Food the whole industry, which was a heavy user of sugar and imported materials, was controlled and rationalised into the Soft Drinks Industry (War Time) Association: all supplies were rationed, prices fixed and many small firms disappeared. By contrast, on America's entry into the war the Coca-Cola Company's President, Robert Woodruff, promised that every US serving man or woman would be able to buy a bottle for five cents anywhere in the world, regardless of the cost. Bottling plants accompanied the American forces to Britain, Europe, North Africa and the Far East, spreading 'coca-colonisation' virtually around the world. In Britain knowledge about the value of fruit juices was promoted by the Ministry of Food, which made allocations of blackcurrant and rosehip syrup to pregnant mothers, infants and children under five, replaced after 1941 by 'lease-lend' supplies of concentrated orange juice.[37]

Revival of the industry dates from 1952 when sugar rationing ended. With practically full employment and rising wages in the 1950s and 1960s, the youth market was now particularly targeted by the mass media as a distinct sector with surplus income, leisure time and the persuasive influence of fashion. By the 1960s Britain was beginning to experience a cultural revolution which included a transformation of drinking habits: in 1970, when estimated consumption of soft drinks had grown to 500 million gallons (about 80 pints/person/year) Derek Cooper could observe,

> No kitchen is complete now without a bottle of Squash, and whereas before the war in 'the Age of Want', if a child was thirsty it went to the tap it now automatically pours out a 'drink', usually orange in colour and flavour if not in content.[38]

Mothers who had reared their children on subsidised orange juice acquiesced in the belief that they were providing a 'health' beverage, though the principal ingredients, often to the extent of 90 per cent or more, were water and sugar (or saccharin): the Soft Drinks Regulations, 1964, allowed the use of a wide variety of acids, preservatives and artificial colours which were believed to be at least not harmful to health.[39]

However, the real explosion of consumption is a recent phenomenon, occurring mainly within the last twenty-five years. In 1995 production stood at 9.6 billion litres: 57.7 per cent of British people drank soft drinks daily, compared with 77 per cent who drank tea and 31.8 per cent who drank alcohol.[40] The reasons why soft drinks have moved from luxuries to near-necessities are complex and under-explored. Consumption is ultimately influenced by the state of the economy and the volume of personal disposable income, and despite recessions and the return of high levels of unemployment, the majority of families have enjoyed greater spending powers than at any previous period. Food now takes less than 20 per cent of household income, almost half as much as in the 1940s, releasing more purchasing power for leisure, holidays and non-essentials. Around three-quarters of all soft drink purchases are now brought home,[41] indicating that they are integrated into the increasingly informal, individualised food patterns of today, where snacks account for 40 per cent of meal occasions. Soft drinks fit conveniently into these, as do cans into packed school lunches, now brought from home by 40 per cent of children.[42]

Robert Goizueta, Chairman of Coca-Cola, recently described the product's phenomenal success as due to 'The Three A's – Availability, Affordability and Acceptability'.[43] Availability has certainly greatly increased in Britain, with sales in supermarkets, newsagents, garage forecourts and vending machines. But soft drinks are to do with more than the mere satisfaction of thirst. Part of their psychological appeal is that they can equally be associated with activity and relaxation, with resting or doing, since their high sugar content provides about 80 calories of quick energy per can. Advertisements relate them to enjoyment, gratification and reward, to sports, holidays, escape from work and routine. Their acceptability has also gained because of distrust of the quality of public water supplies and because of disapproval of drink driving: around twelve per cent of British adults are now estimated to be non-consumers of alcohol. Traditionally targeted at younger consumers, advertising has recently been directed towards adults, offering soft drinks as healthy alternatives to alcohol and, in diet form, as aids to slimming. To the current range of drinks – carbonates (49 per cent of the total market, colas 46 per cent of carbonates), squashes (33 per cent), fruit juices (12 per cent) and bottled water (5 per cent)[44] – manufacturers have recently added a range of 'Adult Soft Drinks', many of which focus on 'energy' or 'sports' attributes. In some respects these represent a return to the earlier 'health' associations of soft drinks, though endowed with exotic names intended to convey sophistication – 'Kiri', 'Kisqua', 'Royal Mystic', 'Aqua Libra' and many others. Some contain up to 30 fruit and herbal extracts and echo traditional therapeutic claims – 'Oasis' 'calms and rejuvenates' while 'Aqua Libra' 'helps to restore alkaline balance'.[45] In 1995 these 'New Age' elixirs were joined by another new category of alcoholic 'soft' drinks containing 4–5.5 per cent of alcohol from a shot of spirits and aimed particularly at the 18–24 year age group, though there is concern that their sweetness also makes them appealing to younger drinkers.[46]

4. A 'soft drinks revolution' in Britain may now be considered an accomplished fact, comparable in many respects to that of the 'hot drinks revolution' experienced in the seventeenth and eighteenth centuries. This paper argues that from their origin as home-made cordials to the present-day, mass-produced products, soft drinks have consistently laid claim to health benefits, either for specific ills or for generalised tonic values. It is as though their consumption has required legitimisation beyond mere enjoyment and the satisfaction of thirst – that they need and acquire 'meanings' which justify their role in modern society. This is, of course, not peculiar to soft drinks: tea, coffee, milk, beer, wine and spirits have all at different times been promoted as healthful, though none more insistently and consistently. One possible explanation is that no other drink depends so importantly on its high sugar content which, as well as its addictive nature, carries meanings of love and reassurance.[47] This makes it difficult to assess the validity of the health claims of soft drinks, since so many of the carbonates and fruit juices which dominate the market are so highly sweetened. Perhaps the

main benefits of soft drinks have been as alternatives to potentially more
harmful drinks – natural mineral waters as preferable to polluted public
supplies, 'temperance' drinks rather than over-indulgence in alcohol. On
the other hand, there has been strong criticism of many soft drinks in recent
years for the wide use of artificial ingredients[48] and for the dangers to children's health of excessive sugar. Their increased consumption has contributed to raising sugar consumption in Britain to over 100 lbs/person/year,
twice the amount recommended by many nutritionists.[49] A recent survey
of children aged 1½–4½ years showed that 86 per cent consumed non-diet
soft drinks at an average of 2092 grams per week, while citrus fruits were
eaten by only a quarter of children[50]: the danger is that heavy consumption of sugars can inhibit the appetite for more nutritious foods as well as
having particularly harmful effects on teeth: a third of British children aged
3½–4½ years have experienced dental decay.[51]

Within a remarkably short space of time soft drinks have come to occupy
a central place in the British diet. They represent a classic example of the
power of advertising to shape demand, particularly that of young consumers influenced by fashion and popular culture. Tastes acquired in youth
have now passed into adulthood and into the home, so that despite a demographic downturn in the proportion of younger generations, total consumption of soft drinks is forecast to continue substantial growth.

BIBLIOGRAPHY

Brears, Peter. *Traditional Food in Yorkshire*, Edinburgh, 1987.
Camporesi, Piero. *Exotic Brew. The art of living in the age of enlightenment*. Trans-
    lated by Christopher Woodall, Oxford, 1994.
Coca-Cola Company, Annual Report, Atlanta, 1995.
Cooper, Derek. *The Beverage Report*, London, 1970.
Davies, Jennifer. *The Victorian Kitchen*, London, 1991.
Dietz, Lawrence. *Soda Pop. The history, advertising, art and memorabilia of soft
    drinks in America*, New York, 1973.
Economic and Social Research Council. The National Diet and Nutrition Survey:
    Children Aged 1½–4½ Years. *Data Archive Bulletin*, 61 (Jan. 1996).
Emmins, Colin. *Soft Drinks, Their Origins and History*, Princes Risborough, 1991.
Fairley, Jan et al. *Chambers Scottish Drinks Book: whisky, beer, wine and soft
    drinks*, Edinburgh, 1990.
Fisher, M F K. *A Cordiall Water*, London, 1983.
Goodman, Jordan et al. *Consuming Habits. Drugs in history and anthropology*,
    London, 1995.
Guardian Education, Dangers of Drink, *Resources*, 13 (16 Jan. 1996).
Hanssen, Maurice and Marsden, Jill. *E For Additives: The complete E number
    guide*, Wellingborough, 1985.
Harrison, Brian. *Drink and the Victorians. The temperance question in England,
    1815–1872*, London, 1971.
Hembry, Phyllis. *The English Spa, 1560–1815. A social history*, London, 1990.

Hughes, R Elwyn. The Rise and Fall of the Antiscorbutics. Some Notes on the Traditional Cures for 'Land Scurvy', *Medical History G B*, 34, vol 1 (1990), 52–64.

Inglis, Brian. *Fringe Medicine*, London, 1964.

Johnstone, G N. The Growth of the sugar trade and refining industry. In Derek Oddy and Derek Miller, eds, *The Making of the Modern British Diet*, London, 1976.

Kahn, E J. *The Big Drink. An unofficial history of Coca-Cola*, London, 1960.

Kirkby, William. *The Evolution of Artificial Mineral Waters*, Manchester, 1902.

Leyel, C S. *Elixirs of Life. Culpeper House herbals*, London, 1948.

Longmate, Norman. *The Waterdrinkers. A history of temperance*, London, 1968.

Mayhew, Henry. *London labour and the London Poor, vol 1. The London Street Folk*, London, 1861.

McIntyre, Sylvia. The mineral water trade in the eighteenth century, *Journal of Transport History*, New Series II, Feb (1973), 1-19.

Mintz, Sidney W. *Sweetness and Power. The place of sugar in modern history*, New York, 1985.

Mitchell, B R and Deane, Phyllis. *Abstract of British Historical Statistics*, Cambridge, 1962.

Morgan, R Harold. *Beverage Manufacture (Non-alcoholic)*, London, 1938.

National Food Survey: *Annual Report on Household Food Consumption and Expenditure*, 1994 (HMSO, 1995).

Nichols, Sue. *Vimto. The story of a soft drink*, Preston, 1994.

On the State of the Public Health During Six Years of War. Report of the Chief Medical Officer of the Ministry of Health, (HMSO, 1946).

Pendergrast, Mark. *For God, Country and Coca-Cola. The unauthorized history of the world's most popular soft drink*, London, 1994.

Porter, Roy. *Health for Sale. Quackery in England, 1660–1850*, Manchester 1989.

Prest, A R and Adams A A. *Consumers' Expenditure in the United Kingdom, 1900–1919*, Cambridge, 1954.

Simmons, Douglas A. *Schweppes. The first 200 years*, London, 1983.

Smith, Eliza. *The Compleat Housewife, or Accomplished Gentlewoman's Companion*, facsimile of 1758 edn, London, 1994.

Soft Drinks Industry Reports, Britvic Soft Drinks Ltd (Chelmsford, 1993, 1995, 1996).

Stevenson and Howell Ltd. *The ABC of the Manufacture of Soft Drinks*, 8th edn, London, 1956.

Stone, Richard. *Measurement of Consumers' Expenditure and Behaviour in the United Kingdom, 1920–1938*, 2 vols, Cambridge, 1954.

Tea Council, Annual Report (1995).

Torode, Angeliki. Trends in Fruit Consumption. In Barker et al eds, *Our Changing Fare. Two hundred years of British food habits*, London, 1966.

Wainwright, David. *Stone's Ginger Wine. Fortunes of a family firm, 1740–1990*, London, 1990.

Walker, Caroline and Cannon, Geoffrey. *The Food Scandal*, London, 1985.

Watt, J, et al, eds. *Starving Sailors. The influence of nutrition upon naval and maritime history*, London, 1981.

Wells, Robert. *Pleasant Drinks. Effervescing mixtures, syrups, cordials, home-made wines, etc*, Manchester, c1900.

Williams, Carol and Ward, Patricia. *School Meals. Report of a survey of parents' attitudes to the school meals service*, Consumers' Association, (May 1993).

Woodroof, J G and Phillips, G F. *Beverages, Carbonated and Noncarbonated*, Westport, Connecticut, revised edn, 1981.

Young, Robin. New Age Elixirs Restore Sparkle to Drinks Trade, *The Times*, (22 April, 1995).

NOTES

1 Soft Drinks Industry Report (1995), 3. Consumption of soft drinks in the UK was 145 litres per person per year, in Germany 230, Italy 200, France 185.
2 Pendergrast, 1994, 10.
3 Inglis, 1964, 67–8.
4 Leyel, 1948, 14. Leyel lists 80 Nutritious Herbs, 52 Tonic Herbs and 22 Bitter Herbs.
5 Smith (sixteenth edn 1758), facsimile 1994, 255 seq. Smith included a number of older folk medicines such as Snail Water (500 snails) and Cock Water (for consumption).
6 Porter, 1989, 107 seq.
7 See, for example Wells, c 1900.
8 Wainwright, 1990, 31, 96.
9 Camporesi, 1994, 71, 83.
10 Hughes, 1990, 52–64.
11 Watt et al, 1981, 31. The daily ration was equivalent to six whiskies, and the rum was gradually reduced until abolished in 1970.
12 Fairley et al, 1990, 22.
13 The term 'small beer' also referred to low-gravity beer which came from the second or third brewing of malt and hops: as an alcoholic drink it is not considered in this paper.
14 Brears, 1987, 133.
15 Fairley et al, 1990, 24.
16 Brears, 1987, 134.
17 Davies, 1991, 156.
18 McIntyre, 1973, 1.
19 The leading tea merchant, Thomas Twining, was importing 7,000 flasks of Spa water in 1721–2: McIntyre, 8.
20 Kirkby, 1902, describes the early history of analysis of natural mineral waters.
21 Simmons, 1983, 11–27.
22 ibid, 42.
23 Kirkby, 1902, 82–3, 101.
24 Mayhew, 1861, vol 1, 186–9.
25 Harrison, 1971, 301, 312; Fairley et al, 1990, 24.
26 Mitchell and Deane, 1962, 356-7.
27 Johnstone, 1976 (Tables II and V), 61, 63. The price of raw sugar fell from 21/6d a hundredweight in 1854 to 11/3d in 1900.
28 Torode, 1966, 125.
29 Prest and Adams, 1954, (Tables 47, 52, 58), 75, 84, 88.
30 Woodroof and Phillips, 1981, 4.

31 Information on the history of American soft drinks is from Kahn, 1960; Dietz, 1973 and Pendergrast, 1994.
32 For the indigenous uses and properties of coca and kola, see Goodman et al, 1995, chs 2 and 5.
33 Simmons, 1983, 45–6. Other British manufacturers produced 'Kola Champagne' and 'Kola Tonic' in the 1880s
34 Fairley et al, 1990, 24–7. It is claimed that 'Irn-Bru' (renamed 1946) was outselling Coca-Cola in Scotland in the 1980s by three to one.
35 Nichols, 1994.
36 Stone, 1954, vol I, (tables 53 and 68) 160, 188.
37 On the State of the Public Health During Six Years of War, 1946, 92–3.
38 Cooper, 1970, 49.
39 Cyclamates and rhodamine B, formerly allowed, were prohibited in the later 1960s.
40 Tea Council, Annual Report 1995.
41 National Food Survey 1995 (Tables 2.10, 2.12, 2.13), 9, 11, 12.
42 Williams and Ward, 1993, 9.
43 The Coca-Cola Company: Annual Report 1995, 3–4.
44 Soft Drinks Industry Report 1993, 2.
45 Young, 1995, 8.
46 *Guardian* Education 1996, 13. Campaigners are anxious that 'alcopops' be removed from soft drinks displays in supermarkets and their advertisement controlled.
47 See Mintz, 1985.
48 Hanssen and Marsden, 1985. Permitted ingredients include 11 preservatives, 8 emulsifiers and stabilisers and 4 colours, besides sweeteners and flavourings which may be natural or artificial.
49 It was estimated in 1985 that a bottle of Coca-Cola contained the equivalent of 7 teaspoons of sugar, a glass of bitter lemon 5, tonic water 4 and orange squash 2. Walker and Cannon, 1985, 227.
50 Economic and Social Research Council, Data Archive Bulletin 1996, 9–10.
51 ibid, 11.

18 The making of health biscuits: interaction between nutritional sciences and industrial interests*

Adel P den Hartog

INTRODUCTION

At the end of the nineteenth and the beginning of the twentieth century, human nutrition emerged as a distinct scientific discipline. At the same time in several European countries the relationship between food and health became a point of public concern. The food industry gradually started to take some of the new nutritional concepts into account in manufacturing food products. At present, the food industry cannot be totally indifferent to the outcome of the nutritional sciences. On the contrary, many food manufacturers use nutrition as one of the means of promoting their foods.

The aim of this study is to get more insight into the interactions between the nutritional sciences and the food industry. This will be demonstrated using as an example the health biscuits made by the Dutch food manufacturer Liga. The later-developed dietary products of the firm are beyond the scope of this paper.

FOOD AND HEALTH

Food plays a crucial role in daily life, and in folk medicine various concepts exist on what is healthy or not healthy to eat. In the nineteenth century scientific concepts on food and health changed drastically. The dietetics of antiquity, which so long dominated concepts of health and food, were replaced by new knowledge and insights into the physiology of man and chemistry of food.[1]

From the middle of the nineteenth century onwards progressive food manufacturers started to incorporate new scientific knowledge in food processing. An early example is the *Liebig's Extract of Meat Company Ltd* of 1865.[2] Gradually the food industry gained a better understanding of the nature of good food, and even began to use scientific facts as part of food promotion activities.[3] Issues of hygiene and results of microbiological research dominated scientific thinking. The term 'hygienically processed and packaged' was an important selling point for promotion activities far into the twentieth century. The food canning industry and later the dairy industry are examples of early introductions of new scientific developments into their food processing activities.[4] This is probably much related to the perishable nature of the food products and food processing techniques compared with products such as biscuits. When, at the end of the nineteenth century, nutrition as a new scientific discipline emerged, some food manufacturers started to use nutritional health aspects for their own specific needs. In the 1920s the food industry, both in the United States and western Europe, began to make more systematic use of what McCollum calls the 'newer knowledge of nutrition' in particular vitamins and health.[5]

RUSKS AND BISCUITS

Before dealing with the biscuits of the firm Liga, it is necessary to treat first the biscuit itself. The biscuit as we know it now is a nineteenth century and most probably a British invention. The biscuit is evolved from the ship's biscuits and became popular in Britain among well-to-do people in the 1860s.[6] In the Netherlands, a maritime nation like Britain, ships' biscuits were produced in great quantities in the seventeenth and eighteenth century. In fact the making of ships' biscuits is a way of preserving bread by baking it twice. Hence the old Dutch name of *tweeback*, 'baked twice' ('biscuit' itself has the same meaning).[7] The river Zaan area, just north of Amsterdam, was the pre-eminent area for ship building and victualling. It is still an area with a sizable food industry, including biscuit and rusk manufacturing.[8] The rusk, the competitor of the biscuit, was developed most likely from the ships' biscuit as a finer and luxury product. The ingredients are not only flour as is the case with the ships' biscuit, but also yeast, eggs, sometimes milk instead of water, sugar or syrup. The rusks were not only used by the well-to-do as a luxury product at breakfast or with afternoon tea, but also as a typical food to be served to sick persons as the rusk is easy to digest. English biscuits of good quality were well known in the Netherlands in the nineteenth century. In the beginning of the twentieth century there was fierce competition on the biscuit market: imported biscuits versus locally produced biscuits, cheaper varieties versus high quality products.[9]

The eating patterns of biscuits are not the same in Europe. In Britain, by the 1860s, meal times altered radically. Breakfast was served earlier and on a far less elaborate scale, and dinner time was put back until 7–8 pm. This allowed room for a set lunch and afternoon tea. At these meals biscuits, both plain and sweet were often served.[10] In the Netherlands biscuits were for a very long time a luxury accompaniment of tea and coffee. They largely replaced the role of the rusk. In the years after 1950 biscuits were increasingly used as a snack between meals. In Italy biscuits are often used as part of breakfast.[11] Frequent snacking is not part of the food culture in Italy as is also the case in France. In the Netherlands the level of biscuit consumption (18 kg per head/year in 1996) is now under pressure. The traditional times for biscuit consumption are tending to fade away. Young consumers prefer the large assortment of crisps and sweets.[12]

HEALTH BISCUITS FOR CHILDREN AND ADULTS

In a paper presented at a symposium on health and food in 1972, the British nutritionist Hugh Sinclair stated that a health food is difficult to define. As a working definition Sinclair's concept still has much validity; a health food is any food that retains all its nutritionally desirable constituents and has not had added to it any substance that is harmful.[13] The definition is, however, too defensive and should be extended: it should contain nutrients and other substances as a contribution to the health of the consumer within a given nutritional context. Basically a food as such can never be healthy, it is the diet that counts. In other words, a health food is a response to a specific nutrition problem.

The firm Liga was originally a biscuit factory, a joint venture of a number of self-employed bakers in the town of Bergen op Zoom, near the Belgian border. After World War I the biscuit firm did not perform well because of the fierce competition on the biscuit market. In 1922 the new director Th Neutelings decided to step out of the production of fancy biscuits and to produce a good quality infant biscuit. During World War I Neutelings had good contacts with the Belgian physicians of the Belgian refugee camp near Bergen op Zoom and learned from them the important relation between food and health. Infant and child mortality were still high and a health biscuit could play an important role in improving nutrition. The innovation of the infant biscuit made the firm well known in the Netherlands as a manufacturer of food products that took nutritional concepts into account.[14] The innovation of the infant biscuit was based on the newest knowledge and insight of the nutritional sciences at that time:

(i)   The biscuit was enriched with the nutrients vitamin A and D. The nutritional sciences were at the time very much concerned with vitamin deficiencies. These problems became apparent among the low income households during World War I.

(ii) Much attention was given to the packaging of the product. Hygiene was still a point of special interest in public health circles. Well packaged food products were not so obvious as is now the case. Biscuits and other food products were mainly sold loose. So the infant biscuits were hygienically wrapped in a red carton box, with a picture of an infant and instructions on how to use it. The whole gave the impression of a medicine rather than a food product.

The application of the infant biscuit was very practical. It could be consumed in the form of a porridge or just as a biscuit. Also it was possible to soak the biscuit in milk or water and to use it in the feeding bottle. At the end of the 1930s the Liga biscuit became a very well known product.

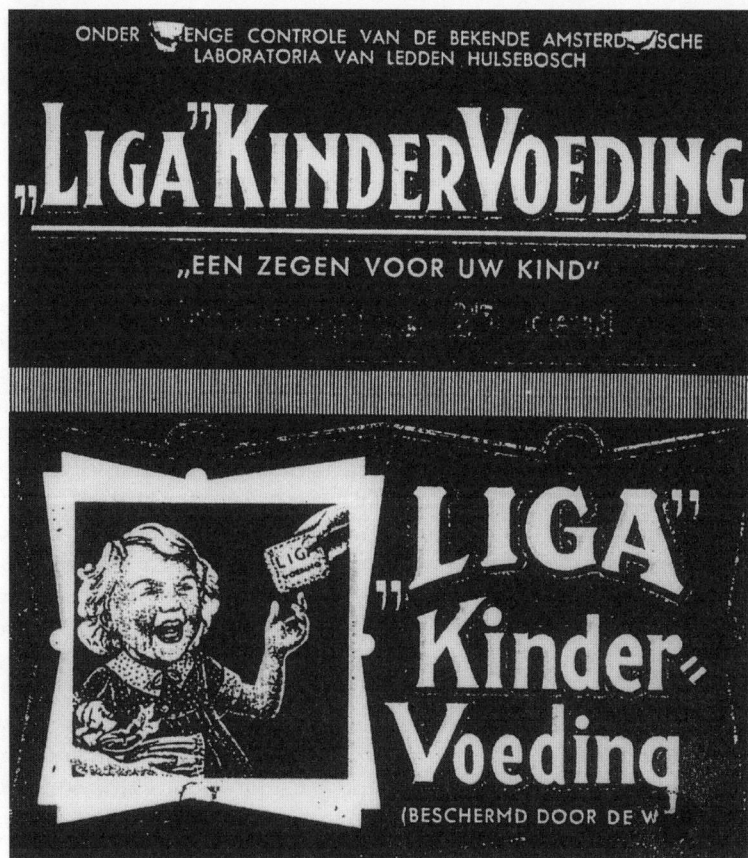

Fig.1. Packaging of the infant biscuit in the 1930s: 'Liga child nutrition. a blessing for your child.'

In order to reach older children and adults, a bread substitute was developed, the biscuit 'Sanovite'. This was done with the scientific support of Professor E C van Leersum, Director of the Netherlands Institute for Public Nutrition (NIVV, *Nederlands Instituut voor de Volksvoeding*). This product was introduced on the market in 1929. In the development of 'Sanovite' much attention was given to minerals, calcium and iron. In the 1930s there was among health authorities a concern for a low calcium intake among the low income groups, despite the presence of a strong dairy industry. Likewise the iron intake was considered to be too low.

NUTRITIONAL THREATS

The relationship between the food industry on the one hand and public health and the nutritional sciences on the other has not been an easy one. The problematic relationship was focused on two major issues: problems of food adulteration and misuse of scientific knowledge and concepts in the manufacturing and promotion of food products. The concept of health has been used very frequently in advertisements, whether it is relevant or not. It was only after 1980 in the Netherlands, as in other European countries, that legislation forbade mentioning the term 'healthy' or 'good for your health' in food advertisements.[15] Misuse of nutritional science is a recurrent theme in the non-specialist Dutch periodical *Voeding en Hygiëne* (Nutrition and Hygiene) in the years 1920 to 1930. In 1933 the periodical stated that the vitamin fashion has lead to swindling with vitamins, misuse in advertisements and unnecessary additions to food products.[16] In the early period of the modern food industry till the 1940s, it was, however, not too difficult to use the results of nutritional research as a positive asset in product development. However, in the 1950s in western Europe nutritional deficiencies for the first time almost disappeared.

Gradually the food industry was faced with two major challenges: a relatively saturated market as people cannot eat more than they already do, and the health implications of overnutrition. From various sides there was a call for policies for a prudent diet.[17] In the 1960s sugar consumption and dental caries became an issue of public debate. National Heart Associations campaigned to reduce the consumption of animal fats and cholesterol. In February 1977 the US Senate Select Committee on Nutrition and Human Needs issued a staff report, Dietary Goals for the United States.[18]

The dietary goals had far reaching effects both in the US and western Europe. The report created widespread discussions between nutritionists, health authorities, and food industry and consumer organisations. Inspired by the dietary goals, some European countries established their own food and nutrition goals. Norway was the first country to do so in Europe.

FOOD INNOVATIONS

The question is how did Liga react to these, at first sight unfavourable, issues? In the 1960s dental caries became a public health issue in several European countries. The consumption of sugar and in particular the frequency of consumption was one of the main aetiological factors of dental caries. In the minds of public health authorities, nutritionists and consumer groups, sugar became a malefactor. Nutrition education started to discourage the consumption of sugar. In the UK the nutritionist John Yudkin (1972) published his provocative book on sugar entitled *Pure, White and Deadly: the problem of sugar.*[19] Biscuits were included in the list of foods of which the intake had to be reduced. Biscuits are cariogenic because of a relative high sugar content and a long lasting plaque on the teeth after consumption.

The Liga infant biscuit, so well promoted as an indispensable health food for infants, came under attack. Health authorities and in particular health centres dissuaded the consumption of the infant biscuit. The effect

of such negative advice was so strong that the production had to be drastically reduced, because of a much lower demand. The dental caries issue
threatened even the very existence of the food manufacturer. So the management turned for advice to the Netherlands Institute for Public Nutrition.
The sugar or saccharose in the biscuit was replaced in 1972 by glucose and
fructose (on the assumption that they were not cariogenic). The new product, Liga-junior, was well received. Soon, however, it became clear from
new findings that glucose and fructose were cariogenic as well. Also the
sticky properties of the biscuits were investigated. The results indicated that
all Liga biscuits were cariogenic regardless of their composition. However,
in the long run the public attention for dental caries faded away, to the relief
of the food manufacturer.

A new topic of nutritional research emerged, that of dietary fibre. In the
1970s nutritional epidemiological studies suggested that a lack of dietary
fibre may be a contributing factor in a number of non-infectious diseases
in the industrialised countries of North America and western Europe, such
as diverticular diseases of the colon, coronary heart disease and colonic
cancer. Various nutritionists recommended that cereal fibre should be added
to food. The food industry picked up these recommendations quickly by
adding dietary fibre, in particular cheap bran, to food products such as
breakfast cereals and biscuits.[20] However, from a technological point of
view, supplementing biscuits with dietary fibre is not easy as the palatability
is easily reduced.[21] It should be realised that the 1970's concept of high
fibre containing biscuits for health reasons was not an entirely new one.
In England in the eighteenth century charcoal biscuits were produced as a
medical agent, an antidote to flatulence and other stomach disorders.[22] Well
known already in the 1920s in the UK were the Digestive Biscuits, prepared
fully or partially from coarse wheat flour.[23]

The management of Liga realised that the Infant biscuit as a core activity was too small a basis for the firm. Apart from losing customers because
of the caries issue there was also a demographic factor. The birth rate in
the Netherlands, as in other European countries decreased. In the period
1960–90, the birth rate in the Netherlands dropped from 20.9 to 12.7
per 1000 of population.[24] This meant fewer potential consumers for the
biscuit. So the management had to look for new promising alternatives.
The opportunity came at the end of the 1970s when the American Dietary
Goals stimulated a fierce debate between food manufacturers, nutritionists, public health authorities and consumer organisations. The food industry was often accused of not operating in the nutritional interests of the
consumer. Again the firm looked for nutrition advice and to see how the
Dietary Goals could be used in the development of a new product. The first
recommendation of the Dietary Goals in food selection and preparation is
to increase consumption of fruit, vegetables and whole grains.[25] Being basically a biscuit manufacturer these recommendations gave promising perspectives. The new product was named 'Evergreen', a wholewheat biscuit

with dietary fibre from fruits. However, at the beginning, the dietary fibre content was still too low and the taste too dry. The biscuit was improved by adding more fibre and currants. The 'Evergreen' was promoted as a sound health snack, to be considered as a mini meal between the daily meal pattern. 'Evergreen' was very successful and new versions were developed under the name of 'Switch'.

In 1989 Liga started to take the Dutch Guidelines for a Good Nutrition (*Richtlijnen Goede Voeding*) as reference for the development of their health biscuits.[26] Basically the Dutch Guidelines do not differ from the Dietary Goals. So for Liga the nutritional ups and downs ended well thanks to wise management and close contacts with the nutrition world. Since 1977 Liga has become part of General Biscuits Nederland, which belongs to the French Food Group BSN (Boussions Souchan Neuvese).

CONCLUDING REMARKS

In a historical perspective the relation between the food industry and the nutritional sciences and related policies is a complex one. The nature of the relationship of food products and nutrition may shift from nutritionally well desired to less desired and even undesired. It all depends on the stages of knowledge in nutrition and the nutritional context of society in a particular period. For instance, milk was hailed as an indispensable drink from the end of the nineteenth century till the 1970s. Then it came much under pressure because of fat and cholesterol as a public health issue. The same applies to meat. It is surprising to see that even products without apparent nutritional qualities, such as tea and wine, are now nutritionally appreciated because of a high content of flavonoids.

The development of the Liga biscuit in the 1920s shows that a positive nutritional image is no guarantee that it will always be the case. The dental caries issue was nearly fatal for the manufacturer. It also demonstrates that picking up new ideas in nutrition, such as the Dietary Goals, can help both manufacturer and consumer.

Table. 1. *The Liga biscuit and developments*
in the nutritional sciences 1922–1990

Developments in the nutritional sciences	The Liga biscuit
1900–1950: Vitamins and minerals	1923: Vitamin A and D, iron and calcium added to the biscuit
1960s: Dental caries issue	1972: Liga-Junior on the market without saccharose
1977: Dietary Goals, US	1979: Development of Evergreen Biscuit, fibre and fruit
1986: Dietary Guidelines Sound Nutrition, NL	1986: Development of assortment of health snacks (biscuits)

BIBLIOGRAPHY

Consudel. Interview United Biscuits, *Consude*, (1996), 8–11.

Corley, T A B. Nutrition, technology and the growth of the British biscuit industry 1820–1900. In Oddy et al, *The Making of the Modern British Diet*, London, 1976, 13–25.

Damen, H J J et al. Interactie tussen voedingswetenschap en bedrijfsleven [Interaction between nutritional sciences and the industry], *Voeding*, 56 (1995), 19–22.

Dreher, Mark L. *Handbook of Dietary Fibre. An applied approach*, New York, 1987.

Efdée, Ria. *Beschuit, een tere juffer* (Rusk, a fragile young lady), Den Haag, 1989.

Hansen, Maurice. The validity of the concept of health foods. In Birch, G G and Parker, K J, eds, *Food and Health, Science and Technology*, London, 1980, 27–41.

Harris, H G, Borella, S P. *All About Biscuits*, (Offices of The British Baker), London, c 1925.

Hartog, den Adel P. The role of nutrition in food advertisements: the case of the Netherlands, in den Hartog, A P ed, *Food Technology, Science and Marketing: European diet in the twentieth century*, East Linton, 1995, 268–280.

Horrocks, Sally M. Nutrition science and the food industry in Britain. In den Hartog, A P, ed, *Food technology, science and marketing: European diet in the twentieth century*, East Linton, 1995, 7–18.

Kasteren, J van. General Biscuits vertaalt Richtlijnen in product (General biscuits translates dietary guidelines into product), *Voeding*, 52 (1991), 231–233.

Kessler, David A. The evolution of national nutrition policy, *Annual Review of Nutrition*, 15 (1995), xiii–xxvi.

Kjaernes, Uni. Milk: nutritional science and agricultural development in Norway, 1890–1990. In den Hartog, A P, *Food Technology, Science and Marketing: European diet in the twentieth century*, East Linton 1995, 103–116.

Lee, Philip R. Nutrition policy from neglect and uncertainty to debate and action, *Journal of the American Dietetic Association*, 72 (1978), 581–588.

Marks, Linda. Policies for a prudent diet, *Food Policy*, 10 (1985), 166–174.

Mol, J. *Van melkinrichting tot levensmiddelenfabriek* (from dairy to food factory), *Voeding* (1980), 166-172.

Morris, T N. Management and preservation of food. In Singer, C et al, eds, *A History of Technology, Vol 5, 1850-1900*, Oxford, 1958, 26–52.

Pyke, Magnus. *Food and Society*, London, 1968.

Seibel, W. Ballaststoffanreicherung bei Lebensmitteln auf Getreidebasis, *Gordian*, 79 (1979), 297–300.

Teuteberg, Hans-Jürgen. *Kleine Geschichte der Fleischbrühe*, Münster, 1989.

Verkade. *Honderd jaar Verkade* (hundred years of Verkade), Wormer, 1986.

Voeding en Hygiëne (Nutrition and Hygiene), 7 (1933), 114

Voedings- en genotsmiddelenindustrie. Een geschiedenis en bronnenoverzicht (Food Industry, a history and survey of sources), Amsterdam, 1933.

Vratanina, Diane L and Zabik, Mary E. Bran as a source of dietary fibre in oatmeal cookies, *Journal of the American Dietic Association*, 77, (1980), 26–30.

Yudkin, John. *Pure, White and Deadly: the problem of sugar*, London, 1972.

NOTES

1 Pyke, 1968.
2 Teuteberg, 1989, 12–15.
3 Horrocks, 1995.
4 Morris, 1958; Mol, 1980; Kjaernes, 1995.
5 Horrocks, 1995, 7; Levenstein, 1988, 147–60.
6 Corley, 1976,13–15, 22–3.
7 Efdée, 1989, 20–3.
8 Voedings- en Genotsmiddelenindustrie, 1993, 7.
9 Verkade, 1986, 21.
10 Corley, 23.
11 Consudel, 1996, 9.
12 NRC 29.01.1997.
13 Hansen, 1980, 28.
14 Damen et al, 1995.
15 Den Hartog, 1995, 273–5.
16 Voeding en Hygiëne, 1933.
17 Marks, 1985.
18 Lee, 1978, 585-7; Kessler, 1995, xvi.
19 Yudkin, 1972.
20 Vratania, 1980; Seibel, 1979.
21 Dreher, 1987, 398, 400.
22 Corley, 16.
23 Harris and Borella, c1925, 160–1.
24 CBS, The Hague.
25 Lee, 1978, 585.
26 Kasteren, 1991.

Part 4
Tobacco

19 The changing perceptions of tobacco: smoking in Germany during the 1930s and 1940s

Christoph Maria Merki

The medical profession looks upon tobacco consumption as the single most important avoidable cause of illness and premature death. Despite all medical warnings, there is no product which goes through so many hands daily as the cigarette – the specifically modern form of tobacco consumption. As the result of medical criticism of smoking, historiography has also gradually discovered tobacco as a theme: one which incidentally has proved to be extremely multi-layered, containing economic, financial, or commercial aspects as well as social and medical ones.[1] The history of tobacco in Germany hardly distinguishes itself from that of the rest of Europe. It spread as an import from the New World, first of all as a medical and ornamental plant before it began to achieve popularity as a semi-luxury item in the seventeenth century. In the course of the twentieth century Germany, too, experienced the triumphal march of the cigarette and the everyday acceptance of consumption by women. However, at least two notable points justify examining German consumption more closely during the first half of the twentieth century and especially in the 1930s and 1940s – namely the prevention policy of Hitler as well as the role of the cigarette as a replacement currency after World War II.

GERMAN CONSUMPTION DURING THE TWENTIETH CENTURY – AN OVERVIEW

For fiscal reasons the state has been interested in tobacco for many years. Although individual statistics can be traced back to the early contemporary period, they tell precious little about secular changes in the prevalence of tobacco. An important measurement for developing consumption is the use of raw tobacco per capita and per year which amounted to about 1.5 kg in the first third of the twentieth century. It can not be independent of the general course of economic and social history. Thus German consumption during World War I increased significantly before shortage-related factors forced drastic limitations, and it sank from 2.1 kg (1915) to 0.8 kg (1918). During the inflationary period (1922–3) as well as during the world economic crisis (1931–2) it declined 10–15 per cent in both cases. Despite rising tax burdens, the consumption level during the second half of the 1920s lay notably higher than in the pre-war period – an unmistakable indicator that tobacco use soon started to establish itself among previously non-smoking or seldom-smoking women as well.

The cigarette succeeded in opening up this new women's market. Introduced during the 1870s, the cigarette was first of all a product for the city and the upper class. Practical in usage and suitable for the hectic pace of modern daily life, it developed within a few decades from a fashion accessory into a standardised article for mass consumption, selling itself through modern market advertising. The cigarette's share of the total German tobacco market rose from 0.2 per cent (1877) to 12 per cent (1912), 25 per cent (1925), and 35 per cent (1935). That the cigarette had still been unable to displace its older sister, the cigar, during the 1920s was above all a result of German taxation policy. The tax authorities preferred cigars in order to support the related handwork required for their production. Finally the pipe had already lost its position as the long-dominant form of tobacco consumption in the last third of the nineteenth century. It celebrated a brief comeback during the inflationary period, since many cigar and cigarette smokers had returned to this the cheapest smoking alternative.

The rise in cigarette consumption was stimulated once more during the 1930s. Average consumption doubled between 1931 and 1940 from 452 to 914 cigarettes per capita, per year. Just as tobacco consumption had accelerated at the outset of World War I, it rose at the beginning of World War II before it began to dwindle in mid-1941. The 1950s and 1960s then saw the decline of pipes and cigars, the upswing in demand for filtered cigarettes, and a further increase in consumption by women. The ratio of women smokers peaked in the 1970s at about 30 per cent. Among German men a dubious record of 84 per cent smoked at the beginning of the 1950s. Today the figure has dipped below 40 per cent.[2]

THE NATIONAL SOCIALIST ANTI-TOBACCO POLICY AND THE TOBACCO INDUSTRY'S COUNTERSTRATEGY

As the 'first Tobacco Science Institute' was opened at the University of Jena in April of 1941, '*Führer*' Adolf Hitler relayed his 'best wishes' to those gathered for the 'task of freeing humanity from one of its most dangerous poisons'.[3] The non- or ex-smoker Hitler, a convinced vegetarian and notorious hypochondriac, seemed during the course of time to have developed a pronounced antipathy to tobacco. In 1940, Martin Bormann, one of his closest confidants, referred to him as 'a strong opponent of smoking'.[4] The extent to which non-smoking lay on Hitler's heart is also illustrated by his custom of presenting a gold watch as a gift to any member of his inner circle who had given up smoking.

Hitler's determined outlook on smoking obviously had an impact on National Socialist tobacco policy, even if it cannot be explained by Hitler's

personal aversion alone. It was rooted too deeply for this in National Socialist reproductive and performance medicine. This is also shown in the example of the Tobacco Science Institute. The idea of founding it came from
athletics team doctor Karl Astel, professor of human eugenics and heredi-
tary research and since 1939 rector of the University of Jena. Moreover,
Astel led the Thüringen Office for Racial Research, created in 1933, which
knew how to promote its programme by focusing on 'racially valuable'
population segments throughout Germany by pushing health and fertility
research promotion.[5] If the discourse criticising tobacco had previously
been a domain of social hygiene, it was now gradually transformed into
racial biology. Tobacco was a 'creeping' and 'addictive' 'racial poison'
which, based on the views of this discourse's protagonists, must be stamped
out. It was an 'underworld vice dragged in by the Jews' which blocked the
goal of the Reich's health leader Leonardo Conti 'to make human beings
more beautiful, healthier, and better'.[6] Medicine had exposed tobacco –
which it once prized as a remedy – as a weed. Anything else was a question
of political will and social technology.

Thus the struggle against tobacco, to use a metaphor of sociologist Zygmunt Bauman,[7] sprang from gardening ambitions – ie correcting and selecting – which National Socialism also propagated in other areas. It was part
of a comprehensive biopolicy[8] in which personal needs and habits had lost
their private character and one had to take public responsibility for them.
'Your health does not belong to you!' ran the related motto, and Astel
explained that refraining from smoking amounted to a 'National Socialist
duty'. Obviously National Socialism did not lead the fight against the weed
tobacco with such murderous consequences as it led the fight against for
example, 'valueless life'. Such a comparison may also seem a bit off the
mark, yet the logic which stood behind this struggle, namely that an object
recognised as socially and racially undesirable should be eliminated, was
similar in its reasoning.

Their anti-tobacco policy permitted National Socialists to link themselves to the preliminary work which the Federation of Tobacco Opponents
had performed since 1912. Morally motivated and critical of existing culture, the Federation was embedded in the temperance and life-reform movement. If it had been moralistic entrepreneurs who had shaped the profile
of the anti-smoking lobby in the 1920s, since the mid-1930s it was medically schooled experts who came into the foreground. They popularised
the knowledge provided by medicine with the help of professional communication methods. In promoting this risk-taking know-how and making it
relevant for everyday use, German scientists had taken a leading position
between the world wars,[9] and research at the end of the 1930s received a
strong impulse, profiting even more from the pronounced support of the
Reich's Office of Health.

The social revolutionary impetus which accompanied the formation of
the Third Reich also invigorated tobacco smoking prevention. National

Socialist police chiefs in the spring of 1933 permitted the display of placards which announced in an imperative tone 'The German woman does not
smoke!' 'National comrades,' they urged, 'women encountered smoking on
the street should be reminded of their duty as German women and mothers'.[10] It was naturally no accident that the only rudimentarily organised
anti-tobacco agitation in 1933 had – of all things – singled out discredited
women's smoking as 'unaesthetic'. The cigarette had served as the symbol
of feminine emancipation since George Sand and Lola Montez had smoked
publicly and demonstratively. To that extent, this agitation had less a
health-care policy touch than an antifeminist one which foiled the symbolic function of the cigarette. In the ideology of fascist male society, cigarette smoking by women was viewed as part of the insignia of a detestable
'bordel culture'; the 'really German' girl was also attractive without cigarettes.[11]

Only during the second half of the 1930s did institutional changes[12] get
off the ground with any great consequences. The Federation of Tobacco
Opponents was annexed to the 'Reich's task force against the danger of
alcohol and tobacco', and from 1938 officials of the Interior Ministry had
reinforced this through their so-called explanatory work, operating hand-
in-hand with other organisations such as the health insurance office, the
Hitler Youth, and the solidarity union *Arbeitsfront*. Warnings about smoking were heard, for instance, at doctors' offices and on school playgrounds.
One found them too in newspapers and on fliers, on radio, and in school
books. Today it is hardly possible to determine if the images related to
changing smoking patterns permanently actually succeeded.

Besides the attempt to bring smoking into disrepute as a health-endanger-
ing vice, it was also possible to identify changes to formalised regulations.
This did not involve a programme decreed and implemented purposefully
by the party but individual campaigns by various bodies in which the dicta-
tor himself intervened now and then with his own arrangements. The smoking ban in the NSDAP 1939 service areas, for instance, carried Hitler's
signature, as did the April 1941 instructions to 'in no way' expand acreage
for tobacco cultivation.[13] When the economics minister complained about
'disparaging the tobacco business' after the opening of the Tobacco Science
Institute, the Office of the Reich's Chancellor let him know in its best
totalitarian manner that, in the *Führer*'s opinion, the peoples' health took
priority over such economic considerations.[14] Constraints on tobacco advertising were sharply disputed. Such advertising was a central theme at
the 'Reich's meeting on National Health and Toxic Consumption', which
brought 15,000 people from all over Germany to Frankfurt am Main in
March 1939. It was emphatically demanded that advertising be 'controlled'. The advertising which appealed to youths and women was forbidden
soon after; also banned were beliefs (eg over the harmlessness of mild cigarettes) as well as motifs (eg from the sporting world).[15] At the end of 1940
the Reich's leader of the press Max Amann stopped 'any advertising for

tobacco products in the text portion of newspapers'.[16] A year later tobacco advertising was all but forbidden from public areas. Neither in public transportation nor on placards, on loud-speaker cars or by mass mailings, could smoking be advertised in the future.[17] Even compared with today's measures, these constraints seem tough; if they were meaningful at a time when demand clearly exceeded supply is another issue.

Obviously the German tobacco industry moved heaven and earth to block these institutional changes or to get around them by prudent adaptation. In 1935 it demonstrated its basically nationalistic attitude on trading cards of German heroes as well as a splendid book glorifying the *Führer*. Yet the preventive policy was never life-threatening for the industry. The tobacco market experienced a unique boom during the first half of the War, and the massive cutback in production during the war's second half was not the result of intended policy but simply reflected war-related conditions.

The industry pursued various strategies to silence the criticism of smoking. Besides political lobbying work, it attempted above all to improve tobacco technically as a means of pleasure. Thus in the 1930s the growth of low-nicotine tobacco sprouted its first blossoms, and the first cigarettes with built-in filters appeared on the market. An obvious and 'scientifically' based ideology of its own served to give assurance to the industry and to the clientele. The Tobacco Science Society had devoted itself to this task since 1938, and little by little most of the branch's enterprises joined it. At the centre of the criticism opposing tobacco[18] stood the addiction-encouraging nicotine substance which was said to lead to an 'uncontrollable' tobacco addiction (above all in the case of 'genetic predisposition'); such addiction was called 'tobaccoism' or 'nicotinism' – analogous to alcoholism. Criticism started out with this substance-centred addiction terminology. The incriminating means of pleasure did not addict; it served only to bring the neurotic disposition of the addict to light. Whoever sought to heal the addict by forbidding the 'means of addiction' subscribed to a 'belief in demons'. 'The effort to fight against addiction through banning the "means of addiction" is practically exorcism, driving out the devil', wrote Helmuth Aschenbrenner,[19] editor of *Monographiae Nicotianae*, publications issued by the Society. Even so, the industry experts also accepted a possible 'misuse' of tobacco. 'Abuse' in their eyes was to be rejected just as was militant 'abstinence'. The psychobiologist Hans Lungwitz put abstinence on a level with abuse and explained both to be a 'perversion'.[20] On the other hand, the 'learned' and 'biologically healthy' tobacco consumer was stylised as normal; this average human being would depend on 'support of a luxury item' until he developed into a 'Superman'.[21]

Corresponding to this ideology, tobacco advertising knew only one vital *leitmotif*: ignore excessive, addictive consumption and popularise conscious, moderate enjoyment. Using such a credo even allowed flirtation with the anti-tobacco movement. As demand for cigarettes in the summer of 1941 could hardly be satisfied, the cigarette firm Brinkmann challenged its customers not to hoard: 'smoking a bit less can only benefit your health'; the important thing after all remained the 'unchanged high quality' of the brand 'Alva'. With this call to moderation, the firm in no way repudiated its own interests. Its goal was not a despicable increase in turnover; its 'unconditional openness' through 'public-interest' styled advertising had picked up something more valuable, as the official responsible for the campaign openly admitted: consumer 'trust'.[22]

SMOKING DURING THE WAR

Tobacco, as Economics Minister Funk put it, had an eminent 'political importance'.[23] In war it proved itself as an outstanding means of suppressing hunger pangs, as a complement to an ever more monotonous menu, or for overcoming the extraordinary emotional tensions of that time. The National Socialists were dependent on this polyvalent and multi-functional psycho-drug which could work as either a sedative or stimulant. To this extent their tobacco policy was contradictory, and it remained – as far as practical prevention was concerned – predominantly ideological. The National Socialist leadership, incidentally, was fully aware of this contradiction. Propaganda Minister Joseph Goebbels put it bluntly and succinctly in an internal ministerial conference in May 1941: 'As useful as it might perhaps be to stamp out smoking generally from a health standpoint, it is inadvisable at the present time.'[24]

Thus effective steps to reduce consumption failed to materialise. The necessary economic policy instrument for it would actually have been available. In the mid-1930s the already heavily cartel-oriented tobacco industry was in a technical group combined with one of the typical compulsory bodies of the National Socialist economy. Without it neither the production quota system nor the guidance of sales could have been realised. From September 1939 – in addition to conventional tax – a massive war surcharge of first 20 per cent and then 50 per cent of the retail price was levied on all tobacco goods. To reduce buying power and stifle threatening inflation, the Finance Ministry also in the years after 1941 pressed for an increase in this and other special taxes. Out of consideration for the public mood, however, these plans were never actually implemented.

Despite the fiscally related rise in cost of tobacco goods, their consumption also increased after 1939, quite in contrast to most other goods whose consumption had already experienced drastic cutbacks during the early phase of the war.[25] The first supply problems with raw tobacco occurred in March and April of 1940 at a time when the German cigarette industry produced 20 per cent more than in the pre-war period.[26] Even the spoils looted in the Balkans hardly relaxed the situation in the raw tobacco market. In May of 1941 the German cigarette industry worked flat out; shortly before the invasion of Russia it produced 50 per cent more than during the pre-war period.

In the summer of 1941 the situation became more acute. Despite the successive cutbacks now introduced for production due to the shortage of raw materials, petrol, and manpower, a steady high demand still increased. In the cities long queues formed in front of tobacco shops, which was noted with concern in the Propaganda Ministry. The armed services, which in 1940 had absorbed less than a sixth of all production, now – in the autumn of 1941 – used a quarter of it. The preventive spirit called for earlier refused to vanish. Consumers simply did not want to hear that delivery of tobacco goods was greater than in the pre-war era. And they incorrectly viewed the anti-tobacco movement as the actual cause of scarcity.[27]

In order to ensure a 'fair' supply, the government finally resorted to a step which the industry had struggled against for a long time: regulating sales by means of cards. The corresponding plans were laid down in a December 1941 meeting chaired by Economics Minister Walther Funk.[28] The most sensitive issue proved to be how large the circle of those entitled to delivery should be. Could one exclude non-smokers from distribution? And, if so, how? Ultimately the control card was issued every four weeks to all applicants aged 18 or older (in the case of men) or between 25 and 55 (in the case of women). The card simply entitled one to claim a specified amount of tobacco but failed to guarantee it. Since non-smokers could also apply, they rapidly became an envied gift and exchange object. And here lay an important reason for the later development of cigarettes as replacement currency.

Sharply disputed by tobacco opponents was the inclusion of women, whose 'fertility for motherhood'[29] became an issue. Yet the critics could not prevail. In determining the minimum-age restrictions, propaganda and health-policy considerations became stuck in a clinch. While health policy demanded a higher age minimum, representatives of the armed forces and the Propaganda Ministry defended as low an age cut-off point as possible. The issue for them was the motivational importance of 'love parcels' from young women to soldiers at the front. Age 25 was rather a high minimum level, but young women could also apply for a tobacco card if they were already married and their husbands were in the field. Women over 55 also finally received a card if they could prove that their husband or at least an unmarried son was in military service, or if she could make a credible claim about her need for tobacco and ensure in writing that she 'needed it for personal use'.[30]

The anger of male smokers directed itself mainly at 'women of "high society"' who often sit for hours in the cafés'.[31] On the other hand, they rather accepted women who worked in industry and who now discovered the cigarette as a new means of pleasure enabling them to cope with their jobs; thus cigarettes mainly substituted for other luxury goods which, like coffee, had practically vanished from everyday use. The Economics Ministry attached great importance to the commitment of these women and for this reason above all held out to the end for allocation to all women, even if distribution to men took priority at the closing phase of the war. Since the autumn of 1944 their cards entitled them to double the number of coupons as women's cards. Only the armed forces had their own rules at the end. They profited from countless privileges covering luxury goods quotas and during the final phase of the war claimed a third of all tobacco production alone. In the Army smoking was part of an entire set of lifestyle norms, self-images, and rituals. The 'last cigarette' was shared before dangerous missions, and it helped evoke a final moment of comradeship, common ground, and security.

The development of German tobacco consumption between 1942 and 1945 can hardly be documented today. Already at the beginning of 1942, only half as many smoking goods should have been available for the civil population as at the outset of summer 1941. If at the beginning of 1942 the civil population had a per capita monthly ration of 48 cigarettes, three cigars, and 19 grams of unpacked smoking tobacco, a German man in spring of 1945 – despite all production and delivery problems – could still claim two cigarettes per day on average. However, this entitlement sometimes simply existed on paper, and production quality also suffered drastically.[32]

It only remains to point out changes in the manner of consumption. Thus – especially among soldiers – the short pipe (in which one could stuff everything) replaced the earlier more popular long pipe. While cigar consumption had already suffered a massive collapse before 1942, the use of cigarettes experienced a powerful boom, and one can speak of a triumphal march of this form of consumption, particularly if one considers the 1940s as a whole.[33] The cigarette was not only the preferred form for feminine consumers but was also extraordinarily attractive for soldiers, quickly available and guaranteeing them 'the most rational nicotine use' in these nerve-wracking times. According to the psychohistoric stimulation insights of neurologist Kurt Pohlisch the 'pleasure complex of smoking' generally lost its significance during the war years while at the same time the pharmaceutical effect of the tobacco began to determine consumption.[34] I would like to sharpen Pohlisch's thesis even more: thus just as at the end of National Socialism it was not the propagated national community which resulted but rather the 'atomising of society' (Peukert), so the Nazis bequeathed not their envisioned tobacco-free society but – on the contrary – a society more than ever reliant on tobacco, if not to say addicted to it. The later reconstruction of prevalence rates show that the war brought with it a significant increase in smoking potential.[35] During this time, whoever entered the final period of socialisation, especially a man in the Army, found in all probability a constant companion in tobacco.

Under these conditions talk of real 'control' of consumption was naturally out of the question. The national socialists had to confine themselves to the administration of the shortage, to keep the dissatisfaction of consumers within bounds. Further implementation of the prevention policy in this situation would only have caused scorn. The campaigns against 'tobacco abuse' were even officially discontinued as 'redundant'[36] in February 1943. That does not mean that the contradiction between the ideological health-care policy attitude and the social system's need for nicotine would be removed once and for all. The contradiction broke out a final time in 1945 over the issue of supplying tobacco to youth. In the last phase of the war, as ever more youths were conscripted into the Reich's civilian service or the armed forces, they too adapted their consumption behaviour to that of adults. Given the choice between sweets or tobacco products, they opted as a rule for cigarettes over bonbons. After the intervention of the Reich's Health Minister Conti, distribution of tobacco products to those below age 18 was discontinued in February 1945. But one could not and *did not want to* forbid smoking to any youths in combat.[37]

SMOKING AFTER THE WAR

When the war was over, most Germans could breathe a sigh of relief. Yet there was hardly any tobacco for a pipe of peace: luxury items remained rare until the currency reform of June 1948, in some cases until the beginning of the 1950s. The grave shortage of raw tobacco, which had already occurred throughout the war, became still more acute and could only be overcome after the introduction of the Marshall Plan. In the Western zones, to which I will confine myself in the following, the shortage of currency prevented any importing of raw tobacco, let alone any finished tobacco products, until the spring of 1948. Of necessity, the industry lived off wartime stocks to the extent that they were not confiscated as looted goods by the Allies. Evasion by use of domestic tobacco only occurred under certain conditions. Shortly before the war it had covered only a quarter of demand. In the British zone the 'tobacco emergency' was especially severe: there, of all places, where the lion's share of the industry was headquartered, one found an almost total lack of commercial tobacco cultivation.

How scarce tobacco was until 1948 is best seen in its massive cultivation in small acreages, ie in backyards and gardens, on embankments, and on balconies. Until 1948 small planters had harvested as much tobacco as the commercial tobacco plantations. There numbers were in the millions. In the British zone alone 930,000 small planters were counted in 1946.[38] Like commercial cultivation, small planting was also taxable. Yet the authorities were not really happy with the taxation. Unregistered tobacco cultivation was the most frequent tax violation of those years, and a large portion of the harvest surely landed on the black market, though all small planters had to give written assurance that this tobacco was only for personal use. Yet the fact that small cultivation was not banned or that the planters were not – as in the French zone – forced to turn over their harvests, was due mainly to social psychological factors. In the vernacular the tobacco gained by domestic cultivation was aptly termed '*Siedlerstolz*' or 'settler's pride', and the tax authorities could not lay claim to this pride.

The overwhelming success of the privately cultivated brand was mainly a result of the state's own poorly managed supply system which also remained precarious as the management system came back into effect. Rationing measures from wartime were retained. The average consumption of a German male aged 15 or older for 1946 was estimated at 0.65 kg of tobacco products per year (13 per cent of the 1937 figure). According to my calculations the average male ration in American-occupied Hesse amounted to about 20 cigarettes per month. In the second half of 1947 it increased to 25 cigarettes or the corresponding number of cigars or unpacked smoking tobacco.[39]

As low as these quantities may appear, tobacco became all the more avidly sought after. One knew other 'colonial goods' such as coffee or tea only from hearsay; beer had almost nothing in common with the beverage of the same name, and one paid fantasy prices for distilled spirits sold on the black-market. Tobacco may have taken over the role of other luxury goods, such as the discontinued coffee. Nonetheless, the number of female temporary smokers provides a clear index. In any case, even after 1945 tobacco retained its 'political importance'.[40] The American zone's Council of States saw a direct link in 1946 between job performance of the 'German worker' and his being supplied with tobacco products he could afford: 'Tobacco in today's Germany is not only a luxury item but largely a means of relaxation and diversion from hunger and worry'. Even the trade journal found evidence of tobacco's 'psychological importance on the job' and declared it a 'drug'. During the winter famine of 1946–7 Paul Schmidt of the Hessian Finance Ministry referred to it as 'the last consolation' which remained for the needy population.[41] These comments recall a nutrition and behaviour model which the Italian historian Piero Camporesi described for pre-industrialised Europe and which now, at least by extension, had arisen once more. In pre-modern Europe hunger and hallucinations marked the world vision of the starving masses; their lot became half-way bearable if a meal was enriched with various consciousness-altering substances such as poppy seeds or ergot.[42] Tobacco had an analogous function in the collapse of German society.

The attractiveness which tobacco enjoyed especially in these starvation years can help clarify behaviour which must otherwise be dismissed as irrational. This is how Pohlisch observed concentration camp prisoners who tried to survive a life-threatening situation by trading food for tobacco.[43] Numerous women engaged in prostitution with the 'Ami' (American soldier) for 'Amis' (American cigarettes). Men begged for cigarettes and collected discarded but not completely smoked stubs at the feet of the occupational forces. Poisonings due to consumption of poorly fermented tobacco were part of daily life. Often everything that would burn was crammed into a smoking pipe: leaves from cherry trees, beech or birch wood, and even coltsfoot, clover, and dandelions. People were even found who reportedly developed a taste for 'cigarettes' produced from peat moss. However, these people were not mainly ill from smoking bad tobacco; on the contrary, they smoked low-quality tobacco because they believed that only in this way could they survive the catastrophic nutrition and health situation.[44]

The government profited from the fact that tobacco had become a product with practically inelastic demand. In May 1946 the Allies Control Council raised the tobacco tax so massively that, depending on the product, one would have had to increase the retail price from eight to 10 times the pre-war level. The cigar industry of the British zone without more ado discontinued production. In December of 1946 the occupied powers gradually gave in to the German protest and reduced the surcharges again.[45] It was the first and only time that the four triumphant powers had brought themselves to revise a law. Indeed even after the reduction, prices still lay about four times as high as before the war. But they were paid willingly. Yet tobacco belonged to the few luxury goods which one could still receive through cards. Because the tobacco tax was raised so sharply, it continued to produce an enviable tax revenue despite the decline in consumption. After the currency reform, step-by-step reduction in the surcharge was compensated for by expanded consumption. Thus taxation retained its fiscal significance. In 1950 a seventh of all Federal Republic of Germany tax revenue stemmed from this source.

To close this chapter, I want to call attention to a development which at the collapse of 1945 also marked a most notable and lasting break in terms of tobacco consumption: the triumphal march of the American blend, the USA cigarette type. This easy-to-inhale cigarette consisted above all of industrially dried Virginia tobacco. After 1945 it replaced the previously dominant taste for Oriental blends. If Oriental cigarettes ruled up to 95 per cent of the German pre-war market, they had to be gratified to hold a 3 per cent market share in the Federal Republic at the end of the 1940s. The basis for this revolutionary change in taste was at first the use of cigarettes as currency: every 'Ami' was smoked as if it were pure gold. It proved to have a high distinctive value and exuded, so to speak, the prestige of a victor. Quite soon it was imitated by the German producers, and one favoured the American blends in cultivation. Since the loss of the Balkans, ie since mid-1944, importing of Oriental tobacco had been held up. Now imports within the framework of the Marshall Plan became pivotal. They fitted beautifully into the trade policy concept of the USA administration, since even during the war large amounts of surplus tobacco had accumulated in national storage depots. While Germany before the war had been an unimportant raw-tobacco customer for the USA, West Germany in 1950 became one of its biggest markets. On the German side importing was organised by the Bremen keg tobacco dealers. Bremen had inherited the Dresden market to where Oriental tobacco had been transported previously. The new orientation of West German trade policy after 1945 could hardly be viewed more clearly than through raw tobacco distribution: from Dresden to Bremen, from Oriental to Virginia blends, from Southeastern Europe to the USA.

As the import of Greek tobaccos rose again after 1950, Oriental cigarettes were denied the comeback they had hoped for. The Federal Republic smokers – especially the young ones – had become too used to the aroma of the great wide world.[46]

PECUNIA OLET: THE RISE AND FALL OF CIGARETTES AS CURRENCY

The rise of the cigarette to become the leading currency on the black market had two central premises: first, the 'tobacco emergency' with the shortage of raw tobacco and tobacco products described earlier; second, repudiation of the official currency which paralleled the ruination of Germany's economy as a result of the excessive military build-up. In contrast to the post-World War I era, rampant inflation could be prevented after World War II, and indeed by forced management of all vital goods as well as by a general freeze on prices and wages which applied until 1948. Yet already in 1941–2 the discrepancy between private income and declining consumer options was so great that the shady grey market developed into a true black market. Despite police-state terror, the underground economy devoured one new sector after another.

The beginning of the cigarette currency[47] can be traced back to those days. The cigarette developed successively from a beloved exchange object to a means of converting value and then into a generally valid measure of value for barter. In the illegal markets one reckoned to a certain extent in cigarettes, since the actual value of the official Reichsmark currency could no longer be estimated. Relations between black-market goods and the new currency unit often had an astounding stability. To fulfil these new money-related functions, the cigarette possessed ideal prerequisites: it was handy, easy to transport, practically packed, fairly imperishable, difficult to counterfeit, and met international norms in weight and size. In contrast to normal money it had the crucial advantage of being resistant to inflation. If the cigarette had served its purpose as a means of barter or a unit of calculation and wound up in the yellow fingers of a smoker, it vanished into thin air. This sort of automatic money supply regulation was more efficient than the work of any bank of issue.

Already in mid-1943 a conventional four-pfennig cigarette cost 60 pfennigs on the Berlin black market. The price inflated in the autumn of 1944 to two Reichsmarks and then in April 1945 up to eight RM per cigarette, a two hundred-fold rise over the official price. After the capitulation the alternative currency stretched further through the influx of foreign cigarettes. In the Western-occupied zones the American cigarette was – analogous to the dollar in the world economy – the new currency leader of the shadow economy. Its possession was forbidden to the Germans yet (in contrast to trading) usually went unpunished. Thus the 'Ami' could establish itself as the most important means of exchange and the central unit of calculation on the black and grey markets. Indeed German tobacco goods also appeared on the black market, but their price remained clearly lower than that of the foreign competition. Because tobacco products represented pure gold, so to speak, one had to guard them accordingly. The German subsidiary of British-American Tobacco (the BAT) even demanded military escort protection for transportation by train.[48]

The buying power of foreign soldiers' cigarettes remained obvious to them. For only 700 'Amis' the 'Ami' could buy a Leica camera. And 70 Chesterfields would purchase a bottle of Cognac – 120 a perfume bottle of Chanel No 5. With this he could then spoil his German lover (the vernacular named her jokingly 'Amilette'). On 26 May 1947 the American military government prohibited private importing of cigarettes. Yet this step failed to kill, as General Lucius D Clay had hoped, 'the heart of the black market'. Prices rose only temporarily until smuggling had become better organised. As Clay believed, one would have to 'deluge' Germany with cigarettes in order to end their role as an alternative currency. Great Britain, which itself suffered from a 'tobacco emergency', was strictly opposed. The cigarette lost its function as an alternative currency after the monetary reform of 20 June 1948. Yet the shadow economy, viewed in aggregate, receded only slowly, and cigarettes remained much sought-after items on the illegal markets. As late as 1950 some 500 million cigarettes a month were brought into the Federal Republic illegally, ie more than a quarter of domestic production. Only reduction in the tax surcharges brought about a graduate decrease in smuggling.[49]

SUMMARY

In contradiction to their official prevention policy, the National Socialists did all they could to assure distribution of tobacco to the German population. Particularly during World War II tobacco was sought after as a calming and hunger-stifling psycho-drug and even after the capitulation remained a product with practically inelastic demand which was even grown by millions of smokers privately. Smoker cards and tobacco goods figured in the standard offers in illegal markets from 1941–2. The 'Ami' or American cigarette demanded peak prices in the years after 1945 when it finally assumed the role of an unofficial currency. At the same time a permanent change in taste occurred: in the Western zones the American blend cigarette replaced Oriental tobacco. Substitution processes also occurred in individual forms of tobacco consumption. Thus despite fiscal disadvantages the cigarette was finally accepted over the cigar. Only after the Germans had satisfied their 'hunger for nicotine' (Pohlisch) did the debate over preventive medicine resume in the mid-1950s.

BIBLIOGRAPHY

Akten der Partei-Kanzlei der NSDAP (Institut für Zeitgeschichte) Part I, Vol 1, München, 1983.

Akten der Partei-Kanzlei der NSDAP (Institut für Zeitgeschichte) Part II, Vol. 4 München, 1992.

Aschenbrenner, Helmuth and Stahl, Günther. *Handbuch des Tabakhandels*, Berlin, 1944, 2nd edn.

Bauman, Zygmunt. *Moderne und Ambivalenz*, Hamburg, 1992, Engl 1991.

Fehér, Ferenc and Heller, Agnes. *Biopolitics*, Aldershot, 1994.

Goodman, Jordan. *Tobacco in History: The cultures of dependence*, London/New York, 1993.

Hengartner, Thomas and Merki, Christoph Maria, eds. *Tabakfragen: Rauchen aus kulturwissenschaftlicher Sicht*, Zürich, 1996.

Hess, Henner. *Rauchen: Geschichte, Geschäfte, Gefahren*, Frankfurt am Main/New York, 1987.

Lungwitz, Hans. *Tabak und Neurose*, Bremen, 1942, typescript.

Merki, Christoph Maria. Die amerikanische Zigarette – das Mass aller Dinge: Rauchen in Deutschland zur Zeit der Zigarettenwährung (1945–1948). In Hengartner and Merki, eds, *Tabakfragen*, Zürich, 1996, 57–82.

Merki, Christoph Maria. Zur Widersprüchlichkeit der nationalsozialistischen Tabakpolitik, *Vierteljahrshefte für Zeitgeschichte*, 46 (1998), 19–42.

North, Douglass C. *Institutions, Institutional Change and Economic Performance*, Cambridge, 1990.

Overy, Richard J. *War and Economy in the Third Reich*, Oxford, 1994.

Pohlisch, Kurt. *Tabak: Betrachtungen über Genuss- und Rauschpharmaka*, Stuttgart, 1954.

Schmölders, Günter. Die Zigarettenwährung. In Brinkmann et al, eds, *Sozialökonomische Verhaltensforschung – Ausgewählte Aufsätze von Günter Schmölders*, Berlin, 1973, 166–71.

Stübner, Gabriele. *Der Kampf gegen den Hunger 1945–1950*, Neumünster, 1984.

Stünzner, Wilfried von. *Psychosoziale Bedingungen des Rauchens*, Frankfurt am Main, 1994.

Weindling, Paul. 'Mustergau' Thüringen: Rassenhygiene zwischen Ideologie und Machtpolitik. In Frei, Norbert, ed, *Medizin und Gesundheitspolitik in der NS-Zeit*, München, 1993, 81–97.

Wenusch, Adolf. *Warum raucht der Mensch?* (Austria Tabakwerke AG), Wien, 1942, typescript.

NOTES

1 See Hess, 1987; Goodman, 1993; Hengartner and Merki, 1996.
2 For developing consumption during recent decades, see Stünzner, 1994; for consumption during the first half of the twentieth century, see Merki, 1998.
3 *Reine Luft*, 2 (1941), (the telegram text).
4 Federal Archives, Berlin, 21.1 / B 9014 (Bormann to Amann).
5 Thüringen ranked as a National Socialist 'model region' in terms of health-care policy, see Weindling, 1993.

6 Quotations from speeches at the opening of the Jena Institute see *Reine Luft*, 2 (1941).
7 Bauman, 1992.
8 Feher and Heller, 1994.
9 See Lickint, Fritz. *Tabak und Organismus. Handbuch der gesamten Tabakkunde*, Stuttgart, 1939.
10 Federal Archives, Berlin, 21.1 / B 9013.
11 *Reine Luft*, 2 (1941).
12 In the sense of Douglass C. North, 1990. Viewed in this manner, National Socialist preventive and prohibitive steps could be seen as an attempt to reinforce the institutional structure which prevented one from smoking.
13 Akten der Partei-Kanzlei, Part I, vol 1, nos 14937 and 17611.
14 ibid, no 14971.
15 *Reichs-Gesundheitsblatt*, 1939, 626–7.
16 Federal Archives, Berlin, 21.1 / B 9014.
17 *Reichs-Gesundheitsblatt*, 1942, 95–6.
18 On the theme, among others: *Der öffentliche Gesundheitsdienst* (1937–8), 385–8, and (1941), 513–6.
19 Aschenbrenner and Stahl, 1944, 533.
20 Lungwitz, 1942.
21 Wenusch, 1942.
22 *Deutsche Werbung* (1941), 516–7.
23 Federal Archives, Berlin, 31.01/11882 (meeting of 5 December 1941).
24 Federal Archives, Berlin, 50.01/lg, 104.
25 See Overy, 1994.
26 Federal Archives, Berlin, 21. 01/B 1911.
27 Federal Archives, Berlin, 50.01/lg and 31.01/11822.
28 Federal Archives, Berlin, 31.01/11882 (protocol).
29 See Bernhard, Paul. *Der Einfluss der Tabakgifte auf die Gesundheit und die Fruchtbarkeit der Frau*, Jena, 1943 with a foreword by Karl Astel.
30 Federal Archives, Potsdam, 31.01/11882 (decree of 3 July 1942 and 14 August 1942).
31 Federal Archives, Berlin, 31.01/11886 and 21.01/B 9127.
32 Federal Archives, Berlin, 31.01/11882, 11885, and 11888.
33 Data from Merki, 1996, 78.
34 Pohlisch, 1954.
35 Von Stünzner, 1994.
36 Akten der Partei-Kanzlei, Part II, Vol 4, no 44010.
37 Federal Archives, Koblenz, R 18, nos 3069 and 3161.
38 Federal Archives, Koblenz, Z 31/559 and 560. Further material on home-made products there too. See also: Koenig, Paul. *Tabakkleinanbau*, Hanover, 1946, 2nd edn.
39 Merki, 1996, 69.
40 In spring of 1949, 37 of 100 women smoked 'constantly'; of those women below age 30, the share of smokers was 54 per cent (from a 1949 Reemtsma survey; Federal Archives, Koblenz, Z 8/1824). Until 1953 the proportion of smoking women had again shrunk to 11 per cent.
41 Citation from: Merki, 1996, 70.
42 Camporesi, Piero. *Il pane selvaggio*, Bologna, 1980.

43 Pohlisch, 1954, 168.
44 For the health situation: Stübner, 1984.
45 For tobacco tax: Federal Archives, Koblenz, among others B 102/73559, Z 31/549/550/571 and Z 8/66.
46 Merki, 1996, 79–80.
47 On this point see Schmölders, 1973.
48 Federal Archives, Koblenz, Z 31/549/550.
49 Merki, 1996, 67–8.

Index